Nuances in the Management of Hand and Wrist Injuries in Athletes

Editor

SANJEEV KAKAR

CLINICS IN SPORTS MEDICINE

www.sportsmed.theclinics.com

Consulting Editor
MARK D. MILLER

April 2020 • Volume 39 • Number 2

ELSEVIER

1600 John F. Kennedy Boulevard ● Suite 1800 ● Philadelphia, Pennsylvania, 19103-2899

http://www.theclinics.com

CLINICS IN SPORTS MEDICINE Volume 39, Number 2
April 2020 ISSN 0278-5919, ISBN-13: 978-0-323-76307-3

Editor: Lauren Boyle
Developmental Editor: Donald Mumford

Clinics in Sports Medicine (ISSN 0278-5919) is published quarterly by Elsevier Inc., 360 Park Avenue South, New York, NY 10010-1710. Months of issue are January, April, July, and October. Business and Editorial Offices: 1600 John F. Kennedy Blvd., Ste. 1800, Philadelphia, PA 19103-2899. Customer Service Office: 3251 Riverport Lane, Maryland Heights, MO 63043. Periodicals postage paid at New York, NY and additional mailing offices. Subscription prices are $364.00 per year (US individuals), $733.00 per year (US institutions), $100.00 per year (US students), $405.00 per year (Canadian individuals), $904.00 per year (Canadian institutions), $100.00 (Canadian students), $475.00 per year (foreign individuals), $904.00 per year (foreign institutions), and $235.00 per year (foreign students). Foreign air speed delivery is included in all *Clinics* subscription prices. All prices are subject to change without notice. **POSTMASTER:** Send address changes to *Clinics in Sports Medicine*, Elsevier Health Sciences Division, Subscription Customer Service, 3251 Riverport Lane, Maryland Heights, MO 63043. Customer Service (orders, claims, online, change of address): Elsevier Health Sciences Division, Subscription Customer Service, 3251 Riverport Lane, Maryland Heights, MO 63043. **Tel: 1-800-654-2452 (U.S. and Canada); 314-447-8871 (outside U.S. and Canada). Fax: 314-447-8029. E-mail: journalscustomerservice-usa@elsevier.com (for print support); journalsonlinesupport-usa@elsevier.com (for online support).**

Reprints. For copies of 100 or more of articles in this publication, please contact the Commercial Reprints Department, Elsevier Inc., 360 Park Avenue South, New York, NY 10010-1710. Tel.: 212-633-3874; Fax: 212-633-3820; E-mail: reprints@elsevier.com.

Clinics in Sports Medicine is covered in *MEDLINE/PubMed (Index Medicus) Current Contents/Clinical Medicine, Excerpta Medica,* and *ISI/Biomed.*

Contributors

CONSULTING EDITOR

MARK D. MILLER, MD
S. Ward Casscells Professor, Head, Department of Orthopaedic Surgery, Division of Sports Medicine, University of Virginia, Charlottesville, Virginia; Team Physician, Miller Review Course, Harrisonburg, Virginia

EDITOR

SANJEEV KAKAR, MD, FAOA
Professor of Orthopaedic Surgery, Mayo Clinic, Rochester, Minnesota

AUTHORS

RYAN P. CALFEE, MD, MSc
Associate Professor, Department of Orthopedic Surgery, Washington University in St. Louis, St Louis, Missouri

DANE DALEY, MD
Assistant Professor, Department of Orthopedics and Physical Medicine, Medical University of South Carolina, Charleston, South Carolina

HANNAH A. DINEEN, MD
Fellow, Indiana Hand to Shoulder Center, Indianapolis, Indiana

JANE M. FEDORCZYK, PT, PhD, CHT
Director, Center for Hand and Upper Limb Health and Performance, Professor, Departments of Physical Therapy and Occupational Therapy, Jefferson College of Rehabilitation Sciences, Thomas Jefferson University, Philadelphia, Pennsylvania

JEFFREY B. FRIEDRICH, MD, MC
Professor, Division of Plastic Surgery, Department of Surgery, University of Washington, Harborview Medical Center, Seattle, Washington

RAYMOND GLENN GASTON, MD
Chief of Hand Surgery, Atrium Musculoskeletal Institute, Fellowship Director, OrthoCarolina Hand and Upper Extremity Fellowship, Charlotte, North Carolina

MICHAEL GEARY, MD
Atrium Musculoskeletal Institute, Charlotte Medical Center, Charlotte, North Carolina

JACOB D. GIRE, MD
Robert A. Chase Hand and Upper Limb Center, Department of Orthopaedic Surgery, Stanford University Medical Center, Redwood City, California

JEFFREY A. GREENBERG, MD, MS
Partner, Indiana Hand to Shoulder Center, Indianapolis, Indiana

WARREN C. HAMMERT, MD
Professor of Orthopaedic and Plastic Surgery, Chief, Division of Hand and Wrist Surgery, Department of Orthopaedics and Rehabilitation, University of Rochester Medical Center, Rochester, New York

B. MATTHEW HOWE, MD
Associate Professor, Department of Radiology, Mayo Clinic, Rochester, Minnesota

THOMAS B. HUGHES, MD
Clinical Associate Professor of Orthopaedic Surgery, University of Pittsburgh School of Medicine, Orthopaedic Specialists, UPMC, Pittsburgh, Pennsylvania

JONATHAN ISAACS, MD
Herman M. and Vera H. Nachman Distinguished Research Professor, Professor and Chief, Division of Hand Surgery, Vice Chairman of Research and Education, Department of Orthopedic Surgery, Virginia Commonwealth University Health System, Richmond, Virginia

ROBIN N. KAMAL, MD
Assistant Professor, Department of Orthopaedic Surgery, Stanford University, Stanford, California

SCOTT H. KOZIN, MD
Clinical Professor of Orthopaedics, The Sidney Kimmel Medical College of Thomas Jefferson University, Shriners Hospitals for Children – Philadelphia, Philadelphia, Pennsylvania

STEVE K. LEE, MD
Associate Professor of Orthopaedic Surgery, Hospital for Special Surgery, New York, New York

BILAL MAHMOOD, MD
Assistant Professor, Department of Orthopaedic Surgery, University of Rochester, Rochester, New York

ERIN A. MILLER, MD, MS
Assistant Professor, Division of Plastic Surgery, Department of Surgery, University of Washington, Harborview Medical Center, Seattle, Washington

NATHAN C. PATRICK, MD
Fellow, Division of Hand and Wrist Surgery, Department of Orthopaedics and Rehabilitation, University of Rochester Medical Center, Rochester, New York

MARC J. RICHARD, MD
Department of Orthopaedic Surgery, Duke University Medical Center, Durham, North Carolina

LAUREN M. SHAPIRO, MD
Department of Orthopaedic Surgery, Stanford University, Stanford, California

SPENCER SKINNER, MD
Division of Hand Surgery, Department of Orthopedic Surgery, Virginia Commonwealth University Health System, Richmond, Virginia

ANDREW D. SOBEL, MD
Hand and Microsurgery Fellow, Department of Orthopedic Surgery, Washington University in St. Louis, St Louis, Missouri

CHRISTIN A. TIEGS-HEIDEN, MD
Assistant Professor, Department of Radiology, Mayo Clinic, Rochester, Minnesota

ELIZABETH P. WAHL, MD
Department of Orthopaedic Surgery, Duke University Medical Center, Durham, North Carolina

JEFFREY YAO, MD
Robert A. Chase Hand and Upper Limb Center, Department of Orthopaedic Surgery, Stanford University Medical Center, Redwood City, California

DAN A. ZLOTOLOW, MD
Professor of Orthopaedics, The Sidney Kimmel Medical College of Thomas Jefferson University, Shriners Hospitals for Children – Philadelphia, Philadelphia, Pennsylvania; Shriners Hospitals for Children – Greenville, Greenville, South Carolina; The Hospital for Special Surgery, New York, New York; The Philadelphia Hand to Shoulder Center, Philadelphia, Pennsylvania

Contents

Imaging plays a key role in the evaluation and treatment planning of hand and wrist injuries in athletes. Depending on the suspected injury, a combination of conventional radiographs, computed tomography, magnetic resonance imaging, magnetic resonance arthrography, and/or ultrasound may be indicated. This article reviews the strengths and limitations of these imaging modalities and how they can be utilized in commonly encountered clinical questions.

Tendinopathies in the hand and wrist are common in athletes. This article reviews some of the common hand and wrist conditions, such as trigger digits, first dorsal compartment tendonitis, and extensor carpi ulnaris tendonitis. In addition, it reviews less commonly seen tendon conditions of the flexor carpi radialis and ulnaris, intersection syndrome, and extensor pollicis entrapment conditions. Diagnosis, nonoperative and operative treatment, and postoperative recommendations and return to play are also discussed.

An athlete's hands are susceptible to a variety of acute and cumulative traumas depending on their chosen sport. Depending on the timing of the injury, the immediate requirements of the athlete, and future aspirations, treatment strategies may need individual customization. This article offers a brief review of the anatomy and complex function of the extensor mechanism, discusses the etiologies of various extensor injuries, and outlines the multiple treatment options and expected outcomes.

Flexor tendon and pulley injuries in athletes present a unique challenge to the treating clinician. An understanding of the anatomy and mechanism of injury helps the clinician appropriately diagnose and treat the injury.

Treatment may become more complicated when associated with delays in diagnosis, in-season considerations, and an athlete's desire to return to play. Two injuries involving the flexor tendon-pulley system, avulsion injuries of the flexor digitorum profundus tendon from its insertion onto the base of the distal phalanx and flexor pulley injuries, are examined in detail in this article.

Although the technical details of distal radius fracture fixation in athletes are largely similar to the general population, the issues surrounding the injury, desire to return to sport, and rehabilitation require specialized attention. Athletes are generally healthy, with a drive to recover and must balance the risk of long-term consequences of returning to play too early with the potential loss of scholarship, salary, or opportunities for advancement. Outcomes after nonoperative and operative treatment of distal radius fractures are generally excellent in athletes and return to the same level of sport occurs in most patients.

The treatment of athletes with carpal ligament injuries provides many challenges. Our initial goals remain to make a timely and accurate diagnosis, provide treatment options, and create an environment for shared decision making. To optimize outcomes and facilitate return to play, early surgical intervention may be warranted. This article reviews common carpal ligament injury patterns in the athlete with a focus on both classic and newer surgical techniques.

Scaphoid fractures are the most common carpal fracture and the most challenging. Although appropriately managing acute scaphoid waist fractures is a priority, it also is of primary importance to make a diagnosis acutely. Scaphoid waist fractures can occur with low-energy trauma and lead to mild symptoms. A tendency to minimize symptoms and low level of initial disability lead to delay in diagnosis. Displaced scaphoid fractures require operative intervention uniformly. Although nondisplaced fractures can heal with nonoperative treatment, management of these injuries is affected by patient demands. In high-level athletes, operative treatment of nondisplaced injuries may lead to earlier return to sport.

Carpal fractures of bones other than the scaphoid occur at a much lower rate than scaphoid fractures. The close relationship between the carpus, intrinsic and extrinsic wrist ligaments, and wrist kinematics makes a thorough history, clinical examination, and interpretation of imaging for carpal malalignment essential. Carpal malalignment should be addressed with reduction and fixation. Nondisplaced fractures are often treated nonoperatively and displaced intraarticular fractures are almost always treatment operatively. The physician should keep in mind the athlete's specific goals and needs. Treatment must be individualized. Options for early return to play should be discussed when possible.

Ulnar-sided wrist pain is a common problem in athletes that can be challenging owing to its frequent combination of overuse in conjunction with acute injury. Repetitive pronosupination, wrist flexion and extension, as well as radial and ulnar deviation can predispose the athlete to injury of ulnar structures. Careful understanding of the sport-specific injuries as well as the underlying biomechanics are key to understanding and treating the athlete. In this article, we discuss the most frequent causes of ulnar-sided wrist pain in the athlete and focus on anatomy and pathophysiology, presentation, and diagnosis, as well as nonoperative and operative treatment options.

Metacarpal and phalangeal fractures are common injuries in athletes and occur frequently in contact and ball-handling sports. They usually result after direct hits from other players or athletic equipment. The fractures often are minimally displaced and require a short period of immobilization followed by early range of motion for expeditious return to play. Unstable or intra-articular fractures may require operative fixation. Open reduction and internal fixation afford the most stability while allowing for early rehabilitation. Athletes represent a unique population, and treatment of these fractures requires consideration of specific sport, timing of injury, and level of play.

Although finger joint dislocations are generally thought of as benign by many athletes and assumed to be a sprain, these injuries represent a spectrum that includes disabling fracture-dislocations. Failure to recognize certain dislocations or fracture-dislocations may result in permanent deformity and loss of motion. Simple dislocations are frequently amenable to early return to play with protection; however, more complex injuries may require specialized splinting or surgery. Delay in diagnosis of unstable proximal interphalangeal fracture-dislocations may require reconstruction or fusion. Early diagnosis and appropriate treatment are essential to ensure optimal functional results.

Thumb metacarpophalangeal collateral ligament injuries are common in athletes and occur via forced abduction or hyperextension. Management primarily depends on the grade of ligamentous injury and the presence of a Stener lesion or large avulsion fracture. Surgeons should consider the athlete's position, hand dominance, duration of season remaining, and goals. Shared decision making regarding timing of surgery is imperative. Acutely, primary ligamentous repair with or without augmentation is achievable. Chronic collateral ligament injuries are effectively treated with ligament reconstruction. Numerous surgical techniques have been described without 1 showing superiority. Postoperative rehabilitation protocols vary based on repair quality and sports-specific considerations.

This article examines the most common problematic hand and wrist injuries in the pediatric athlete. Hand and wrist injuries in the growing skeleton pose a different diagnostic and therapeutic challenge than in the mature skeleton. Ligaments are stronger than bone, and unossified cartilaginous sections of the skeleton are yet more susceptible to injury than bone. Although remodeling can correct for even moderate deformities if sufficient growth potential exists, remodeling cannot return the child to normal anatomy in many cases. Remodeling depends on intact periosteum, a nearby growing physis, and competent ligaments to direct remodeling via Hueter-Volkmann and Wolff's laws.

During the protective phase of treatment, therapy for hand and wrist injuries in athletes is similar to the plan of care provided to all patients. The nuances in the care provided to athletes become apparent during the transition to the postprotective phase of rehabilitation when the focus has shifted to return to play. Therapy following a sports injury should address the individual needs of the athletes in their everyday lives as well as the specificity of their training and sports-specific activities. The factors that influence return to play are discussed.

CLINICS IN SPORTS MEDICINE

SERIES OF RELATED INTERESTED

Orthopedic Clinics
Foot and Ankle Clinics
Hand Clinics
Physical Medicine and Rehabilitation Clinics
Clinics in Podiatric Medicine and Surgery

THE CLINICS ARE AVAILABLE ONLINE!
Access your subscription at:
www.theclinics.com

Foreword

Athletic Hand and Wrist Injuries Return to Play

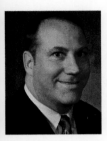

Mark D. Miller, MD
Consulting Editor

As I look back at my early career as a team physician, I recall some of my most challenging injuries involved the hand and wrist. Fortunately, I had experienced colleagues that I could (and did) call, even from the sidelines. My good fortune continued throughout my career, and recently, one of my colleagues literally came down from the stands in a championship football game to devise a splint to allow one of our star players to safely return to play.

My good friend, Dr Sanj Kakar, is one of the best and brightest hand surgeons that I know. He has done a fantastic job teaching hand surgery at the Miller Review Course, and I felt that he would be the perfect person to edit this issue of *Clinics in Sports Medicine*. He has put together a superb treatise on the treatment of hand and wrist injuries with an emphasis on return to play. This issue covers the entire gamut of these injuries in a very systematic and thorough manner. I have to hand it to him, this is an excellent issue, and I encourage you to keep a copy in your training room…and maybe on the sidelines!

Mark D. Miller, MD
Division of Sports Medicine
Department of Orthopaedic Surgery
University of Virginia
James Madison University
400 Ray C. Hunt Drive, Suite 330
Charlottesville, VA 22908-0159, USA

E-mail address:
mdm3p@virginia.edu

Clin Sports Med 39 (2020) xiii
https://doi.org/10.1016/j.csm.2020.01.003
0278-5919/20/© 2020 Published by Elsevier Inc.

Preface

Nuances in the Management of Hand and Wrist Injuries in Athletes

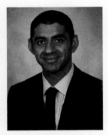

Sanjeev Kakar, MD, FAOA
Editor

The management of patients with sports-related injuries can be confusing. Do I manage these patients in the same way as other non-athletes? Is there a role for non-operative treatment? Should I fix the fracture, and does the rehabilitation of these patients vary to get the patient back to play sooner? Given this, I have had the privilege to solicit the opinions from some of the thought-leaders within the hand and wrist community to provide their expertise in managing these patients. I hope the readers will find these articles stimulating, informative, and helpful in the care of the injured athlete.

Sanjeev Kakar, MD, FAOA
Mayo Clinic
200 1st St SW
Rochester, MN 55905, USA

E-mail address:
Kakar.Sanjeev@mayo.edu

Clin Sports Med 39 (2020) xv
https://doi.org/10.1016/j.csm.2020.01.002
0278-5919/20/© 2020 Published by Elsevier Inc.

sportsmed.theclinics.com

Imaging of the Hand and Wrist

Christin A. Tiegs-Heiden, MD*, B. Matthew Howe, MD

KEYWORDS

• Imaging • Radiograph • CT • MRI • Ultrasound

KEY POINTS

• Radiographs are the primary initial diagnostic tool for hand and wrist injuries, particularly in the setting of osseous injury.
• Computed tomography offers improved contrast resolution compared with radiographs and the benefit of multiplanar reconstruction and is particularly useful in the setting of suspected osseous injuries with negative or equivocal radiographs.
• Magnetic resonance imaging and magnetic resonance arthrogram are the modalities of choice for evaluating soft tissue injuries of the hand and wrist and occult fractures.
• Ultrasound provides good visualization of superficial structures, such as tendons, peripheral nerves, the digital pulley system, and ganglion cysts. Ultrasound excels in the ability to dynamically evaluate structures and to compare with the contralateral anatomy.

INTRODUCTION

Hand and wrist injuries are common in athletes, accounting for 9% to 25% of sports injuries.[1,2] The hand and wrist anatomy is complex and often requires the evaluation of small structures that have significant implications on clinical and surgical management. Conventional radiographs, computed tomography (CT), magnetic resonance imaging (MRI), MR arthrography, and ultrasound are all commonly used in the evaluation of hand and wrist injuries. This article reviews strengths and limitations of these imaging modalities and how they can best be utilized in commonly encountered clinical questions.

IMAGING MODALITIES
Conventional Radiographs

Osseous injuries of the hand and wrist often are diagnosed based on a combination of clinical examination and plain radiographs.[1] Even with the availability of advanced imaging modalities, conventional radiographs remain cost effective, offering a large amount of information to help guide further evaluation and treatment.[3] Initial

Department of Radiology, Mayo Clinic, 200 1st Street Southwest, Rochester, MN 55905, USA
* Corresponding author.
E-mail address: tiegsheiden.christin@mayo.edu

Clin Sports Med 39 (2020) 223–245
https://doi.org/10.1016/j.csm.2019.10.003
0278-5919/20/© 2019 Elsevier Inc. All rights reserved.

sportsmed.theclinics.com

radiographs should consist of 3 views of the affected area: posteroanterior (PA), oblique, and lateral, although specialized views also may be requested.[4–6]

Conventional radiographs of the hand and wrist are best evaluated with an organized approach. All radiographic interpretations should first include an evaluation of positioning and technique. Positioning in patients with an acute injury and pain may be challenging, and it is important to ensure that the radiographs are adequate to answer the clinical question. Particular attention should be paid to osseous alignment. This is important in the evaluation of acute injuries to identify not only dislocations but also more subtle alignment abnormalities that may indicate a soft tissue injury. It also is important to identify old osseous injuries, anatomic variants, and accessory ossicles that may confound the interpretation of radiographs in an acute injury (**Fig. 1**).

In the setting of a suspected acute hand or wrist fracture, radiographic examination is the initial test of choice.[4,7] Radiographs also remain the primary modality for fracture follow-up to confirm healing.[8] Due to overlapping structures and lack of dedicated views in some cases, some fractures of the hand and wrist are not well seen radiographically.[4] Fractures of the lunate, triquetrum, capitate, and hamate are particularly challenging to diagnose on radiographs.[4] Conventional radiographs also have low sensitivity in the detection of early stress fractures.[9]

Digital radiography offers the benefit of improved dynamic range over conventional radiographs with better visualization of the soft tissues. Radiographs of the hand and wrist should be evaluated carefully for areas of soft tissue swelling or abnormalities that may suggest a soft tissue injury better evaluated with advanced imaging (**Fig. 2**).

Computed Tomography

CT of the hand and wrist should be obtained using thin slices (<1 mm) with isometric voxels that subsequently can be reformatted in any plane.[4] This also allows for the creation of 3-dimensional (3-D) reformatted images and 3-D printed models for operative planning.[6] Although 3-D printed models are not routinely used in clinical practice, they are a tool that likely will become more available in the future and may be beneficial in the treatment of complex injuries, such as scaphoid malunion.

Noncontrast CT often is indicated in the evaluation of suspected hand or wrist fractures with negative or equivocal radiographs, but the cost benefit of the exposure to ionizing radiation and added cost should be considered.[3] CT also can be used for

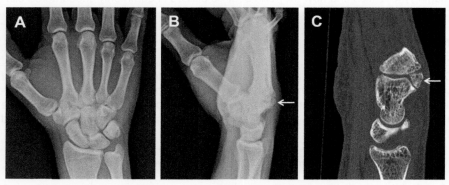

Fig. 1. PA (*A*) and lateral (*B*) radiographs in a 30-year-old man with dorsal wrist pain and swelling after a direct blow. A small osseous fragment along the third metacarpal base (*arrows*) should be recognized as an os styloideum (an accessory ossicle), as confirmed on sagittal CT (*C*).

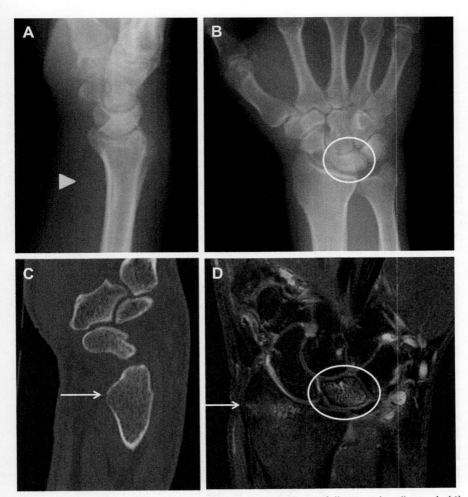

Fig. 2. A 41-year-old man presented with wrist pain after a fall. Lateral radiograph (*A*) demonstrated elevation of the pronator quadratus fat pad (*arrowhead*). There was no radiographic evidence of acute fracture; however, a nondisplaced intra-articular distal radial fracture was seen on sagittal CT (*C* [*arrow*]). Coronal T2FS MRI (*D*) obtained several months later demonstrated faint residual bone marrow edema along the healing fracture line (*arrow*). Also noted on PA radiograph (*B*) and MRI are sclerosis and increased signal within the lunate due to AVN (*circles*).

further characterization of known fractures, to aid in preoperative planning, and to evaluate fracture healing not well depicted on conventional radiographs.[1,4,6,7] Displacement of fracture fragments, comminution, intra-articular extension, and articular surface step-off and gap are better demonstrated on CT than conventional radiographs (**Fig. 3**).[3]

The superior contrast resolution of CT compared with conventional radiographs also allows for gross evaluation of the surrounding soft tissues, including the tendons of the wrist.[6] As with conventional radiographs, it is important to evaluate the soft tissues because injuries sometimes are identified (**Fig. 4**).

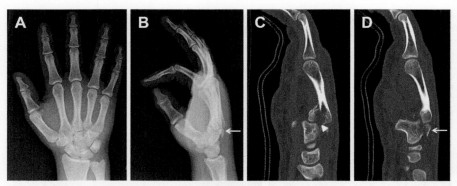

Fig. 3. AP (*A*) and lateral (*B*) radiographs in an 18-year-old man with wrist pain after punching a wall demonstrate a displaced fracture of the dorsal hamate (*arrows*). A concomitant fracture dislocation of the fourth metacarpal base was better seen on sagittal noncontrast CT (*C* [*arrowhead*]). The hamate fracture was also well evaluated on sagittal CT (*D*). For both fractures, CT better demonstrates the intra-articular extension and articular surface step-off (*C, D*).

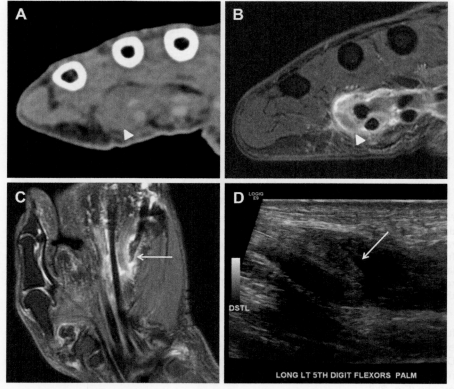

Fig. 4. A 59-year-old woman who previously competed in wheelchair marathons presented with inability to flex her fifth digit. Corresponding axial CT image (*A*) and T2FS MRI (*B*) demonstrate absence of the fifth digit flexor tendons at the level of the distal metacarpal shafts (*arrowheads*). Coronal T2FS MRI (*C*) and longitudinal ultrasound (*D*) confirm complete rupture of the tendons (*arrows*).

CT arthrography has been shown to be at least as accurate as MR arthrography in the diagnosis of intrinsic ligament and triangular fibrocartilage complex (TFCC) tears, although it is relatively limited in the evaluation of bone marrow and other extra-articular structures.[10–12] CT arthrography may be useful for ligamentous evaluation in patients with contraindication to MRI.

Dynamic (4-dimensional) CT allows for noninvasive assessment of osseous alignment during wrist motion and may guide surgical treatment in situations, such as scapholunate ligament (SLL) and distal radioulnar joint (DRUJ) instability.[13,14]

Dual-energy CT (DECT) is performed by obtaining images at 2 different energy levels.[15] Musculoskeletal applications for DECT include creating virtual noncalcium images, reducing metal artifact, creating iodine maps in contrast-enhanced studies, identifying monosodium urate deposition in gout, and assessing tendons.[15] Virtual noncalcium images are created by subtracting calcium from cancellous bone, allowing for the identification of bone marrow lesions, such as edema, which can aid in the diagnosis of acute fracture.[15] DECT techniques that reduce beam hardening artifact from metal allow improved visualization of tissues surrounding prostheses and hardware.[15]

Cone beam CT is a technique available on certain x-ray units that provides similar information to standard CT technique (**Fig. 5**). In the hand and wrist, cone beam CT

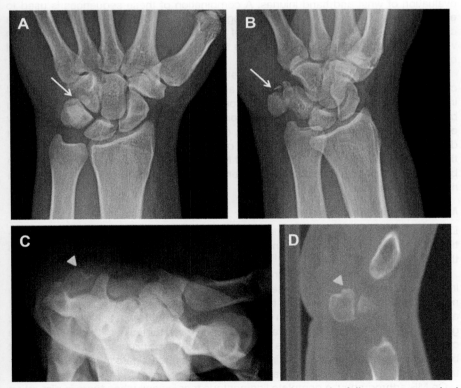

Fig. 5. AP (*A*) and oblique (*B*) radiographs in a 26-year-old man who fell on an outstretched hand. A displaced and mildly comminuted fracture of the pisiform (*arrows*) is better demonstrated on the oblique view. Carpal tunnel view radiograph (*C*) and sagittal cone beam CT (*D*) obtained 3 months later show that the fracture is healing (*arrowheads*).

offers the benefit of superior accuracy in the detection of carpal region fractures compared with standard radiographs, with lower radiation dose than conventional CT.[16] Additionally, positioning is easier compared with the traditional superman position, which may be difficult in a patient with concomitant shoulder injury. Cone beam CT may serve as an alternative to conventional CT for the evaluation of acute osseous injury as well as follow-up of fracture healing that is not well depicted on conventional radiographs.

Magnetic Resonance Imaging

The superior contrast resolution of MRI makes it the modality of choice for evaluation of suspected soft tissue injuries in the hand and wrist.[1,6] Subtle bony abnormalities, such as occult fracture, osteonecrosis, and abutment syndromes, also are best evaluated by MRI.[17] MRI also can play an important role in the assessment of arthritis and articular cartilage.[17]

Given the intricate anatomy of the wrist, it is critical to obtain images with high spatial resolution, high-contrast resolution, and high signal-to-noise ratio.[17,18] A dedicated coil, small field of view, and thin contiguous slices are important technical considerations.[17] 3T MRI, has been shown to provide significant diagnostic benefit relative to 1.5T MRI.[10,19,20] T1-weighted (T1), T2-weighted fat-saturated (T2FS), proton density (PD), and gradient sequences are the sequences typically used for the evaluation of wrist and hand injuries. A combination of these sequences is used to evaluate for a wide possibility of pathologic processes. Isotropic 3-D MRI may be considered to allow for the reformatting of images into any plane, which may help in visualizing anatomy that runs oblique to the standard axial, sagittal, and coronal orientations.[18]

MRI is ideal in the setting of occult wrist fractures due to its ability to image both cortex and bone marrow.[1,4] On MRI, an acute fracture is identified as a low-signal intensity line extending through the bone on all sequences with surrounding bone marrow edema (**Fig. 6**).[1,17] Bone contusion is seen as areas of bone marrow edema (high signal within the marrow on fluid-sensitive sequences) without a discrete fracture line.[1,17] At least 1 plane of T1-weighted images without fat saturation is recommended in all wrist and hand MRI examinations because it provides the best depiction of a fracture and helps differentiate nondisplaced fractures from bone marrow contusions.

Magnetic Resonance Arthrography

Direct MR arthrography is a minimally invasive technique that provides higher sensitivity in the detection of scapholunate and lunotriquetral ligament and TFCC injuries than conventional MRI (**Fig. 7**).[10,19]

It is critical for radiologists performing the contrast injection to have an understanding of the clinical question because the compartments injected and order of injection may be altered to better answer the specific clinical question. Triple-compartment arthrography refers to the injection of 3 compartments of the wrist under fluoroscopic guidance prior to MRI (midcarpal, radiocarpal, and distal radioulnar). Depending on the clinical question, any number of the 3 compartments can be injected and all 3 might not be required for the diagnosis. The findings at injection under fluoroscopy can be particularly helpful in the diagnosis and are an important portion of the entire examination.

On MR arthrography, a complete ligamentous tear is seen when there is disruption of the ligament and communication of contrast between the radiocarpal and midcarpal joints.[21] Fluid within a small ligamentous defect, but no communication between these joints, indicates a partial tear.[21]

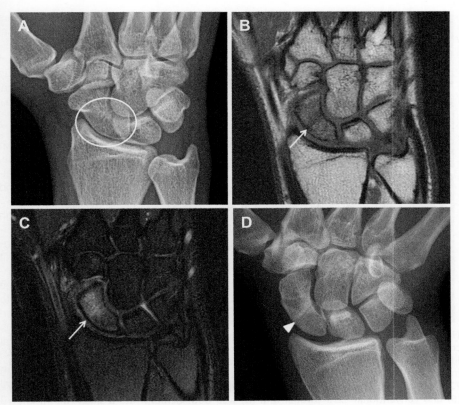

Fig. 6. An 18-year-old man developed wrist pain during rehabilitation after a traumatic spinal cord injury. Oblique radiograph at the time of presentation (*A*) demonstrated questionable lucency in the scaphoid waist (*circle*). Coronal T1 (*B*) and T2FS (*C*) MRIs better demonstrate a stress fracture of the scaphoid (*arrows*), with hypointense fracture line and surrounding bone marrow edema, but no cortical disruption. Follow-up radiograph (*D*) obtained 2 months later demonstrates sclerosis about the healing fracture (*arrowhead*).

Ultrasound

Ultrasound is a useful tool in the evaluation of hand and wrist pathologies, particularly given its dynamic nature, ability to compare with the contralateral side, relative accessibility, relatively low cost, and lack of ionizing radiation.[22]

Use of a high-resolution linear array transducer with a broad bandwidth is recommended for musculoskeletal applications.[23] A high-frequency transducer (10–15 MHz) should be used for the evaluation of superficial structures.[24] Color and power Doppler imaging allow for the assessment of vascularity, which may be increased in the setting of tenosynovitis or injury.[22]

The tendons, digital pulley system, and peripheral nerves of the hand and wrist can be well assessed sonographically.[22,24] Some superficial ligamentous injuries also can be identified, and the ability to stress the joint under direct visualization can provide information regarding the severity of the injury.[22] Ultrasound is a useful tool for the evaluation of soft tissue masses, such as ganglion cysts, or in the identification of radiolucent foreign bodies.[22] In the setting of inflammatory or osteoarthritis,

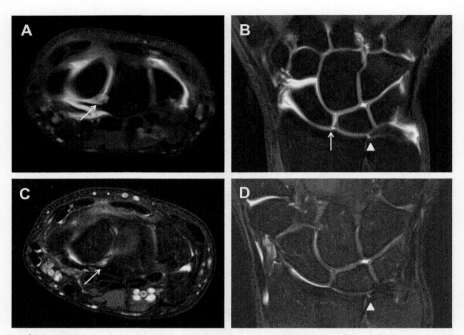

Fig. 7. Axial (*A*) and coronal (*B*) T1 MR arthrogram images obtained after injection of contrast into the radiocarpal joint in a 26-year-old male patient with wrist pain after heavy lifting. Both images demonstrate gadolinium extending through the scapholunate interval into the midcarpal joint, compatible with SLL tear (*arrows*). This tear also is seen on axial T2FS nonarthrographic MRI obtained 6 months later (*C* [*arrow*]). Coronal T1 MRA image (*B*) and conventional T2FS coronal MRI (*D*) also both demonstrate a small full-thickness tear of the triangular fibrocartilage disk (*arrowheads*).

ultrasound also be can used to detect synovitis, joint space narrowing, erosions, and/ or joint effusions.[22]

When intervention, such as aspiration or injection, is indicated, ultrasound can safely guide these procedures.[22]

Limitations of ultrasound are the difficulty in imaging intrinsic structures of the wrist, such as the TFCC and intrinsic ligaments, and the inability to visualize subtle bony pathology.[1,22]

COMMONLY ENCOUNTERED PATHOLOGIES IN THE ATHLETE'S HAND AND WRIST
Distal Radial and Ulnar Fractures

Standard PA, oblique, and lateral views are necessary for complete assessment of distal radial fractures and for detecting associated fractures.[5,25] One study found that the semisupinated oblique view of the wrist was the most sensitive radiographic view for the detection of radial fractures, possibly because it displays the dorsal cortex most clearly (**Fig. 8**).[5] Key features to assess radiographically include the degree of displacement, degree of comminution, extension into the distal radioulnar and/or radiocarpal joints, radial length, inclination, tilt, and the presence of associated injuries.[25] CT may provide better detail of the fracture and aid in treatment planning.[25] MRI is useful if there is suspicion for associated soft tissue injury or in the setting of suspected radiographically occult fracture.[25]

Fractures of the ulnar styloid are readily diagnosed on PA radiographs of the wrist.[21] Both size and degree of displacement of the ulnar styloid fracture are risk factures for DRUJ instability.[26]

Carpal Fractures

The scaphoid is the most commonly fractured carpal bone, representing approximately 70% of carpal fractures.[2,4,21,27] Initial radiographs should include PA and lateral radiographs of the wrist in neutral, an oblique view at 45° to 60° pronation, and a PA view with the wrist in 45° ulnar deviation and pronation.[21,27] Because approximately 20% of scaphoid fractures are occult on initial radiographs, either repeat radiographs in 10 days to 14 days or CT or MRI should be obtained if there is clinical suspicion.[17,27] CT may be used to better assess the 3-D anatomy of the fracture, evaluate displacement, and plan the operative approach.[27] The sensitivity and specificity of MRI in the diagnosis of scaphoid fractures have both been reported at 100%.[28] MRI has the added benefit of evaluating for associated soft tissue injuries

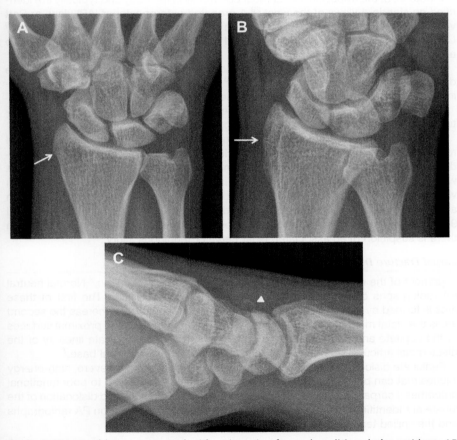

Fig. 8. A 43-year-old man presented with wrist pain after a demolition derby accident. AP (*A*) and oblique (*B*) radiographs of the wrist show a nondisplaced fracture of the distal radius (*arrows*), better demonstrated on the oblique view. A dorsal triquetral avulsion fracture is seen on the lateral view (*C* [*arrowhead*]).

concurrently.[17] Stress fractures of the scaphoid are best diagnosed with MRI (see **Fig. 6**).[1]

Lunate fractures account for approximately 1% of all carpal fractures.[29] Small fractures may not be detected on plain radiographs due to overlapping bone; therefore, CT or MRI is indicated if the clinical examination is suggestive.[29]

The triquetrum is the second most commonly fractured carpal bone, with the vast majority being dorsal chip fractures.[29] Triquetral body fractures make up the majority of the remaining fractures and often are seen in high energy injuries.[29] Triquetral fractures often can be diagnosed with PA, lateral, and 45° pronated oblique radiographs of the wrist; the lateral view is particularly useful for dorsal chip fractures (see **Fig. 8**).[29]

Pisiform fractures are rare; however, they may be underestimated because they are challenging to diagnose on radiographs.[29,30] The semisupinated oblique view highlights the pisiform and pisotriquetral joint (see **Fig. 5**).[30] Injury to the pisotriquetral joint is demonstrated by a joint width of greater than 3 mm or if the bone surfaces are more than 20° from parallel.[29] The carpal tunnel view also may be useful to diagnose pisiform fractures (see **Fig. 5**).[29]

Fractures of the trapezium occur most commonly in the body and typically are identified on standard views of the wrist.[29] A pronated anteroposterior (AP) view, or Bett view, can be used to improve visualization of the trapeziometacarpal articulation.[29] CT may be useful to identify more unusual fractures, such as occult trapezial ridge and coronal fractures.[29]

Trapezoid fractures are rare, and most fractures and fracture dislocations should be diagnosed on standard views of the wrist.[29] Dislocation of the trapezoid allows proximal migration of the second metacarpal, best identified on the PA view.[29]

Capitate fractures also are typically well seen on standard views of the wrist.[29] Fractures in the coronal plane, however, are more easily identified by CT scan.[29]

Hook of the hamate fractures are the most common fractures of the distal carpal row (**Fig. 9**).[21,31] Hamate fractures are challenging to diagnose on standard wrist radiographs due to overlapping bones but may be suspected when the hook is not well visualized on the PA view.[21,30] Specialized views, such as the carpal tunnel view or lateral view with the hand radially deviated and the thumb abducted, can aid in diagnosis.[21,31] CT has demonstrated sensitivity and specificity of 100% and 94%, respectively, and is considered the test of choice.[2,31,32] MRI is indicated when there is suspicion of an associated ulnar nerve or tendinous injury.[30]

Carpal Fracture Dislocations

Alignment of the wrist should be assessed carefully on radiographs.[7] Normal neutral PA radiographs demonstrate continuity of the 2 arcs of Gilula.[7] The first of these arcs is formed by the proximal scaphoid, lunate, and triquetrum, whereas the second arc is the distal margins of these bones.[7] The third is formed by the proximal surfaces of the capitate and hamate.[7] Lateral radiograph should demonstrate linearity of the distal radial articular surface, lunate, capitate, and third metacarpal base.[7]

Perilunate dislocations and perilunate fracture dislocations are severe, high-energy injuries that can be overlooked on initial radiographs and may lead to poor functional outcomes if carpal alignment is not assessed carefully.[7] Volar tilt and dislocation of the lunate are identified by the piece-of-pie appearance of the lunate on PA radiographs and the spilled teacup appearance on lateral view (**Fig. 10**).

Metacarpal and Phalangeal Fractures

Radiographic evaluation of metacarpal and phalangeal fractures should be performed prior to attempted reduction in order to demonstrate the fracture and/or dislocation

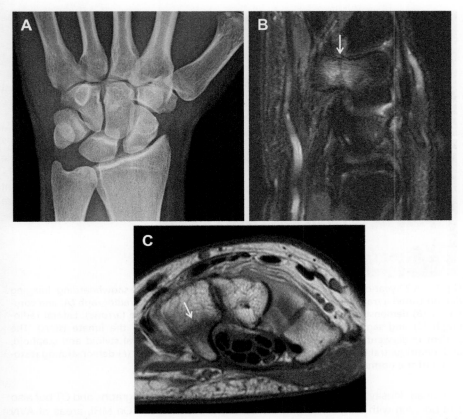

Fig. 9. A 19-year-old man with wrist pain after falling off his bike. Initial radiographs (*A*) were negative. Sagittal T2FS (*B*) and axial T1 (*C*) MRIs obtained the same day demonstrate a linear hypointense line through the base of the hook of the hamate, consistent with non-displaced fracture (*arrows*) with surrounding T2 hyperintense bone marrow edema. This fracture was radiographically occult, even at follow-up.

pattern.[33] CT is useful when further fracture characterization is needed, such as the evaluation of intra-articular involvement.[33]

Fractures of the metacarpal base can be associated with carpometacarpal joint dislocations, can be overlooked on the frontal view of the hand, and are better demonstrated on the lateral projection but still may be challenging to diagnose given overlapping structures (see **Fig. 3**).[33] Pronated oblique view may assist in evaluation of the long and index finger metacarpals, whereas a supinated view better demonstrates the fifth metacarpal and carpometacarpal joint.[6,33]

Avascular Necrosis

In the wrist, avascular necrosis (AVN) is seen most commonly in the proximal pole of the scaphoid after a scaphoid fracture but also occurs in the lunate, capitate, and hook of the hamate.[1] In athletes with injuries, the presentation can be early or late in the disease process. Although plain radiographs or CT may be sufficient for diagnosis and treatment planning, MRI can make the diagnosis earlier in the disease process.[1]

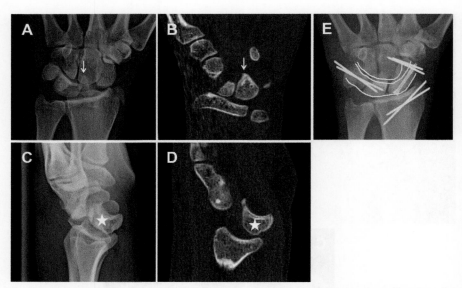

Fig. 10. A 22-year-old man who fell on his outstretched hand while snowboarding. Imaging demonstrated a trans-scaphoid perilunate fracture dislocation. PA radiograph (*A*) and coronal CT (*B*) demonstrate the piece-of-pie appearance of the lunate (*arrows*). Lateral radiograph (*C*) and sagittal CT (*D*) demonstrate volar dislocation of the lunate (*stars*). The patient underwent open reduction, internal fixation of the radial styloid and scaphoid, and lunotriquetral ligament repair, with postoperative radiograph (*E*) demonstrating restoration of the normal arcs of Gilula (*curved lines*).

Increased density of the affected bone is a sign of AVN on radiographs and CT but also can be seen with early healing in the setting of a fracture.[34] On MRI, areas of AVN demonstrate low signal intensity in the affected bone, particularly on T1-weighted non-FS images, although there may be bone marrow edema in the acute phase (**Fig. 11**).[1,35] Osseous fragmentation and collapse are seen in advanced disease.[1]

Both dynamic and delayed gadolinium-enhanced MRI may be used to assess osseous vascularity in the setting of scaphoid fracture; however, the reported utility of these methods is variable. One study showed that delayed contrast-enhanced images had the best diagnostic performance in the diagnosis of scaphoid AVN, followed by dynamic imaging and then conventional MRI.[36] Similarly, a study of MRI with delayed enhancement in 28 patients showed this to be superior to dynamic contrast-enhanced MRI.[37] A different study, however, found unenhanced MRI more sensitive and accurate than enhanced MRI.[35] Contrast-enhanced MRI did not show benefit in predicting the outcome of bone graft and internal fixation surgery in the setting of scaphoid nonunion in another study.[38]

Kienböck disease, or osteonecrosis of the lunate, is seen most commonly in the dominant hand of athletes who perform repetitive wrist loading.[21] MRI demonstrates diffuse bone marrow edema, sclerosis, and/or cystic changes throughout the lunate (see **Fig. 2**).[21]

Impaction Syndromes

Impaction or abutment syndromes may occur as a result of trauma or activities that lead to excessive carpal loading, particularly in the setting of certain anatomic variants.[1] These syndromes typically are diagnosed with clinical evaluation and

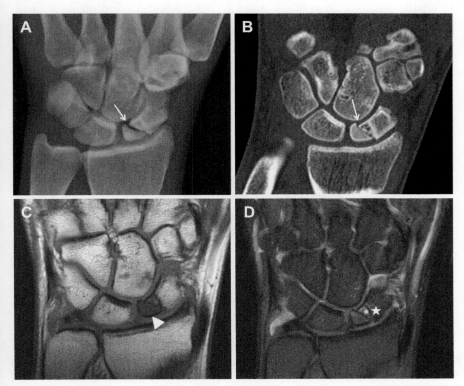

Fig. 11. A 26-year-old woman developed wrist pain after trying to catch a softball with her ungloved hand. PA radiograph (*A*) at the time of injury demonstrated a chronic-appearing ununited fracture of the scaphoid waist (*arrow*). On further questioning, she recalled wrist pain after a head-on go-cart collision approximately 10 years previously, for which she did not seek treatment. Coronal CT image (*B*) demonstrates the chronic fracture with cystic change about the distal fracture margin (*arrow*). There also is increased density of the proximal pole, suspicious for AVN. Coronal T1 MRI (*C*) demonstrates complete replacement of the normal bone marrow fat in the proximal pole (*arrowhead*), confirming the diagnosis of AVN. There is no fragmentation or collapse of the proximal pole. Coronal T2FS image (*D*) again demonstrates cystic change along the fracture (*star*).

radiographs.[1] MRI is useful for earlier diagnosis or to characterize the full extent of injuries, including associated chondral injury, bone marrow edema, and subchondral irregularity or cystic change (**Fig. 12**).[1]

Ulnar impaction syndrome, or ulnolunate abutment, may be seen in the setting of positive ulnar variance.[1,39] If dynamic ulnar impaction is suspected, the power grip PA view can be used to demonstrate maximal ulnar-positive variance radiographically (**Fig. 13**).[12] Additional imaging features include triangular fibrocartilage thinning or tear, chondral damage along the proximal lunate and distal ulna, bone marrow edema and subchondral cystic change and sclerosis in the proximal lunate, and lunotriquetral ligament tear (see **Fig. 12**).[17,39] Subchondral bone marrow edema is strongly associated with clinical symptoms.[39]

Ulnar impingement syndrome also can be seen in the setting of negative ulnar variance, when the distal ulna impinges on the distal radius, and can cause a painful pseudarthrosis.[1,17]

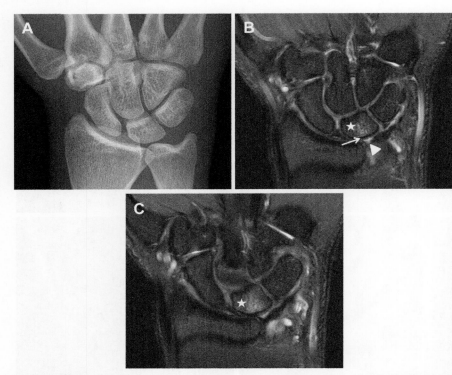

Fig. 12. A 20-year-old college baseball player presented with a history of chronic ulnar-sided wrist pain. PA radiograph (*A*) demonstrates positive ulnar variance. Coronal T2FS MRIs (*B, C*) demonstrate bone marrow edema within the medial lunate (*stars*), overlying chondral irregularity (*arrow*), and a full-thickness tear of the triangular fibrocartilage disc (*arrowhead*). These imaging findings are compatible with ulnar impaction syndrome.

Degenerative Arthritis

Age is the primary factor in the development of osteoarthritis; however, prior hand or wrist injuries, such as sprain, fracture, and osteonecrosis, also are risk factors.[39] Radiographic and CT hallmarks of osteoarthritis include joint space narrowing and irregularity, osteophyte formation, subchondral sclerosis, and subchondral cysts or geodes.[39] MRI is useful to demonstrate associated chondral damage, synovitis, and bone marrow edema.[39] In the assessment of intracarpal chondral lesions, CT arthrography has demonstrated higher sensitivity and specificity than both MRI and MR arthrography.[40]

Ligament Injury

Ligaments of the wrist are divided into 2 main types: intrinsic, or between carpal bones, and extrinsic, which extend beyond the carpal bones.[7] The scapholunate and lunotriquetral interosseous ligaments are the 2 key intrinsic ligaments of the wrist.[7]

The SLL complex is composed of 3 segments: the strongest dorsal, the weak fibrocartilaginous intermediate (central), and the volar components.[7,21] Imaging is important to assess the severity of SLL injuries and guide management.[21] Static scapholunate instability is demonstrated by widening of the scapholunate interval (≥3 mm) on neutral PA radiograph.[7,21] Dynamic scapholunate instability is identified by widening of the scapholunate interval only on clenched fist or ulnar deviation

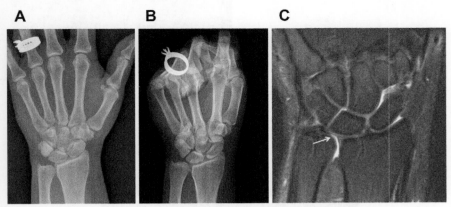

Fig. 13. Standard AP (*A*) and power grip (*B*) views in this patient with wrist pain demonstrate ulnar positive variance, which develops on the grip view. Coronal T2FS MRI (*C*) shows a full-thickness tear of the triangular fibrocartilage (*arrow*), with fluid in the DRUJ.

views.[21] Radiographs are normal in predynamic SLL injuries, which are best seen on MRI or CT arthrographic examinations.[21] Conventional arthrography can confirm an SLL tear but does not demonstrate which components of the ligament are torn. On MRI examinations, the SLL is best evaluated on axial and coronal sequences.[21] Thinning, irregularity, and increased signal intensity are features of partial tear.[21] A complete tear of the SLL is seen as discontinuity or nonvisualization of the ligament or injected contrast extending through a gap in the ligament on MR arthrography (see **Fig. 7**; **Fig. 14**).[21] A recent literature review evaluated the diagnostic performance of MRI in the detection of SLL tears and demonstrated the following sensitivities and specificities: MRA (82.1% and 92.8%, respectively), 3.0T MRI (75.7% and 97.1%, respectively), and 1.5T MRI (45.7% and 80.5%, respectively).[19]

In the setting of SLL injury, the scaphoid tends to palmar flex, and the lunate tends to dorsiflex.[7] Dorsal intercalated segment instability develops when the secondary stabilizers are also injured and may ultimately lead to scapholunate advanced collapse wrist.[21] This can be evaluated by measuring the scapholunate angle or the angle taken from a line drawn along the long access of the scaphoid and a line drawn along the short axis of the lunate.[7] Normally, this angle measures between 30° and 60°.[7] Dorsal intercalated segment instability deformity is defined as a scapholunate angle greater than 60° and typically occurs in the setting of both SLL and extrinsic dorsal intercarpal ligament injuries.[7]

The smaller lunotriquetral ligament also has 3 bands, the dorsal, central, and, most important, volar bands.[7] Volar intercalated segment instability is seen in the setting of complete lunotriquetral ligament tear plus disruption of 1 of the secondary stabilizers of the lunotriquetral joint.[21] It is diagnosed by a scapholunate angle of less than 30° and typically is seen in the setting of lunotriquetral and extrinsic dorsal radiocarpal ligament tear.[7] Lunotriquetral ligament tears are challenging to diagnose on nonarthrographic MRI, with sensitivity and specificity of 50% and 94%, respectively, at 3T and 22% and 94%, respectively, at 1.5T[20]

The ulnotriquetral ligament extends from the palmar radioulnar ligament to the volar triquetrum and is a component of the TFCC.[41] As with other ligament injuries, the MRI findings of disruption of the ligament or focal full-thickness increased signal are seen in the setting of a full-thickness tear.[41] Longitudinal split tears of the ulnotriquetral

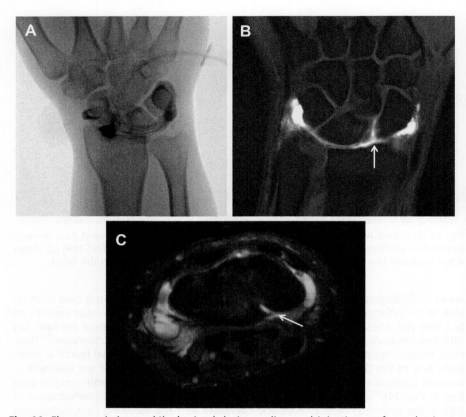

Fig. 14. Fluoroscopic image (*A*) obtained during radiocarpal injection performed prior to MR arthrogram in a 22-year-old woman with wrist pain, most bothersome when doing push-ups. Coronal T1FS (*B*) and axial T2FS (*C*) images demonstrate gadolinium contrast extending through the volar portion of the SLL (*arrows*), compatible with a tear.

ligament are challenging to diagnose on noncontrast MRI, with 1 study reporting sensitivity of 30% to 58% and specificity of 60% at 3T (**Fig. 15**).[41]

Injury to the extrinsic ligaments of the wrist can occur in isolation or in combination with intrinsic ligament injury.[21] The palmar extrinsic ligaments of the wrist are thicker and stronger than the dorsal extrinsic ligaments.[7] Similar to injury of other ligaments, MR findings of injury are T2 hyperintensity, irregularity, and fraying of the involved ligament.[21]

Collateral ligament injuries may be seen at the metacarpophalangeal and interphalangeal joints of the fingers.[21] Both MRI and ultrasound can identify these injuries, demonstrating thickening of the affected ligament with increased T2 signal or hypoechogenicity and/or either a partial or complete tear (**Fig. 16**).[21] MRI and ultrasound also can identify a suspected Stener lesion of the thumb metacarpophalangeal joint, in which the torn ulnar collateral ligament is retracted, allowing for interposition of the adductor aponeurosis.[42] Volar plate injuries may result after hyperextension of a joint, are best seen with MRI or ultrasound, and typically occur at the distal aspect of the volar plate.[21]

Triangular Fibrocartilage Complex Injury

The TFCC is a key stabilizer of the DRUJ, and injury results in ulnar-sided wrist pain.[2,21] Its components include the triangular fibrocartilage proper, the

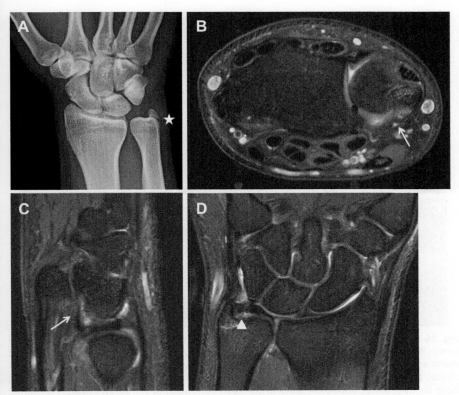

Fig. 15. AP radiograph (*A*) in a 17-year-old male patient who fell on his outstretched hand while riding his skateboard demonstrates a minimally displaced fracture of the ulnar styloid (*star*). Axial (*B*) and sagittal (*C*) T2FS MRIs demonstrate a split tear of the ulnotriquetral ligament (*arrows*). On coronal T2FS image (*D*), a tear of the foveal insertion of the triangular fibrocartilage is seen (*arrowhead*). The ulnar styloid fracture line also is seen.

volar and dorsal radioulnar ligaments, the meniscal homolog, the volar ulnocarpal ligaments, the ulnar collateral ligament, and the extensor carpi ulnaris tendon sheath.[21]

Radiographs often are normal in the setting of TFCC injury; therefore, assessment with MRI or MR arthrography is beneficial (see **Figs. 7, 12,** and **13**).[2] Radiographic evaluation remains important, however, particularly for the assessment of ulnar variance and widening/stability of the DRUJ.[12,32] The foveal attachment is an important stabilizing structure of the DRUJ that is difficult to evaluate with standard MRI (see **Fig. 15**).[43] The secondary MRI feature of subluxation of the ulnar head in relation to the distal radius has been shown to be associated with injuries of the foveal attachment.[43] At 3T, the sensitivity and specificity for the diagnosis of TFCC tears have been reported as 90% and 74%, respectively, compared with 82% and 59%, respectively, at 1.5T[20]

Tendon Injury

Both ultrasound and MRI are important tools in the assessment of the tendons of the hand and wrist.[24]

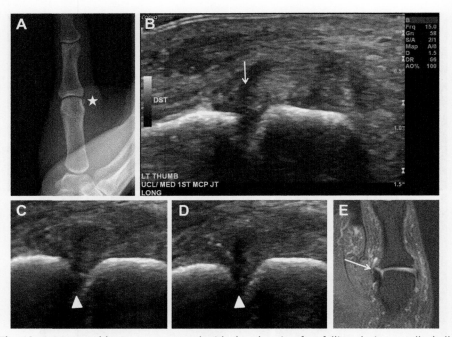

Fig. 16. A 37-year-old woman presented with thumb pain after falling during a volleyball game. PA radiograph (*A*) demonstrates soft tissue swelling along the ulnar aspect of the first metacarpophalangeal joint (*star*). Longitudinal gray-scale ultrasound image (*B*) demonstrates avulsion of the distal ulnar collateral ligament from the first proximal phalangeal base (*arrow*), with hypoechoic fluid in the tear. Longitudinal ultrasound images obtained at rest (*C*) and with valgus stress (*D*) show instability of the joint, with widening of the joint space and fluid extending through the tear with stress (*arrowheads*). Complete avulsion of the distal UCL was confirmed at surgery. Coronal T2FS MRI (*E*) in a different patient also shows complete avulsion of the distal UCL at the first metacarpophalangeal joint (*arrow*).

With ultrasound, the tendons should be assessed along their length and in both the axial and longitudinal planes.[24] Ultrasound examination can be focused to the specific area of a patient's symptoms and should include a dynamic examination.[24] Normal tendons are echogenic with fibrillated pattern, appearing as individual dots in cross-section and parallel fascicles in long axis.[24] Tendinopathy appears as thickening, enlargement, and hypoechogenicity of the involved tendon, whereas tenosynovitis is hypoechoic or anechoic fluid surrounding the tendon.[22] The ultrasound beam should always be perpendicular to the tendon being evaluated, or anisotropy causes the tendon to appear falsely hypoechoic and may mimic a tear.[22,24]

On MRI, the tendons should be evaluated in multiple planes on both T1 and fluid-sensitive sequences.[24] Normal tendons should be low in signal intensity on both T1 and fluid-sensitive images.[24,44] Thickening and increased T2 signal are signs of tendinopathy.[24] Increased fluid surrounding a tendon, apparent as increased signal on fluid-sensitive sequences, signifies tenosynovitis.[24]

de Quervain stenosing tenosynovitis is the most common tendinopathy in athletes.[21] Imaging often demonstrates hypertrophy of the first extensor compartment tendon sheath, thickening of the underlying tendons, and surrounding inflammatory changes.[21]

Intersection syndromes also can be diagnosed on ultrasound or MRI.[24] Proximal intersection syndrome occurs where the first extensor compartment tendons cross over the second, approximately 4 cm to 8 cm proximal to the Lister tubercle (**Fig. 17**).[24] Distal intersection syndrome occurs just distal to the Lister tubercle, where the third extensor compartment tendon crosses over the second.[24] Imaging findings in both syndromes include tendon thickening, tenosynovitis, and peritendinous edema and hypervascularity.[21,24]

The flexor and extensor tendons of the fingers also are vulnerable to athletic injuries.[42] Avulsion injuries are some of the most common injuries, occurring in the setting of forced flexion or hyperextension.[44] It is important to assess the location of these tears and degree of retraction, because these features have treatment implications.[44]

The pulley system, consisting of 5 annular and 3 cruciate pulleys about the flexor tendons of the fingers, keeps the flexor tendons in close proximity to the underlying bones.[44] On ultrasound and MRI, the annular pulleys are seen as regions of slight thickening along the volar tendon sheath, best assessed in the axial and sagittal planes.[44] Imaging signs of a complete tear of the annular pulleys include a discrete gap in the pulley fibers or bowstringing of the flexor tendon away from the underlying bones, particularly with flexion of the finger (**Fig. 18**).[42,44]

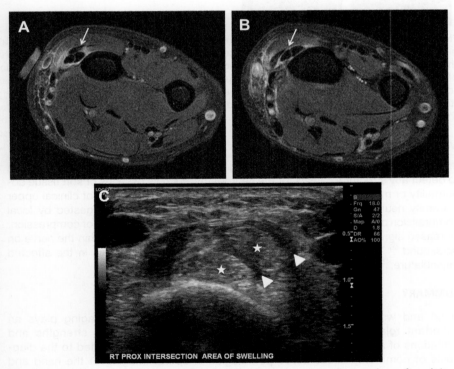

Fig. 17. A 30-year-old man presented with forearm pain and swelling 2 days after doing heavy lifting. Axial T2FS images at the intersection of the first extensor compartment over the second (*A, B*) demonstrate hyperintense fluid and edema about the intersection (*arrows*). Transverse gray-scale ultrasound image (*C*) demonstrates hypoechoic fluid (*arrowheads*) about the crossing tendons (*stars*), compatible with proximal intersection syndrome.

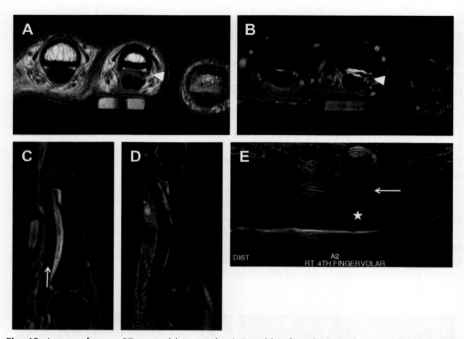

Fig. 18. Images from a 27-year-old man who injured his fourth digit during a flag football game. Axial T1 (*A*) and T2FS (*B*) MRIs demonstrate tear of the A2 pulley with dislocation of the flexor tendons through the tear (*arrowheads*). Coronal T2FS MRI (*C*) shows bowstringing of the flexor tendons away from the proximal phalanx at the level of the pulley tear (*arrow*), compared with the normal third digit (*D*). Dynamic ultrasound examination (*E*) also demonstrated tendon bowstringing, which increased during flexion (*arrow*), with fluid between the tendon and the underlying bone (*star*).

Neuropathy

Imaging is useful to confirm the clinical diagnosis of entrapment neuropathy as well as to detect any structural causes for the neuropathy, such as osseous or soft tissue abnormality or mass.[45] In 1 study, MRI was able to identify the cause of clinical upper extremity neuropathy in 93% of cases.[46] Nerve entrapment is suggested by focal compression of a nerve, enlargement of the nerve proximal to the site of compression, increased signal within the nerve on MRI, and hypoechoic signal within the nerve on ultrasound.[45] There may be acute or chronic denervation changes in the affected musculature.[45]

SUMMARY

Hand and wrist injuries often are seen in the athlete, and imaging plays an important role in assessing these injuries. This article reviews strengths and limitations of available imaging modalities and how these are applied to the diagnosis of commonly encountered pathologies in sports imaging of the hand and wrist.

DISCLOSURE

The authors have nothing to disclose.

CONFLICT OF INTEREST

None.

REFERENCES

1. Lisle DA, Shepherd GJ, Cowderoy GA, et al. MR imaging of traumatic and overuse injuries of the wrist and hand in athletes. Magn Reson Imaging Clin N Am 2009;17(4):639–54, vi.
2. Avery DM 3rd, Rodner CM, Edgar CM. Sports-related wrist and hand injuries: a review. J Orthop Surg Res 2016;11(1):99.
3. Torabi M, Lenchik L, Beaman FD, et al. ACR Appropriateness Criteria® acute hand and wrist trauma. Reston (VA): American College of Radiology; 2018. Available at: https://acsearch.acr.org/docs/69418/Narrative/. Accessed November 26, 2019.
4. Welling RD, Jacobson JA, Jamadar DA, et al. MDCT and radiography of wrist fractures: radiographic sensitivity and fracture patterns. AJR Am J Roentgenol 2008;190(1):10–6.
5. Russin LD, Bergman G, Miller L, et al. Should the routine wrist examination for trauma be a four-view study, including a semisupinated oblique view? AJR Am J Roentgenol 2003;181(5):1235–8.
6. Sundaram N, Bosley J, Stacy GS. Conventional radiographic evaluation of athletic injuries to the hand. Radiol Clin North Am 2013;51(2):239–55.
7. Scalcione LR, Gimber LH, Ho AM, et al. Spectrum of carpal dislocations and fracture-dislocations: imaging and management. AJR Am J Roentgenol 2014; 203(3):541–50.
8. Ricci WM, Black JC, Tornetta P 3rd, et al. Current opinions on fracture follow-up: a survey of OTA members regarding standards of care and implications for clinical research. J Orthop Trauma 2016;30(3):e100–5.
9. Fredericson M, Jennings F, Beaulieu C, et al. Stress fractures in athletes. Top Magn Reson Imaging 2006;17(5):309–25.
10. Lee RK, Ng AW, Tong CS, et al. Intrinsic ligament and triangular fibrocartilage complex tears of the wrist: comparison of MDCT arthrography, conventional 3-T MRI, and MR arthrography. Skeletal Radiol 2013;42(9):1277–85.
11. Theumann N, Favarger N, Schnyder P, et al. Wrist ligament injuries: value of post-arthrography computed tomography. Skeletal Radiol 2001;30(2):88–93.
12. Sachar K. Ulnar-sided wrist pain: evaluation and treatment of triangular fibrocartilage complex tears, ulnocarpal impaction syndrome, and lunotriquetral ligament tears. J Hand Surg Am 2012;37(7):1489–500.
13. Kakar S, Breighner RE, Leng S, et al. The role of dynamic (4D) CT in the detection of scapholunate ligament injury. J Wrist Surg 2016;5(4):306–10.
14. Squires JH, England E, Mehta K, et al. The role of imaging in diagnosing diseases of the distal radioulnar joint, triangular fibrocartilage complex, and distal ulna. AJR Am J Roentgenol 2014;203(1):146–53.
15. Fukuda T, Fukuda K. The role of dual-energy computed tomography in musculoskeletal imaging. PET Clin 2018;13(4):567–78.
16. Edlund R, Skorpil M, Lapidus G, et al. Cone-Beam CT in diagnosis of scaphoid fractures. Skeletal Radiol 2016;45(2):197–204.
17. Hayter CL, Gold SL, Potter HG. Magnetic resonance imaging of the wrist: bone and cartilage injury. J Magn Reson Imaging 2013;37(5):1005–19.
18. Chang AL, Yu HJ, von Borstel D, et al. Advanced Imaging Techniques of the Wrist. AJR Am J Roentgenol 2017;209(3):497–510.

19. Hafezi-Nejad N, Carrino JA, Eng J, et al. Scapholunate interosseous ligament tears: diagnostic performance of 1.5 T, 3 T MRI, and MR arthrography-a systematic review and meta-analysis. Acad Radiol 2016;23(9):1091–103.

20. Anderson ML, Skinner JA, Felmlee JP, et al. Diagnostic comparison of 1.5 Tesla and 3.0 Tesla preoperative MRI of the wrist in patients with ulnar-sided wrist pain. J Hand Surg Am 2008;33(7):1153–9.

21. Cockenpot E, Lefebvre G, Demondion X, et al. Imaging of sports-related hand and wrist injuries: sports imaging series. Radiology 2016;279(3):674–92.

22. Olubaniyi BO, Bhatnagar G, Vardhanabhuti V, et al. Comprehensive musculoskeletal sonographic evaluation of the hand and wrist. J Ultrasound Med 2013;32(6): 901–14.

23. American College of R, Society for Pediatric RSociety of Radiologists in U. AIUM practice guideline for the performance of a musculoskeletal ultrasound examination. J Ultrasound Med 2012;31(9):1473–88.

24. Plotkin B, Sampath SC, Sampath SC, et al. MR Imaging and US of the Wrist Tendons. Radiographics 2016;36(6):1688–700.

25. Porrino JA Jr, Maloney E, Scherer K, et al. Fracture of the distal radius: epidemiology and premanagement radiographic characterization. AJR Am J Roentgenol 2014;203(3):551–9.

26. May MM, Lawton JN, Blazar PE. Ulnar styloid fractures associated with distal radius fractures: incidence and implications for distal radioulnar joint instability. J Hand Surg Am 2002;27(6):965–71.

27. Fowler JR, Hughes TB. Scaphoid fractures. Clin Sports Med 2015;34(1):37–50.

28. Gaebler C, Kukla C, Breitenseher M, et al. Magnetic resonance imaging of occult scaphoid fractures. J Trauma 1996;41(1):73–6.

29. Marchessault J, Conti M, Baratz ME. Carpal fractures in athletes excluding the scaphoid. Hand Clin 2009;25(3):371–88.

30. Blum AG, Zabel J, Kohlmann R, et al. Pathologic conditions of the hypothenar eminence: evaluation with multidetector CT and MR imaging. Radiographics 2006;26(4):1021–44.

31. Andresen R, Radmer S, Sparmann M, et al. Imaging of hamate bone fractures in conventional X-rays and high-resolution computed tomography. An in vitro study. Invest Radiol 1999;34(1):46–50.

32. Henderson CJ, Kobayashi KM. Ulnar-sided wrist pain in the athlete. Orthop Clin North Am 2016;47(4):789–98.

33. Cotterell IH, Richard MJ. Metacarpal and phalangeal fractures in athletes. Clin Sports Med 2015;34(1):69–98.

34. Smith ML, Bain GI, Chabrel N, et al. Using computed tomography to assist with diagnosis of avascular necrosis complicating chronic scaphoid nonunion. J Hand Surg Am 2009;34(6):1037–43.

35. Fox MG, Wang DT, Chhabra AB. Accuracy of enhanced and unenhanced MRI in diagnosing scaphoid proximal pole avascular necrosis and predicting surgical outcome. Skeletal Radiol 2015;44(11):1671–8.

36. Larribe M, Gay A, Freire V, et al. Usefulness of dynamic contrast-enhanced MRI in the evaluation of the viability of acute scaphoid fracture. Skeletal Radiol 2014; 43(12):1697–703.

37. Donati OF, Zanetti M, Nagy L, et al. Is dynamic gadolinium enhancement needed in MR imaging for the preoperative assessment of scaphoidal viability in patients with scaphoid nonunion? Radiology 2011;260(3):808–16.

38. Singh AK, Davis TR, Dawson JS, et al. Gadolinium enhanced MR assessment of proximal fragment vascularity in nonunions after scaphoid fracture: does it predict the outcome of reconstructive surgery? J Hand Surg Br 2004;29(5):444–8.
39. Feydy A, Pluot E, Guerini H, et al. Role of imaging in spine, hand, and wrist osteoarthritis. Rheum Dis Clin North Am 2009;35(3):605–49.
40. Moser T, Dosch JC, Moussaoui A, et al. Wrist ligament tears: evaluation of MRI and combined MDCT and MR arthrography. AJR Am J Roentgenol 2007; 188(5):1278–86.
41. Ringler MD, Howe BM, Amrami KK, et al. Utility of magnetic resonance imaging for detection of longitudinal split tear of the ulnotriquetral ligament. J Hand Surg Am 2013;38(9):1723–7.
42. Clavero JA, Alomar X, Monill JM, et al. MR imaging of ligament and tendon injuries of the fingers. Radiographics 2002;22(2):237–56.
43. Ehman EC, Hayes ML, Berger RA, et al. Subluxation of the distal radioulnar joint as a predictor of foveal triangular fibrocartilage complex tears. J Hand Surg Am 2011;36(11):1780–4.
44. Gupta P, Lenchik L, Wuertzer SD, et al. High-resolution 3-T MRI of the fingers: review of anatomy and common tendon and ligament injuries. AJR Am J Roentgenol 2015;204(3):W314–23.
45. Miller TT, Reinus WR. Nerve entrapment syndromes of the elbow, forearm, and wrist. AJR Am J Roentgenol 2010;195(3):585–94.
46. Andreisek G, Burg D, Studer A, et al. Upper extremity peripheral neuropathies: role and impact of MR imaging on patient management. Eur Radiol 2008;18(9): 1953–61.

Hand and Wrist Tendinopathies

Nathan C. Patrick, MD, Warren C. Hammert, MD*

KEYWORDS

- Tendinopathy • Tendonitis • Tendinopathies in athletes
- Sports-related injuries of the wrist and hand • Flexor tendon injures
- Extensor tendon injuries • Overuse injuries of the hand and wrist

KEY POINTS

- Sports-related tendinopathies of the hand and wrist are common and are predominantly related to overuse.
- Most cases can be diagnosed with history and physical examination alone, with the need for advanced imaging in recalcitrant cases.
- Nonoperative management, consisting of rest, activity modification, antiinflammatory medications, temporary splinting or bracing, hand therapy, and possibly steroid injections, plays a pivotal role. Surgical intervention may be offered in those patients who fail nonoperative treatment.

INTRODUCTION

Hand and wrist tendinopathies are commonly seen in athletes, ranging from contact to noncontact racquet/stick sports. Many of these typically do not cause the athletes to lose time from their sports because treatment is symptomatic and rarely time specific. Diagnosis for tendinopathies in the hand and wrist is predominantly made on clinical examination. If the diagnosis is uncertain or the patient fails nonoperative treatment, advanced imaging may help. Most of these conditions respond to nonoperative treatment with activity modification, antiinflammatory medications, hand therapy, and corticosteroid injections. Although the level of steroid used for injection is typically very low, athletes in competitive leagues, in which testing is performed for performance-enhancing medications, should be aware of possible testing parameters for banned substances before having an injection. Although the authors do not believe these injections will improve overall performance, sports vary regarding their specific testing parameters and banned substances, and thus the medical personnel and the athletes should be aware of the specifics for their sports. When symptoms persist in spite of nonoperative treatment, clinicians offer surgical treatment. This surgery can

Division of Hand and Wrist Surgery, Department of Orthopaedics and Rehabilitation, University of Rochester Medical Center, 601 Elmwood Avenue, Box 665, Rochester, NY 14612, USA
* Corresponding author.
E-mail address: warren_hammert@urmc.rochester.edu

Clin Sports Med 39 (2020) 247–258
https://doi.org/10.1016/j.csm.2019.10.004
0278-5919/20/© 2019 Elsevier Inc. All rights reserved.

typically be done under local anesthesia (WALANT [wide awake local anesthesia no tourniquet]) or local anesthesia with sedation. Following operative treatment, a structured rehabilitation program to resume motion and tendon gliding is imperative under the guidance of a hand therapist and then athletic trainer/coach.

EXTENSOR TENDINOPATHIES
De Quervain Tenosynovitis

Tendinopathy involving the first dorsal extensor compartment, or de Quervain tenosynovitis, is a notable source of radial-sided wrist pain in athletes participating in racquet sports, rowing, golf, volleyball, and bowling.[1–4] In tennis,[3] golf,[4] and rowing,[1] the condition has been attributed to varied grips, altered swing mechanics, and tight grips with poor technique, respectively. In contrast, in volleyball, repetitive microtrauma from impact of the ball on the dorsal radial wrist and increased training time has been implicated with the risk of developing de Quervain tenosynovitis.[2] Regardless of the proposed sport-specific mechanisms, the end result is restricted, painful motion of the tendons of the abductor pollicis longus (APL) and extensor pollicis brevis (EPB) within the fibro-osseous sheath in which they travel immediately proximal to the radial styloid.[5] The tendon sheaths of those affected may be up to 5 times thicker as a result of accumulation of mucopolysaccharides and increased vascularity, consistent with myxoid degeneration rather than acute inflammation.[6,7]

A higher rate of de Quervain tenosynovitis has been shown in women, with a slight predilection for individuals more than 40 years of age or of African American decent.[8] Affected individuals invariably have some degree of swelling in the vicinity of the radial styloid and tenderness with palpation to the first extensor compartment tendons. The Eichhoff and Finkelstein maneuvers (**Fig. 1**) have been described to clinically confirm the diagnosis of de Quervain tenosynovitis. They are commonly thought of as the same maneuver; however, there are differences.[9–11] The Eichhoff maneuver is performed by asking the patient to gently grasp the thumb in the palm while the wrist is ulnarly deviated by the examiner. Pain over the region of the first extensor compartment is considered a positive maneuver and considered consistent with de Quervain tenosynovitis. The Finkelstein maneuver, as originally described, has the examiner passively flex the thumb and ulnarly deviate the wrist, with a positive maneuver producing pain over the first extensor compartment. Wu and colleagues[12] compared these maneuvers on 72 wrists (36 patients) and found the Finkelstein maneuver was more accurate, with fewer positive results and less discomfort for the patients.

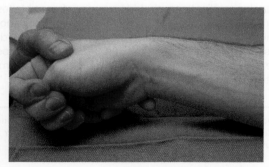

Fig. 1. Eichhoff maneuver. The patient is asked to gently grasp the thumb in the palm as the wrist is ulnarly deviated by the examiner. Reproduction of the patient's pain is a positive maneuver.

More recently, the wrist hyperflexion and abduction of the thumb (WHAT) maneuver (**Fig. 2**) has been described as an additional diagnostic tool with better sensitivity (0.99 vs 0.89) and specificity (0.28 vs 0.14).[13] A positive maneuver is reproduction of symptoms with resisted thumb abduction with the wrist maximally flexed.

As with most tendinopathies, conservative treatment begins with avoiding the inciting event. A short course of immobilization, hand therapy, and nonsteroidal anti-inflammatory medications can be an effective adjunct to limit pain and symptoms. Injection of corticosteroid and local anesthetic into the tendon sheath of the first dorsal compartment is often combined with these conservative modalities. Earp and colleagues[14] reported on the effectiveness of a single injection and determined that 82% of patients are symptom free for the first 6 weeks and more than half were without symptoms at 1 year. A more recent study by Oh and colleagues[15] found that more than 70% of patients who responded to 1 or 2 injections had resolution of symptoms. Surgical release may be warranted in cases of recalcitrant symptoms; however, patients are counseled about the possibility of an extended recovery, incomplete relief, and transient numbness in the superficial radial nerve distribution.[16] In our practice, new patients with de Quervain tenosynovitis are offered a corticosteroid injection in combination with a forearm-based thumb spica orthosis. If possible, athletes are encouraged to await return to play until symptoms have resolved, but no formal restrictions are placed. When symptoms persist, we offer first extensor compartment release, which is done through a transverse incision, taking care to protect the sensory

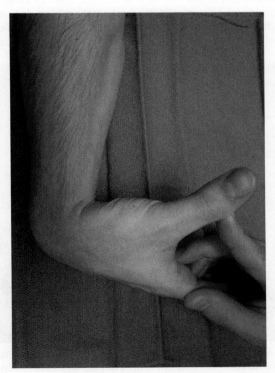

Fig. 2. WHAT maneuver. The patient's wrist is maximally flexed and the thumb is radially abducted against resistance provided by the examiner. Reproduction of the patient's pain is a positive maneuver.

branches of the radial nerve and lateral antebrachial cutaneous nerves, under local anesthesia. The incision in the extensor retinaculum is along the dorsal/ulnar aspect of first extensor compartment in order to minimize the chance of tendons subluxing in a volar direction with wrist flexion and thumb motion. The EPB often has a separate subcompartment that must be recognized and released. A soft dressing is applied, and early movement of the thumb is encouraged to promote tendon gliding. Return to activities depends on wound healing and comfort, but is generally at 2 to 3 weeks after surgery.

Intersection Syndrome

Intersection syndrome is characterized by radial-sided wrist pain, swelling, tenderness, and occasional crepitus in an area approximately 4 cm proximal to the Lister tubercle (**Fig. 3**). Controversy remains with regard to the precise location of the syndrome: the intersection of the muscle bellies of the APL and EPB and the extensor tendons of the second compartment, or stenosing tenosynovitis within the second compartment itself. One of the few reports on this condition, provided by Grundberg and Reagan[17] in 1985, concluded that the disorder was stenosing tenosynovitis of the sheath of the common radial wrist extensors, suggesting that space limitations within this compartment lead to accumulation of reactive tissue beneath the APL and EPB. In their limited cohort, all patients improved with surgical release of the second compartment, indicating its role with this condition.

As with other tendinopathies of the hand and wrist, this has been associated with repetitive use and may be seen in athletes participating in rowing, weightlifting, and cycling. Pain is often elicited with resisted wrist extension and radial deviation, and careful attention should be paid to the location of tenderness because this can be

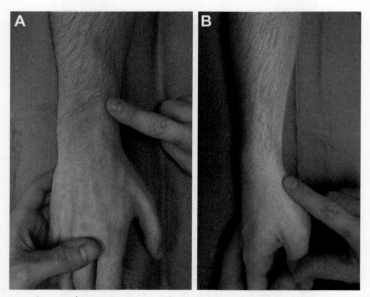

Fig. 3. Intersection syndrome. Patients with intersection syndrome have symptoms approximately 4 cm proximal to Lister tubercle in the area of intersection between the first and second extensor compartments (*A*). In contrast, the location of pain with de Quervain tenosynovitis is more distal, in the area of the radial styloid (*B*). (*Courtesy of* Stephen R. Thompson and Dan A. Zlotolow.)

misdiagnosed as de Quervain tenosynovitis. Treatment involves a combination of activity modification, temporary immobilization with a wrist splint in neutral extension, stretching exercises, and antiinflammatory medications. Steroid injections into the tendon sheath of the second compartment in the area of maximal tenderness may be provided in refractory cases. It has been our experience that most cases resolve with conservative modalities, hence the paucity of reported cases in the literature. In the event that symptoms persist in spite of nonoperative treatment, we release the second extensor compartment and debride any inflamed tenosynovium. This operation is typically performed out of season, with a short period of immobilization and therapy to regain motion and strength. Four to 6 weeks is expected to return to full activities.

Extensor Carpi Ulnaris Conditions

Disorder involving the extensor carpi ulnaris (ECU) tendon is a common source of ulnar-sided wrist pain, particularly in athletes using a club or racquet.[18–20] A broad spectrum of modalities have been described, including stenosing tenosynovitis; tendinosis; bony erosion of the sixth compartment floor; subluxation; and, rarely, rupture.[21] Given the anatomy of the ulnar side of the wrist, thorough physical examination is imperative. Tenderness about the ECU tendon sheath and pain or weakness with resisted wrist extension and ulnar deviation is invariably present. The ECU synergy maneuver (**Fig. 4**), described by Ruland and Hogan,[22] provides another tool to help better differentiate tendon versus intra-articular disorder. To perform this maneuver, the patient's elbow is flexed to 90° with the forearm fully supinated. The patient is then asked to radially abduct the thumb against resistance as the examiner places a counterforce on the middle digit. In doing so, the second extensor compartment tendons activate and to keep the wrist in neutral position, and the ECU fires. The maneuver is deemed positive if the patient's ulnar-sided wrist pain is recreated. The investigators noted symptomatic relief in all patients with a positive test following an ECU tendon sheath lidocaine injection, whereas those with a negative test were found to have intra-articular disorder on either MRI or wrist arthroscopy. ECU subluxation, or snapping ECU, can be evaluated by having the patient flex and ulnarly deviate the wrist with the forearm in supination because that creates the greatest angulation of the ECU tendon with respect to the ulna.

In the setting of stenosing tenosynovitis or ECU tendinopathy, initial treatment is primarily conservative, with activity modification, antiinflammatories, and rest with a short course of immobilization. Although some clinicians prefer above-elbow immobilization, the authors prefer a short-arm orthosis with fingers and thumb free and the wrist in ulnar deviation. The authors are aware of no data to suggest one is more effective than the other, but, from our experience, patients are more comfortable with the elbow free. A trial steroid injection into the ECU tendon sheath may be considered as an adjunct for both diagnostic as well as therapeutic purposes; however, the longevity of such an injection is not known. Care should be given when injecting the ECU tendon sheath to ensure that it is at the appropriate depth to guard against skin hypopigmentation and atrophy from superficial injection. Surgical decompression is reserved for chronic cases that have failed to improve with a minimum of 2 to 3 months of conservative treatment and is typically performed during the off-season. Our preferred operative treatment, in the absence of instability, involves radial incision of the fibroosseous canal of the sixth compartment, debridement of any inflamed tissue within the ECU subsheath, and repair of the overlying extensor retinaculum; however, controversy exist as to the importance of the retinacular repair in preventing ECU tendon instability.[23] Anomalous tendon slips between the ECU and the extensor digiti minimi

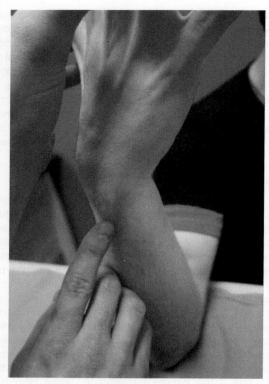

Fig. 4. ECU synergy maneuver. The patient's elbow is flexed to 90° with the forearm in a fully supinated position. The patient is then asked to radially abduct the thumb against resistance as the examiner places a counterforce on the middle digit. Reproduction of pain in the area of the ECU is a positive maneuver.

have been reported and current, limited research suggests excision at the time of decompression.[20] Montalava and colleagues[18] describe their experience in treating 28 professional tennis players, 14 of whom had ECU tendinosis. They were able to manage this condition with orthoses with the athletes continuing to play. Symptoms resolved between 2 and 24 weeks and none of the athletes required surgery. Treatment of ECU instability is largely the same, with the exception of immobilization. In these patients, the wrist is immobilized above the elbow in pronation, wrist extension, and slight radial deviation in order to limit the provocative position of the ECU, typically with a modified Munster orthosis. Montalava and colleagues[18] also described nonoperative treatment of ECU instability, with some patients showing instability and some with subluxation of the ECU completely out of the groove. Symptoms resolved with 3 to 4 months of nonoperative treatment in all 12 patients. When detachment of the extensor retinaculum occurred (3 patients), ultrasonography was used to monitor healing. Immobilization is discontinued when reattachment occurs or at 12 weeks. Surgical management of these patients in the setting of failed conservative treatment entails imbrication of the subsheath in acute cases (<6 months), or reconstruction using a radially based flap of the extensor retinaculum that is passed beneath the ECU and secured to itself, or ECU groove deepening. Our preferred treatment (**Fig. 5**) involves ECU groove deepening. A longitudinal incision is made over the sixth extensor

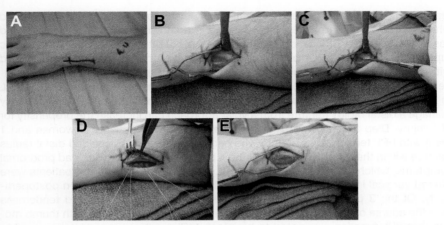

Fig. 5. Example of reconstruction of ECU instability with ulnar groove deepening. (*A*) Location of incision, (*B*) appearance of ulna after elevation of ECU and subsheath, (*C*) Freer elevator placed by ECU groove before deepening, (*D*) appearance after placement of suture anchors in ulna before reattachment of subsheath, and (*E*) appearance after closure of extensor retinaculum.

compartment, taking care to protect the sensory branch of the ulnar nerve. The retinaculum is opened along the ulnar aspect and tagged for later repair. The subsheath is evaluated and dissected off the ulna. If there is notable synovitis, the subsheath is opened and debrided. The groove in the ulna is then evaluated. Using a barrel-shaped bur, the groove is deepened to roughly the depth of a freer elevator. The subsheath is then imbricated and reattached to the ulna using suture anchors, followed by repair of the retinaculum. MacLennan and colleagues[24] reported on 21 patients with ultrasonography confirmation of subluxation treated in this manner, with improvements in grip strength, wrist motion, pain, satisfaction, and DASH (Disabilities of the Arm, Shoulder, and Hand) scores. Alternatively, an ulnarly or radially based strip of extensor retinaculum can be used to stabilize the ECU.[25] Allende and Le Viet[20] reported on 27 patients, 17 of whom were injured playing sports, who had stabilization of the ECU using a radially based sling of extensor retinaculum secured to the ulnar head. Of these patients, 23 were noted to have a good to excellent result based on a composite score of strength, motion, and pain improvement in addition to return to preinjury activities. Twenty-two of the 27 patients returned to previous activities, 10 of whom were professional athletes who were able to perform at their previous level by a mean of 8 months (range, 3–21 months). There are no comparative studies showing that 1 method is superior. Postoperatively, patients are immobilized for 6 weeks in an above-elbow cast or orthosis, followed by a therapy program, with emphasis on regaining wrist motion and forearm rotation. Approximately 2 weeks later, we begin strengthening and allow racquet or stick handling once the patient has painless passive and active motion. We expect return to play between 8 and 10 weeks.

Extensor Pollicis Longus Entrapment

Tendon entrapment of the extensor pollicis longus (EPL) tendon is a rare cause of pain or injury in athletes. Despite the infrequency of this condition, early identification and intervention is vital because cases of spontaneous rupture have been reported.[26] The condition is characterized by pain with active or passive thumb flexion, swelling, tenderness, and crepitus at a level immediately distal to the Lister tubercle, around which the EPL tendon passes. This position is a known watershed area of limited vascularity with the EPL tendon, thus making it potentially vulnerable to ischemic rupture following local trauma.[27] Classically, rupture of the EPL has been associated with nondisplaced distal radius fractures treated with immobilization, with an incidence as high as 5% (**Fig. 6**).[28] In addition, given the intimate proximity of the EPL to the Lister tubercle, any violation of the dorsal cortex when attempting to operatively manage a distal radius fracture from a volar approach can increase the propensity for EPL injury. Diep and Adams[29] retrospectively identified 7 patients (6 women and 1 man) with EPL tendonitis or rupture who had sustained a nondisplaced distal radius fracture within the prior year. Only 2 of the 4 patients with EPL rupture had prodromal symptoms, which included tenderness, snapping, and weakness. All 4 patients were offered surgical intervention and were satisfied with their thumb function postoperatively. Of the 3 patients without rupture, clinical examination revealed tenderness over the course of the EPL tendon and Lister tubercle and wrist pain with thumb motion, but EPL function was noted to be intact. MRI or ultrasonography was used to confirm the diagnosis of EPL tendonitis. Decompression of the EPL tendon was subsequently completed with tendon rupture not experienced in all 3 patients. In lieu of other available evidence, the authors recommend early decompression and transposition for cases of suspected EPL entrapment to prevent the possibility of attritional rupture, a complication that may require an extensor indicis proprius transfer. Steroid injections are avoided in these patients, given the vulnerable watershed zone of the EPL and the potential increased propensity for rupture.

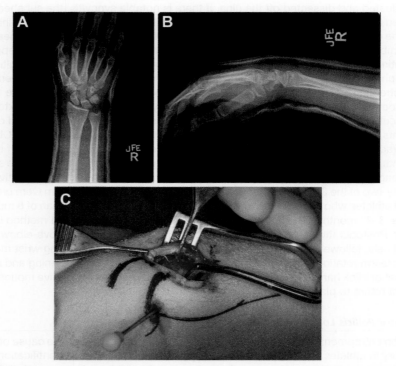

Fig. 6. A patient with a nondisplaced distal radius fracture (*A*, *B*) who developed EPL tendinopathy that required decompression (*C*). (*Courtesy of* Sanjeev Kakar.)

FLEXOR TENDINOPATHIES
Flexor Carpi Radialis Tendinopathy

Although a rare source of tendinopathy, the sharp angulation of the flexor carpi radialis (FCR) tendon across the ridge of the trapezium and tight fibro-osseous sheath through which it passes makes it prone to stenotic tendinopathy. Bishop and colleagues[30,31] reported on10 patients, in whom the primary symptom was pain localized to the proximal aspect of the trapezium and accentuated by resisted flexion and radial deviation (**Fig. 7**). Activities that involve repetitive flexion of the wrist, such as basketball, volleyball, and racquet sports, may increase the susceptibility for this condition, although the risk for development is not completely understood. Use of a lidocaine injection placed into the FCR sheath may aid in the diagnosis of FCR tendinopathy; however, Bishop and colleagues[30] only appreciated an improvement in pain in 5 of their patients, despite complete resolution in 9 patients following decompression. Given the proximity of the trapezium, which encircles the FCR tendon, from 61% to 80% at the level of the trapezial tubercle, and the scaphoid, radiographs of the wrist should be obtained to rule out occult fracture or early degenerative changes.[31] Conservative treatment by means of activity modification, a short course of wrist and basal thumb immobilization, stretching and strengthening exercises, and oral antiinflammatory medications are the main treatment modalities. A corticosteroid injection into the FCR sheath may be considered; however, current literature is lacking in terms of

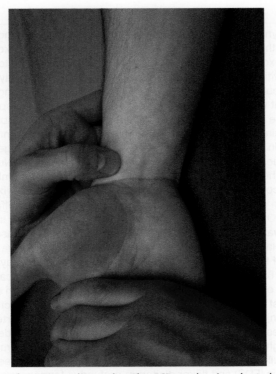

Fig. 7. Examination for FCR tendinopathy. The FCR tendon is palpated as the patient attempts to flex and radially deviate the wrist against resistance provided by the examiner. Reproduction of pain is a positive maneuver.

symptom resolution with this modality. Refractory cases may improve with FCR tunnel decompression, particularly in cases of isolated tendinopathy.

Flexor Carpi Ulnaris Tendinopathy

Tendinopathy of the flexor carpi ulnaris (FCU) are uncommon. Similar to the palmaris longus and unlike other tendons of the wrist and hand, the FCU does not pass through an enclosed sheath during its course. Presentation therefore differs from other tendon disorders in that triggering does not occur. Clinically, athletes may present with activity-related pain localized to the FCU tendon. Examination shows palpable tenderness approximately 2 to 3 cm proximal to the pisiform, in addition to pain localized to the same location with resisted wrist flexion and ulnar deviation. Budoff and colleagues[32] reported on 5 patients (6 wrists) diagnosed with FCU tendinopathy who failed nonsurgical management consisting of antiinflammatory medications, splinting, therapy, and steroid injections (4 patients). Angiofibroblastic hyperplasia (ie, tendinosis) was found in all patients, a finding that has not been described with other tendinopathies of the hand and wrist. This intrasubstance degenerative tissue was excised and the tendon subsequently repaired in a side-to-side manner, with complete to near-complete symptom relief reported in all patients at a minimum of 1-year follow-up. In light of this, the investigators concluded that this type of degenerative tendinopathy may be better treated by strengthening and stretching rather than by modalities aimed at inflammation, similar to recommendations for lateral epicondylosis or tennis elbow.

Trigger Digits

Stenosing tenosynovitis, or trigger digit, is a common cause of hand pain. This phenomenon is a pathologic disproportion of available space in the flexor tendon sheath and the digital flexor tendons. The underlying cause is often difficult to ascertain; however, sports activities involving repetitive gripping or mild trauma may result in relative tendon or retinacular thickening, thus resulting in mechanical impingement. Patients invariably present with pain and tenderness overlying the palmar aspect of the metacarpal head (in the area of the A1 pulley). In addition, they may describe digit snapping, catching, or locking. To minimize symptoms, patients often limit motion of affected digits, resulting in flexion deformities of the proximal interphalangeal joint, and an inability to fully flex the digit into the palm may be appreciated. Numerous studies have evaluated the efficacy of steroid injections, including the number of injections that should be considered before surgery.[25] Kerrigan and Stanwix[33] performed a cost-minimization analysis to identify the least costly strategy for effective treatment of trigger finger. Of the 5 algorithms included, management with 2 steroid injections before surgery was the least costly, with immediate surgical release costing 248% to 340% more. Halim and colleagues[34] more recently evaluated the cost of nonsurgical treatment of trigger finger in terms of dollars reimbursed by payers. In their prospective study of 82 patients, offering up to 3 injections before surgical release yielded potential savings of $72,730 ($826 per digit) or 43% of the cost, with the first injection having the highest component of cost savings ($15,956). In our practice, patients are offered up to 2 injections, with a 60% to 70% success rate reported. In refractory cases, decompression is performed under local anesthetic. This decompression is performed through a longitudinal incision for fingers and a transverse incision in the thumb. The A1 pulley is released and, in the fingers, adhesions between the flexor digitorum superficialis (FDS) and flexor digitorum profundus tendons are separated. This procedure is performed under WALANT so the patient can actively move the finger to ensure the triggering has resolved. In the event that triggering persists following A1 pulley release, the authors excise 1 slip of the FDS. There does not seem to be a difference between the radial and ulnar slips, so we tend to excise the one that has the most fraying or tendon degeneration if present. The incision is closed with absorbable sutures and a surgical glue. A soft dressing in applied following surgery and immediate motion with tendon gliding exercises are performed. Athletes are restricted from gripping and heavy lifting activities until the skin has healed, with return to sport typically in 2 to 3 weeks.

SUMMARY

Tendinopathies of the hand and wrist are a common source of injury in athletes given the repetitive nature of most sports. Diagnosis can often be made with a thorough history and physical examination alone, minimizing the need for advanced imaging. As a whole, this group of injuries responds well in the early or acute phase to conservative measures such as rest and activity modification, temporary immobilization, therapy, and antiinflammatory medications. For recalcitrant cases, steroid injections can be effective. With the exception of EPL entrapment, surgical intervention is reserved for chronic cases that have failed to respond to these conservative modalities.

DISCLOSURE

There are no financial conflicts of interest to disclose.

REFERENCES

1. Rumball JS, Lebrun CM, Di Ciacca SR, et al. Rowing injuries. Sports Med 2005; 35(6):537–55.
2. Rossi C, Cellocco P, Margaritondo E, et al. De Quervain disease in volleyball players. Am J Sports Med 2005;33:424–7.
3. Tagliafico AS, Ameri P, Michaud J, et al. Wrist injuries in nonprofessional tennis players: relationships with different grips. Am J Sports Med 2009;37:760–7.
4. Woo SH, Lee YK, Kim JM, et al. Hand and wrist injuries in golfers and their treatment. Hand Clin 2017;33:81–96.
5. Ilyas A, Ast M, Schaffer AA, et al. De Quervain tenosynovitis of the wrist. J Am Acad Orthop Surg 2007;15:757–64.
6. Kutsumi K, Amadio PC, Zhao C, et al. Gliding resistance of the extensor pollicis brevis tendon and abductor pollicis longus tendon within the first dorsal compartment in fixed wrist positions. J Orthop Res 2005;23(2):243–8.
7. Clarke MT, Lyall HA, Grant JW, et al. The histopathology of de Quervain's disease. J Hand Surg Br 1998;23(6):732–4.
8. Wolf JM, Sturdivant RX, Owens BD. Incidence of de Quervain's tenosynovitis in a young, active population. J Hand Surg Am 2009;34:112–5.
9. Elliott BG. Finkelstein's test: a descriptive error that can produce a false positive. J Hand Surg Br 1992;17(4):481–2.
10. Finkelstein H. Stenosing tendovaginitis at the radial styloid process. J Bone Joint Surg Am 1930;1(2):509–40.
11. Chung K. Optimizing the treatment or upper extremity injuries in athletes. Hand Clinic 2017;33(1):xiii–xiv.
12. Wu F, Rajpura A, Sandher D. Finkelstein's test is superior to Eichhoff's test in the investigation of de Quervain's disease. J Hand Microsurg 2018;10(2):116–8.
13. Goubau JF, Goubau L, Van Tongel A, et al. The wrist hyperflexion and abduction of the thumb (WHAT) test: a more specific and sensitive test to diagnose de

Quervain tenosynovitis than the Eichhoff's test. J Hand Surg Eur Vol 2014;39(3): 286–92.

14. Earp BE, Han CH, Floyd WE, et al. de Quervain Tendinopathy: survivorship and prognostic indicators of recurrence following a single corticosteroid injection. J Hand Surg Am 2015;40(6):1161–5.

15. Oh J, Messing S, Hyrien O, et al. Effectiveness of corticosteroid injections for treatment of de Quervains Tenosynovitis. Hand (NY) 2017;12(4):357–61.

16. Pensak MJ, Wolf JM. Current treatment of de Quervain tendinopathy. J Hand Surg Am 2013;38(11):2247–9.

17. Grundbreg AB, Reagen DS. Pathologic anatomy of the forearm: intersection syndrome. J Hand Surg Am 1985;10(2):299–302.

18. Montalvan B, Parier J, Brasseur JL, et al. Extensor carpi ulnaris injuries in tennis players: a study of 28 cases. Br J Sports Med 2006;40:424–9.

19. Carneiro RS, Fontana R, Mazzer N. Ulnar wrist pain in athletes caused by erosion of the floor of the sixth dorsal compartment: a case series. Am J Sports Med 2005;33:1910–3.

20. Allende C, Le Viet D. Extensor carpi ulnaris problems at the wrist—classification, surgical treatment and results. J Hand Surg Br 2005;30B:265–72.

21. McAuliffe JA. Tendon disorders of the hand and wrist. J Hand Surg Am 2010;35A: 846–53.

22. Ruland RT, Hogan CJ. The ECU synergy test: an aid to diagnose ECU tendonitis. J Hand Surg Am 2008;33A:1777–82.

23. Kip PA, Peimer CA. Release of the sixth dorsal compartment. J Hand Surg Am 1994;19:599–601.

24. MacLennan AJ, Nemechek NM, Waitayawinyu T, et al. Diagnosis and anatomic reconstruction of extensor carpi ulnaris subluxation. J Hand Surg Am 2008; 33(1):59–64.

25. Wolfe SW. Tenosynovitis. In: Green DP, Hotchkiss RN, Pederson WC, et al, editors. Green's operative hand surgery. 5th edition. New York: Churchill Livingstone; 2005. p. 2137–58.

26. Dawson WJ. Sports-induced spontaneous rupture of the extensor pollicis longus tendon. J Hand Surg Am 1992;17A:457–8.

27. Engkvist GL. Rupture of the extensor pollicis longus tendon after fracture of the lower end of the radius—a clinical and microangiographic study. Hand 1979;1: 76–86.

28. Roth KM, Blazar PE, Earp BE, et al. Incidence of extensor pollicis tendon rupture after nondisplaced distal radius fractures. J Hand Surg Am 2012;37(5):942–7.

29. Diep GK, Adams JE. The prodrome of extensor pollicis longus tendonitis and rupture: rupture may be preventable. Orthopedics 2016;39(5):318–22.

30. Bishop AT, Gabel G, Carmichael SW. Flexor carpi radialis tendinitis. Part I: operative anatomy. J Bone Joint Surg 1994;76A:1009–14.

31. Gabel G, Bishop AT, Wood MB. Flexor carpi radialis tendinitis. Part II: results of operative treatment. J Bone Joint Surg 1994;76A:1015–8.

32. Budoff JE, Kraushaar BS, Ayala G. Flexor carpi ulnaris tendinopathy. J Hand Surg Am 2005;30A:125–9.

33. Kerrigan CL, Stanwix MG. Using evidence to minimize the cost of trigger finger care. J Hand Surg Am 2009;34(6):997–1005.

34. Halim A, Sobel AD, Eltorai AEM, et al. Cost-effective management of stenosing tenosynovitis. J Hand Surg Am 2018;43(12):1085–91.

Extensor Tendon Injuries in the Athlete

Spencer Skinner, MD, Jonathan Isaacs, MD*

KEYWORDS

- Extensor tendon injuries • Athletes • Mallet finger • Swan neck • Central slip
- Boutonniere • Sports injuries

KEY POINTS

- Extensor tendon injuries can be difficult to treat given the high demands and expectations of the athlete.
- Delaying treatment until completion of a season is a viable option in certain circumstances.
- Neglected mallet injuries in patients with hyperlax joints can lead to a swan neck deformity.
- Boutonniere injuries and tendon lacerations should be definitively treated without delay whenever possible.
- Tendinitis and overuse syndromes can often be treated conservatively.

INTRODUCTION

Athletes are not only prone to sport-specific hand and wrist injuries but often have unique short- and long-term goals that often necessitate tailored treatment plans. The specific sport, position played, competition level, and future expectations and aspirations must all be considered as the consulting physician guides the athlete toward realistic and mutually acceptable treatment strategies. Definitive treatment postponement until after the current season or return to play with protective devices may be reasonable in certain circumstances. This approach should be applied in a more guarded manor in the skeletally immature athlete and avoided if long-term outcomes could be unacceptably compromised.

The authors have not received or will not receive benefits for personal or professional use from a commercial party related directly or indirectly to the subject of this article.
Division of Hand Surgery, Department of Orthopedic Surgery, Virginia Commonwealth University Health System, 1200 East Broad Street, PO Box 980153, Richmond, VA 23298, USA
* Corresponding author.
E-mail address: jonathan.isaacs@vcuhealth.org

Clin Sports Med 39 (2020) 259–277
https://doi.org/10.1016/j.csm.2019.12.005
0278-5919/20/© 2019 Elsevier Inc. All rights reserved.

sportsmed.theclinics.com

ANATOMY
Extrinsic Contributions

Muscles of the extensor system
The extensor tendons of the fingers and thumb are comprised of the extensor digitorum communis (EDC), extensor indicis proprius, extensor digiti minimi, extensor pollicis longs, and extensor pollicis brevis. Wrist extension is produced through functions of the extensor carpi radialis longus, extensor carpi radialis brevis, and extensor carpi ulnaris (ECU).

Dorsal wrist compartments
The musculotendinous junctions of the wrist and finger extensors lie several centimeters proximal to the wrist with the exception of the extensor indicis proprius, whose muscle belly frequently continues to the level of the wrist joint. At the level of the radial metaphysis, the tendons are separated into 6 synovial lined fibro-osseous sheaths (**Fig. 1**), save the fifth, which has no osseous connections. The sixth extensor compartment is also unique as its subsheath is intimately involved with the dorsal aspect of the triangular fibrocartilage complex.

Juncturae tendinum and sagittal bands
Proximal to the metacarpophalangeal (MCP) joint are stout interconnections between the tendons of the EDC. These connections limit independent ring and middle finger extension when the other digits remained flexed. The sagittal bands are expansions over the extensor tendons at the level of the MCP, which originate from the volar plate and insert onto the extensor hood. The sagittal bands maintain the centralized position of the extensor tendons throughout the arc of motion and facilitate MCP extension by a lasso effect transmitted via the volar plate connections.

Intrinsic Contributions

Anatomy of the extensor hood: Metacarpophalangeal to fingertip
The anatomy of the extensor system distal to the MCP joint is a complex system of converging and separating components that change position and geometry during flexion and extension of the digit, resulting in synergistic and balanced movement. The tendons of the lumbricals lie on the volar radial aspect of the proper digits and flex the MCP and extend the interphalangeal joints when activated. The interossei produce digital adduction/abduction and coalesce with the lumbricals to form the lateral bands.[1] The lateral bands bifurcate and join the extrinsic extensor system at the level

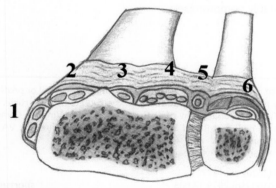

Fig. 1. Cross-section through the wrist demonstrating the 6 dorsal compartments.

of the proximal phalanx.[2] The EDC trifurcates just proximal to the proximal interphalangeal (PIP) joint. The central branch terminates as the central slip, which inserts on the base of the middle phalanx, and the lateral components join the lateral bands to form the conjoined lateral bands, which continue distally, eventually becoming the terminal tendon and inserting at the base of the distal phalanx[3] (**Fig. 2**).

The lateral bands exhibit some physiologic translation, but are maintained in their appropriate position by the balance of tension between the triangular ligament and the transverse retinacular ligament. The triangular ligament unites the lateral bands together on the distal dorsal aspect of the middle phalanx and prevents volar subluxation during PIP flexion, and the transverse retinacular ligaments constrain the lateral bands via their connections to the flexor tendon sheath to prevent excessive dorsal translocation.

The oblique retinacular ligament (ORL) originates from the volar sheath of the flexor system at the PIP joint and inserts dorsally into the terminal tendon. The ORL tightens during PIP extension, leading to concomitant extension of the distal interphalangeal (DIP).[4] The importance and consistency of this structure has been debated in the literature.[5]

ZONES OF INJURY

Extensor tendon injuries are classified from distal to proximal. Injuries overlying joints are given odd numbers: zone 1 over the DIP joint, 3 over the PIP joint, 5 over the MCP joint, and 7 over the wrist. The thumb is labeled differently so the interphalangeal joint is zone 1 and the MCP joint is zone 3. Injuries over nonarticulating segments are labeled with even numbers: zone 2 over the middle phalanx, 4 the proximal phalanx, 6 the metacarpals, and 8 in the forearm (**Fig. 3**).

Zone One Mallet Finger Injury

The mallet, baseball, or droop finger indicates terminal tendon discontinuity and resultant extensor lag at the DIP joint. The mechanism of injury is most often forced flexion

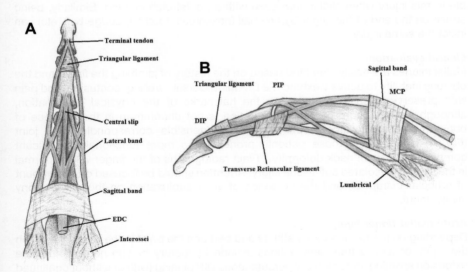

Fig. 2. (*A, B*) Anatomy of the digital extensor system.

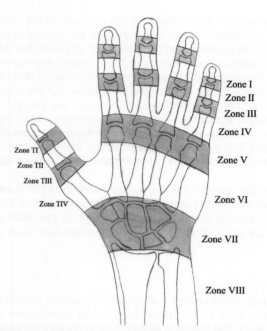

Zone I
Zone II
Zone III
Zone IV
Zone V
Zone VI
Zone VII
Zone VIII

Zone TI
Zone TII
Zone TIII
Zone TIV

Fig. 3. The zones are classified from distal to proximal with the odd numbers overlying the joints. The DIP joint is zone 1, PIP joint zone 3, MCP joint zone 5, and the carpus zone 7. The thumb is similar with the interphalangeal joint zone 1 and the MCP joint zone 3.

of an extended finger[6] and failure can occur through the tendon itself or the distal phalanx. Offering a similar clinical presentation, forced hyperextension through the DIP joint can impact and fracture the dorsal articular surface resulting in a more severe fracture/dislocation injury pattern.[7] Baseball/softball players are particularly susceptible to this injury when sliding into base with an outstretched hand. Similarly, being struck on the end of the finger by any ball (basketball, football, dodge ball, etc) can inflict the same injury.

Clinical evaluation
Mallet injuries are easily identified based on the history of jamming the finger and the obvious inability to actively extend the DIP joint. Dorsal swelling, contusion, and pain with preserved passive motion are the hallmarks of the physical examination, although a much more benign presentation is not uncommon in the absence of bony involvement. Recognition of a hyperextensible corresponding PIP joint (**Fig. 4**) may identify those patients prone to the more functionally significant compensatory swan neck deformity.[8] Plain radiographs of the finger will be normal in the setting of isolated soft tissue injury. Attention should be focused on the amount of articular disruption and the presence of volar subluxation on those with bony involvement.

Acute mallet finger injury
Depending on the desires of the athlete and perhaps the point in the season in which the injury occurs, 3 treatment options include temporary benign neglect, full-time extension splinting, or temporary percutaneous DIP pinning (with or without continued play).

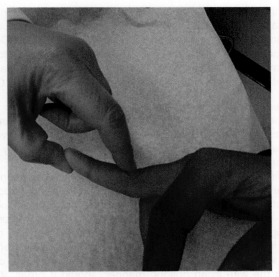

Fig. 4. Hyperlaxity noted in the PIP of a football player who developed a swan neck deformity after sustaining a mallet injury.

Delayed treatment

Late presentation soft tissue mallet injuries can still be treated successfully.[9] Splinting acute and chronic mallet fingers within 3 to 4 months achieved restoration of DIP extension and a residual extensor lag of less than 10° noted in 1 study.[10] An athlete could reasonably opt to complete their season without the hindrance of a restrictive splint or invasive surgery, although they should be made aware that, intuitively, the greater the delay in treatment, the less likely a full restoration of function. Particularly in athletes with hyperlaxity, the development of a swan neck deformity resulting from focused tension at the central slip insertion is a real possibility. Swan neck posturing may be substantially more debilitating than a mallet finger with painful snapping as the PIP moves from the hyperextended to flexed position, loss of dexterity, and loss of grip strength. Additionally, surgical correction of both the DIP extensor lag and PIP hyperextension may be necessary if this sequelae of mallet undertreatment develops.

Extension splinting

Extension splinting is the preferred treatment in nonathletes and compliant athletes, which offers predictable outcomes without the inherent risks of surgery. The DIP joint is held in full extension with the PIP joint left free of immobilization unless substantial laxity is noted.[8] Bony involvement of 30% to 40% of the articular surface can still be effectively treated in a similar manner with satisfactory results at 2 years.[11] Athletes can return to sport immediately if the splint wear can be tolerated during competition. Of the many different methods of immobilization described, none have shown superiority, so splint choice should be based on comfort and compatibility with return to play.[8,12] Alternating between 2 different style splints can alleviate dorsal skin maceration from perspiration. One useful technique is the use of a combination of kinesiotape in association with the orthosis to assist in maintaining the DIP in extension.[13] After 6 to 8 weeks of full-time splinting, the patient is weaned to 6 weeks of night splinting.[14] PIP hyperextension addressed by extending the splint proximally to maintain the

PIP joint in slight flexion could further hinder athletic participation. A slight post-treatment residual extension lag is not uncommon or unexpected, considering that as little as 0.5 mm lengthening can lead to a 10° extension lag.[15] Despite this, with proper compliance, a more substantial deficit is rare,[16,17] and return to previous levels of competition can be anticipated.[18] For less compliant patients, Crawford[19] noted a 20% incidence of a potentially bothersome deformity greater than 10°.

Operative intervention

Surgical indications for the treatment of an acute mallet finger in an athlete include fracture fragments of greater than 40% of the articular surface with volar subluxation of the distal phalanx, or inability to adhere to full-time splinting therapy despite a desire for acute treatment and rapid return to play.

Simple mallet finger injuries, soft tissue or bony without subluxation, can be treated with transarticular Kirschner wire placement yielding expected postoperative mobility ranging from approximately 5° from full extension to 65° to 80° of flexion.[20] The wire, typically a 0.062-inch Kirshner wire (if continued athletic participation is planned), is placed in a retrograde fashion, obliquely across the DIP joint and cut beneath the skin for removal in 6 to 8 weeks, followed by 6 additional weeks of night splinting. Continued splint wear is recommended during competition for fear of hardware failure.[20] By placing the wire in an oblique manner, should it break, it can be readily retrieved.

Bony mallet injuries with volar subluxation generally require surgical treatment by one of several different options, including extension block pinning.[21] Some authors believe that these large fragments can be treated in an analogous fashion to simpler mallet injuries with no increased morbidity other than a dorsal bump.[11] Postoperatively, however, the exposed dorsal Kirschner wire's susceptibility to infection (around 14% incidence[22]) or migration complicates immediate return to sport, a minimal extension lag of less than 5° and near normal flexion can be expected.[22]

Chronic mallet finger injury

A chronic mallet finger or secondary swan neck deformity may result from a neglected or underappreciated injury. Although defined as an injury more than 4 weeks old, the guidelines for acute treatment can be applied for up to 4 months after injury.[7,23] Older injuries affecting only the DIP joint are often well-tolerated and surgical intervention is often not desired.[1] Secondary swan neck deformity from proximal tendon retraction and dorsal subluxation of the lateral bands,[24] in contrast, is poorly tolerated during competition.

ORL reconstruction[25,26] or central slip (Fowler) tenotomy[27] are the 2 primary reconstructive surgeries. Central slip tenotomy is the simpler of the 2 procedures, but is only effective with mild deformities involving less than 30° extension lag at the DIP joint and less than 20° hyperextension at the PIP joint.[28] The central slip is released just proximal to the PIP joint allowing proximal migration of the extensor mechanism and reestablishment of tension at the attenuated terminal slip assuming that the healed pseudotendon has matured and is stable—typically around 6 months.[29] ORL reconstruction, in contrast, can reliably correct swan neck deformities with more severe PIP hyperextension and an average of 42° of DIP extensor lag.[25]

Oblique retinacular ligament reconstruction technique

A curvilinear incision is made on the dorsum of the finger extending from the MCP to the insertion of the terminal tendon. The ulnar lateral band is chosen to preserve the radially based lumbrical. The lateral band is isolated and divided at the level of the MCP joint. A plane is developed at the level of the PIP joint deep to the neurovascular bundle but volar to the flexor tendon sheath and the isolated lateral band is shuttled from an ulnar to radial direction. A 2-mm unicortical hole is drilled in the proximal phalanx shaft and diverging Keith needles are driven across the far cortex and used to pull the tendon into the bone (**Fig. 5**). While securing the tendon in place, tension should be pulled until a position of 30° of flexion across the PIP joint and extension across the DIP is obtained. Sutures through the tendon stump can now be secured down over the far cortex bony bridge. A retrograde 0.045 Kirschner wire is then placed across the DIP joint. Postoperatively, gentle range of motion of the PIP joint from 30° to 60° of flexion can be initiated at 3 weeks, and the Kirschner wire across the DIP joint is left in place for 6 weeks (**Fig. 6**).

Zones 2, 4, and 6 Extensor Tendon Injuries

Zones 2, 4, and 6 injuries are due to open trauma involving 1 or both lateral bands and/ or the triangular ligament, central slip, or EDC tendon, respectively. In the athletic population these are uncommon injuries but still occur from cleats or skates that could potentially lacerate the hand.

Clinical evaluation and treatment
The initial evaluation should always assess contamination and risk of infection and include formal debridement as indicated. For zones 2 and 4 injuries if full extension

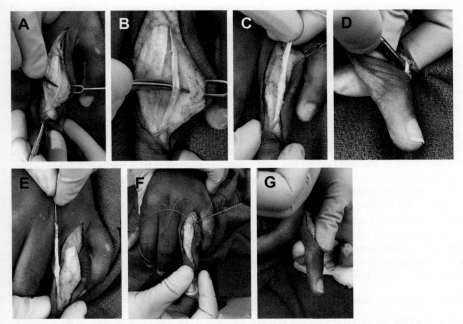

Fig. 5. (A) The surgical exposure with the ulnar based lateral band exposed. (B) The ulnar based lateral band dissected free from the remainder of the extensor system. (C) The lateral band released from the proximal aspect of the extensor hood. (D) Tension pulled through the lateral band demonstrating an extension force through the DIP joint. (E) Suture placed in the proximal aspect of the lateral band in preparation for rerouting. (F) Keith needles used to drill through the far cortex and pass the sutures to be tied down over a boney bridge of the proximal phalanx. (G) Resting position of the finger after completion of ORL reconstruction.

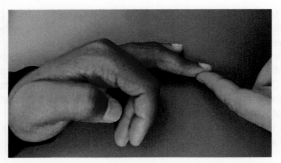

Fig. 6. Patient 3 months postoperative correction of swan neck deformity.

against resistance is preserved or if the injury involves less than 50% of the tendon, the athlete can return to activity with buddy taping for 3 to 4 weeks, although the digit should be monitored for delayed extensor lag.[1,23]

A zone 2 partial laceration with loss of active extension, complete laceration, or developing extensor lag can be directly repaired with equivalent results of an acute mallet finger.[12] If immediate repair is undertaken, protection with DIP pinning will allow early return to play if an extended DIP position can be tolerated during competition.

For zone 6 injuries, partial active extension may still be possible via the junctura and the examiner should maintain a high index of suspicion. A complete zone 4 or 6 injury should be treated with immediate direct surgical repair. Our preferred technique is a running interlocking horizontal mattress repair with a 4-0 nonabsorbable braided stich as described by Lee and colleagues[30] (**Fig. 7**). This technique is easy and quick and has been shown to be stiffer while minimizing tendon shortening compared with other more complex patterns.[30] Unfortunately, delayed presentation or treatment is not amenable to direct repair and will require more complex reconstructive options.

Postoperatively, athletic participation would be limited to conditioning or sports where the hand can be protected. For zone 6 repairs, a postoperative volar splint extending just past the MCP joints maintains extension while allowing interphalangeal motion. This is transitioned at the first postoperative visit to a relative motion splint, which effectively unloads the repair while allowing motion.[31] Zone 4 repairs are treated with temporary splinting in extension for 4 to 6 weeks and both groups are transitioned to buddy taping to encourage range of motion while continued to offer some protection. Unrestricted activity is allowed at 3 months.

More proximal injuries seem to have fewer adhesions and tendon imbalance problems,[32] as reflected in the observation that 50% of zone 4 injuries suffer a residual extensor lag through the PIP joint of less than 10° as well as a loss of flexion of less than 20°.[33] Zone 6 repairs usually regain 80% or more of preoperative motion.[34]

Zone 3 Extensor Tendon Injury

Zone 3 extensor tendon injuries involve disruption of the central slip or its insertion most commonly related to forced hyperflexion of the PIP joint, but also seen with lacerations and volar dislocations.[35] Like mallet fingers, acute injuries are categorized by soft tissue versus bony involvement. Left untreated, proximal migration of the disrupted central slip, attenuation of the triangular ligament, and volar subluxation of the lateral bands leads to progressive flexion deformity of the PIP joint and hyperextension at the DIP joint—the classic Boutonniere posture.[1,36] With time, this deformity becomes rigid and fixed[37] so early recognition and intervention is important.

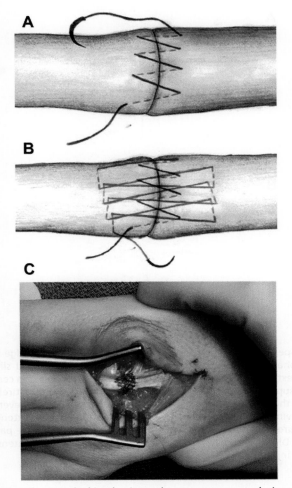

Fig. 7. (*A, B*) The running interlocking horizontal mattress suture technique. (*C*) Repair of an extensor tendon using this technique.

Clinical evaluation

As with other closed tendon injuries, dorsal PIP tenderness to palpation preceded by a history of jamming a finger is typical. Intact extension through the PIP via the intact lateral bands can obscure the diagnosis making the Elson test a valuable diagnostic maneuver (**Fig. 8**A, B).[38] Standard radiographs, or minifluoroscopic imaging, should be incorporated into the workup to assess degree of bony involvement[39] and when necessary, MRI, ultrasound examination,[40] and even the demonstration of radiopaque dye leakage after a fluoroscopic guided intra-articular injection can demonstrate central slip disruption.[41] Delayed presentation with established PIP contracture must be distinguished from pseudo-boutonniere deformity related to volar plate scarring, although typically with preserved DIP motion.[4]

Treatment of acute injuries

A stable soft tissue injury or nondisplaced fracture at the central slip insertion can be approached similarly to a stable mallet finger. In select situations, reasonable

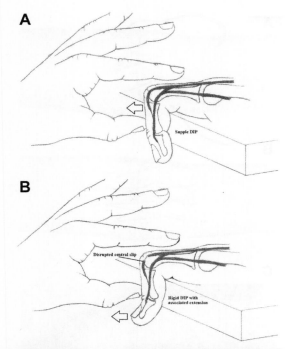

Fig. 8. (*A, B*) To perform the Elson test, bend the PIP 90° over the edge of a table and extend middle phalanx against resistance. In the presence of central slip injury, there will be weak PIP extension, and the DIP will go rigid. In the absence of a central slip injury, the DIP remains supple because the extension force is now directed entirely on maintaining extension of the PIP joint. The lateral bands are not activated. A reverse Elson test is performed by having the patient turn their palm up and have them extend against resistance with pressure to the middle phalanx; a negative test is when the patient is able to extend with the DIP joint remaining supple, a rigid DIP joint with extension is positive for a central slip injury.

treatment deferment can be offered but, the goal of treatment—to achieve tendon healing before secondary deformity develops—should be emphasized.[42] Unlike the undertreated mallet injury, established boutonniere deformity can be much more disabling and difficult to address, and this risk must be carefully weighed against the desire to continue athletic participation even if temporarily. The treatment of choice, splinting with the PIP in full extension and the DIP free to move,[43] may be difficult to accommodate during athletic participation. Active and passive DIP motion maintains joint mobility and pulls the lateral bands dorsally and distally to their normal position. Full-time extension splinting of the PIP joint for 6 weeks followed by 6 weeks of night splinting[1] can be adhered to in sports such as track, lacrosse, or soccer. The published outcomes of conservative treatment are limited but show approximately 70% satisfactory results,[44,45] although the occasional residual 5° to 20° PIP extension lag[46] is usually well-tolerated in this population.

Associated fractures involving greater than 50%, more than 2 mm of displacement and subluxation, or dislocation[47] should be reduced and secured in place with pin or screw. Alternatively, the fragment can be excised and the central slip repaired to bone.[48]

Treatment for chronic injuries

Athletes are more likely to dismiss or underappreciate central slip injuries. Nonoperative treatment can still be successful for supple joints if initiated within 6 weeks.[49,50] Once this window is missed, PIP flexion contracture still needs to be prevented (or corrected with therapy),[51] but surgery can be postponed until convenient. Fixed deformities need to be addressed before addressing the tendon imbalance with serial splinting or casting, or surgically with a dynamic external fixator or volar plate release[50] to ensure full passive range of motion of the PIP joint.

Supple boutonniere injuries are surgically treated using a 4-stage algorithmic approach[50]: (1) extensor tendon tenolysis and transverse retinacular ligament mobilization, (2) transverse retinacular ligament release, (3) extensor tenotomy (over the middle phalanx), and (4) central slip reconstruction.[44,50,52] After each stage, the quality and degree of correction is evaluated to determine if the next step is necessary. Multiple techniques for central slip reconstruction[53,54] have been described including rerouting of the lateral bands[55] or recreating a central slip with a proximal central tendon turn down flap[54,56] (Fig. 9). Restoring tendon balance and avoiding loss of PIP flexion[57,58] are challenges that can compromise the result[58] and an athlete's return to previous level of competition. Reconstruction outcomes depend on the initial deformity, but typically result in an average 10° to 20° extensor lag and only 70° of PIP flexion.[50,59] Loss of PIP flexion may be more performance limiting than the initial deformity.[58]

Zone 5 Extensor Tendon Injury

Injury at zone 5 frequently involves the sagittal bands and has been given the mechanism specific name, the boxer's knuckle.[60] Focal trauma over the MCP joint with the hand in a clenched fist[61] can be the result of sanctioned or nonsanctioned fighting as well as accidental contact against another players helmet, forehead, tooth, and so on. The central fingers are most commonly affected owing to a thinner superficial layer of the sagittal band and more prominent bone.[62,63] With fight bites (owing to tooth penetration), any tendon treatment becomes secondary to infection risk mitigation through irrigation, debridement, and antibiotic administration.[64]

Clinical evaluation and classification

Depending on the extent of injury, the afflicted knuckle may demonstrate pain and swelling only, extensor lag with weakness, or tendon subluxation.[65] Isolated sharp

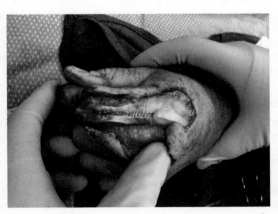

Fig. 9. An extensor tendon turn down technique for reconstruction of a central slip injury.

tendon lacerations (typically related to tooth penetration!) can be masked by the remaining intact sagittal bands and present with a slight loss of extension and weakness. Sagittal band injuries can occur from open or closed injures and are classified into 3 groups: type I injuries involve a partial stable tear; type II, enough disruption to allow subluxation; and type III, a more substantial injury with frank dislocation of the tendon.[62] Although the radial band is more susceptible to rupture,[66] the central tendon will sublux to the opposite side of the injury. Stable injuries can be localized by point tenderness. Tendon dislocation may be obvious, but the classic examination finding is inability to initiate extension from a flexed position while able to actively maintain an extended posture following passive correction. Repetitive trauma resulting in attenuation of the sagittal band may present with chronic pain and swelling exacerbated during boxing competition and can be a career threatening problem.[61] MRI offers a useful imaging modality when the diagnosis is not clear.[67]

Acute and chronic treatment

The central tendon at this level may be thick enough to accommodate a core suture repair analogous to those applied to the flexor tendons though analogous repair to zones 2, 4, and 6 is acceptable as well. A prominent suture knot over the MCP joint can be quite irritating and this should be of absorbable material or carefully buried within the tendon.

Type I closed injuries are treated with buddy taping to the adjacent digit for 4 to 6 weeks but may cause residual pain for up to 1 year.[62] For type II and III injuries, delayed treatment will typically eliminate nonoperative treatment options[68,69] and compromise the prognosis. Relative motion splinting to maintain the MCP joint in 25° to 30° of relative hyperextension for 6 weeks is a good option[70] and, owing to the splint's low profile, many athletic activities can be continued. Sports requiring gripping, grasping, and clenched fist activities (tennis, wrestling, judo, boxing, etc) will be more problematic.

Early surgical intervention does not circumvent the splinting regimen but allows direct repair and the predictable restoration of preinjury strength and range of motion with probable unrestricted return to sport within 5 months.[60] Repair of associated capsular tears is not necessary and, in fact, restricts motion if the capsule cannot be closed with the MCP joint at 90° of flexion.[61] With chronic sagittal band injuries, scarring and tissue retraction may preclude direct repair and a variety of local tissue options have been described, although most commonly a distally based slip of the extensor tendon, passed around the collateral ligament opposite the instability, can be secured back to itself to centralize the tendon.[71] Chronic boxer's knuckle can be treated by surgical excision of the scarred and attenuated extensor hood followed by reconstruction using a transplanted piece of extensor retinaculum. Successful return to professional boxing with full MCP range of motion and no residual tendon subluxation or pain during punching was reported in 5 athletes though after a prolonged average 9-month rehabilitation period.[71]

Zones 7 and 8 Extensor Tendon Injury

More proximal tendon problems are typically related to rupture, attenuation of the extensor compartments, or tendon irritation. Overuse tendinopathies comprise 25% to 50% of athletic injuries[72] and commonly occur in racquet sports, rowing, volleyball, and gymnastics.[73]

De Quervains tenosynovitis

Forceful grasping and repetitive ulnar deviation predispose many fly fishermen, golfers, and tennis players to tenosynovitis of the first dorsal compartment, the most common sports-related extensor tendinitis.[74] Characterized by sharp shooting pains associated with wrist motion, the diagnosis is confirmed by the presence of swelling (**Fig. 10**) and point tenderness over the first dorsal compartment with pain exacerbation during Eichhoff,[75] Finkelstein's[76] and Brunelli's tests[77] (**Fig. 11**). Not all cases are symptomatic enough to warrant treatment but simple interventions, including local ice massage and nonsteroidal anti-inflammatory drugs can be helpful. More symptomatic cases can be resolved in up to 90% of cases with a corticosteroid injection,[78] although rest and immobilization can successful alleviate symptoms (at least temporarily) in about 30% of cases.[79] Symptoms may recur with resumption of activities, but the temptation to inject multiple times should be tempered by the risks of depigmentation and subcutaneous fat atrophy leading to the much more debilitating superficial radial nerve neuritis.

Failed conservative treatment and persistent activity limiting discomfort can be addressed with surgical release of the first dorsal compartment though treatment delay has no adverse consequences. Release along the dorsal aspect limits the risk of tendon subluxation[80] and attention to the commonly missed extensor pollicis brevis subsheath will decrease the chance of surgical failure. Postoperative pain relief and return to preinjury capacity can be anticipated in approximately 90% of patients.[81]

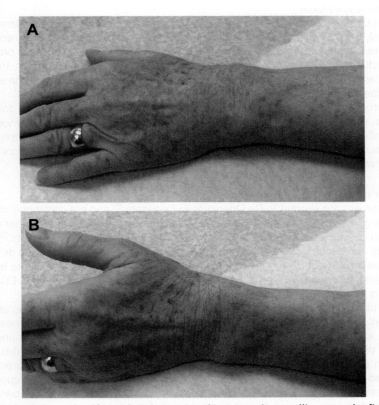

Fig. 10. (*A, B*) An avid golfer with Dequervain's demonstrating swelling over the first dorsal compartment.

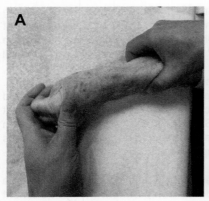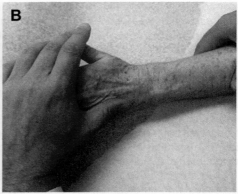

Fig. 11. (*A*) Eichhoff's test, which is commonly confused with Finkelstein's test, consists of the patient grasping their thumb within the palm and having the examiner ulnarly deviate the wrist that, if positive, will reproduce pain in the first dorsal compartment. (*B*) The Brunelli's test produces friction and pain by asking the patient to abduct and extend the thumb with the wrist held in radial deviation. Not shown is the Finkelsteins's test, which is accomplished by placing the wrist in a supported ulnar deviated position while the examiner pulls longitudinal traction and ulnar deviation through the thumb.

Intersection syndrome

Inflammation at the crossing point of the first and second dorsal compartments is commonly seen in rowing, skiing, and racquet sports or any sport requiring repetitive wrist extension.[82] Dorsal-radial distal forearm pain approximately 4 to 8 cm proximal to the radial styloid[83] can be elicited with resisted wrist and thumb extension. In more severe cases, the area is often swollen, and crepitus can be palpated over the area of discomfort.[74]

Symptom relief can be obtained with immobilization in 15° extension for 2 to 3 weeks, nonsteroidal anti-inflammatory drugs, ice, massage, and activity modification. Limited steroid injections have a role and, in rare cases, surgical decompression of the second-compartment tendons and debridement of the local inflammatory bursa are indicated.[83,84]

Extensor carpi ulnaris tendonitis and subluxation

ECU disorders are second to De Quervains in frequency[85] and are commonly seen in baseball, golf, hockey, and racquet sports. They are most likely related to either repetitive or an isolated episode of forced supination and ulnar deviated wrist flexion.[86] ECU instability can occur along a spectrum from subluxation to gross dislocation depending on the severity of tissue disruption, although pain and swelling along the tendon without instability can be seen in ECU tendinitis. MRIs can be helpful when ECU pathology is in the differential diagnoses.

In the absence of severe instability, which is often too painful for continued athletic participation, conservative treatment can range from symptom-alleviating measures such as icing and nonsteroidal anti-inflammatory drugs to temporary splinting.[87] If desired, especially in acute injuries, a trial of immobilization in a long arm splint positioned in pronation and extension for 6 weeks[87] can be successful, but precludes continued athletic participation. An alternative strategy has been described depending on the severity of inflammation and instability[88] in which a much shorter period of immobilization, only ranging from 5 to 14 days, is followed by early range of motion. Strengthening is not introduced until 75% of painless range of motion has been obtained and is only advanced to sport-specific rehabilitation when 75% recovered. Corticosteroid injections can facilitate progress along this protocol. In 1 case series, conservative treatment of prolonged immobilization was successfully used in 5 tennis players with gross ECU instability who were able return to play with no residual symptoms at 5 to 6 months.[86]

Acute repair (which also precludes athletic participation) may be more reliable and is usually the recommended option for an athlete eager to minimize total down time.[89] Surgical reconstruction is determined during initial exploration once the exposed the subsheath is inspected for the location of injury. Debridement of the torn or inflamed tendon may be necessary. Acute and subacute tears can be managed with direct repair or suture anchors to stabilize the sheath within the ulnar groove, taking care to avoid overtightening. Attenuated tissue can be reinforced using pants-over-vest techniques. More chronic tears may require reconstruction using a strip of extensor retinaculum.[90] An ulnar-based 1-cm flap of the central extensor retinaculum is raised to the septum between the fourth and fifth extensor compartments before being passed under the ECU tendon and folded back over and sutured to the proximal retinaculum to create a loose sling. The remainder of the retinaculum is repaired anatomically volar to the ECU tendon. Significant improvement in pain and function with return to sport without recurrent subluxation was reported in 20 of 21 patients in 1 series.[91] Postoperative immobilization in a long arm cast is still necessary for 4 to 6 weeks followed by a progressive rehabilitation program over the next 3 to 4 weeks, including active and passive wrist flexion, extension, and forearm supination and pronation. Progressive strengthening beginning once range of motion is restored, and return to competition is usually delayed for 3 or 4 months to allow full healing.[86]

SUMMARY

The goal of all athletes is to either avoid withdrawal from competition or to at least return to sport and conditioning as rapidly as possible. When approaching an extensor tendon injury or condition, the physician must help the athlete balance the distress of short-term sacrifice against the long-term implications and risks associated with delayed or undertreatment. Legitimate situations in which treatment can be delayed with acceptable harm must be acknowledged and this information incorporated into the decision process.

REFERENCES

1. Chauhan A. Extensor tendon injuries in athletes. Sports Med Arthrosc Rev 2014; 22(1):45–55.
2. Moore JR, Weiland AJ, Valdata L. Independent index extension after extensor indicis proprius transfer. J Hand Surg Am 1987;12(2):232–6.
3. Schultz RJ, Furlong J II, Storace A. Detailed anatomy of the extensor mechanism at the proximal aspect of the finger. J Hand Surg Am 1981;6(5):493–8.
4. Landsmeer JM. Anatomy of the dorsal aponeurosis of the human finger and its functional significance. Anat Rec 1949;104:31–44.
5. Scheittzer TP, Rayan GM. The terminal tendon of the digital extensor mechanism: part I, anatomic study. J Hand Surg Am 2004;29:898–902.
6. Cheung JP, Fung B, Ip WY. Review on mallet finger treatment. Hand Surg 2012; 17(3):439–47.
7. Lange RH, Engber WD. Hyperextension mallet finger. Orthopedics 1983;6: 1426–31.

8. Handoll HH, Vaghela MV. Interventions for treating mallet finger injuries. Cochrane Database Syst Rev 2004;(3):CD004574.

9. Patel MR, Desai SS, Bassini-Lipson L. Conservative management of chronic mallet finger. J Hand Surg Am 1986;11:570–3.

10. Garberman SF, Diao E, Peimer CA. Mallet finger: results of early versus delayed closed treatment. J Hand Surg Am 1994;19(5):850–2.

11. Kalainov DM. Nonsurgical treatment of closed mallet finger fractures. J Hand Surg Am 2005;30(3):580–6.

12. Pike J, Mulpuri K, Metzger M, et al. Blinded, prospective, randomized clinical trial comparing volar, dorsal, and custom thermoplastic splinting in treatment of acute mallet finger. J Hand Surg Am 2010;35:580–8.

13. Devan D. A novel way of treating mallet finger injuries. J Hand Ther 2014;27(4):325–8 [quiz: 329].

14. Simpson D, McQueen MM, Kumar P. Mallet deformity in sport. J Hand Surg Br 2001;26(1):32–3.

15. Scheittzer TP, Rayan GM. The terminal tendon of the digital extensor mechanism: part II, kinematic study. J Hand Surg Am 2004;29:903–8.

16. Okafor B, Mbubaegbu C, Munshi I, et al. Mallet deformity of the finger: five-year follow-up of conservative treatment. J Bone Joint Surg Br 1997;79(4):544–7.

17. Foucher G, Binhamer P, Cange S, et al. Long-term results of splintage for mallet finger. Int Orthop 1996;20:129–31.

18. Stern PJ, Kastrupp JJ. Complications and prognosis of treatment of mallet finger. J Hand Surg 1988;13A:329–33.

19. Crawford GP. The molded polythene splint for mallet finger deformities. J Hand Surg Am 1984;9(2):231–7.

20. Nakamura K, Nanjyo B. Reassessment of surgery for mallet finger. Plast Reconstr Surg 1994;93(1):141–9.

21. Pegoli L. The Ishiguro extension block technique for the treatment of mallet finger fracture: indications and clinical results. J Hand Surg Br 2003;28(1):15–7.

22. Hofmeister EP, Mazurek MT, Shin AY, et al. Extension block pinning for large mallet fractures. J Hand Surg Am 2003;28:453–9.

23. Makhlouf VM, Deek NA. Surgical treatment of chronic mallet finger. Ann Plast Surg 2011;66(6):670–2.

24. McKeon K, Lee D. Posttraumatic boutonniere and swan neck deformities. J Am Acad Orthop Surg 2015;23:623–32.

25. Kanaya K, Wada T, Yamashita T. The Thompson procedure for chronic mallet finger deformity. J Hand Surg Am 2013;38(7):1295–300.

26. Kleinman WB, Petersen DP. Oblique retinacular ligament reconstruction for chronic mallet finger deformity. J Hand Surg Am 1984;9:399–404.

27. Asghar M, Helm RH. Central slip tenotomy for chronic mallet finger. Surgeon 2013;11(5):264–6.

28. Bellemère P. Treatment of chronic extensor tendons lesions of the fingers. Chir Main 2015;34(4):155–81.

29. Suh N, Wolfe SW. Soft tissue mallet finger injuries with delayed treatment. J Hand Surg Am 2013;38(9):1803–5.

30. Lee SK, Dubey A, Kim BH, et al. A biomechanical study of extensor tendon repair methods: introduction to the running-interlocking horizontal mattress extensor tendon repair technique. J Hand Surg Am 2010;35:19–23.

31. Sharma JV, Liang NJ, Owen JR, et al. Analysis of relative motion splint in the treatment of zone VI extensor tendon injuries. J Hand Surg Am 2006;31(7):118–1122.

32. Matzon JL, Bozentka DJ. Extensor tendon injuries. J Hand Surg Am 2010;35: 854–61.
33. Newport ML, Blair WF, Steyers CM. Longterm results of extensor tendon repair. J Hand Surg Am 1990;15:961.
34. Littler JW. Restoration of the oblique retinacular ligament for correcting hyperextension deformity of the proximal interphalangeal joint. In: Tubiana R, editor. La main rheumatoide. Paris: Expansion Scientifique Francaise; 1966. p. 159–67.
35. Spinner M, Choi BY. Anterior dislocation of the proximal interphalangeal joint. J Bone Joint Surg Am 1970;52A:1329–36.
36. Massengill JB. The Boutonniere deformity. Hand Clin 1992;8:787–801.
37. Marino JT, Lourie GM. Boutonniere and pulley rupture in elite athletes. Hand Clin 2012;28(3):437–45.
38. Rubin J, Bozentka DJ, Bora FW. Diagnosis of closed central slip injuries. A cadaveric analysis of non-invasive tests. J Hand Surg 1996;21B:614–6.
39. Imatami J. The central slip attachment fracture. J Hand Surg Br 1997;22(1): 107–9.
40. Rosner JL, Zlatkin MB, Clifford P, et al. Imaging of athletic wrist and hand injuries. Semin Musculoskelet Radiol 2004;8:57–79.
41. Carducci AT. Potential boutonniere deformity its recognition and treatment. Orthop Rev 1981;10:121–3.
42. Smith DW. Boutonnie're and pulley rupture in elite basketball. Hand Clin 2012; 28(3):449–50.
43. Peterson JJ, Bancroft LW. Injuries of the fingers and thumb in the athlete. Clin Sports Med 2006;25(3):527–42.
44. To P, Watson JT. Boutonniere deformity. J Hand Surg Am 2011;36(1):139–42.
45. Souter WA. The Boutonniere deformity. J Bone Joint Surg Am 1967;49B:710–21.
46. Saldana MJ, Choban S, Westerbeck P, et al. Results of acute zone III extensor tendon injuries treated with dynamic extension splinting. J Hand Surg 1991; 16A:1145–50.
47. Kang R, Stern PJ. Fracture dislocations of the proximal interphalangeal joint. J Am Soc Surg Hand 2002;2:47–59.
48. Cluett J, Milne AD, Yang D, et al. Repair of central slip avulsions using Mitek Micro Arc bone anchors. An *in vitro* biomechanical assessment. J Hand Surg 1999;24B: 679–82.
49. Weiland AJ. Boutonnie're and pulley rupture in elite baseball players. Hand Clin 2012;28(3):447.
50. Curtis RM, Reid RL, Provost JM. A staged technique for the repair of the traumatic boutonniere deformity. J Hand Surg Am 1983;8(2):167–71.
51. El-Sallakh S. Surgical management of chronic boutonniere deformity. Hand Surg 2012;17(3):359–64.
52. Dolphin JA. Extensor tenotomy for chronic boutonnie're deformity of the finger; report of two cases. J Bone Joint Surg Am 1965;47A:161–4.
53. Urbaniak JR, Hayes MG. Chronic boutonniere deformity—an anatomic reconstruction. J Hand Surg 1981;6:379–83.
54. Snow JW. A method for reconstruction of the central slip of the extensor tendon of a finger. Plast Reconstr Surg 1976;57:455–9.
55. Matev I. Transposition of the lateral slips of the aponeurosis in treatment of longstanding "boutonniere deformity" of the fingers. Br J Plast Surg 1964;17:281–6.
56. Snow JW. Use of a retrograde tendon flap in repairing a severed extensor in the PIP joint area. Plast Reconstr Surg 1973;51:555–8.

57. Rothwell AG. Repair of the established post traumatic boutonnie're deformity. Hand 1978;3:241–5.

58. Grundberg AB. Anatomic repair of boutonniere deformity. Clin Orthop Relat Res 1980;153:226–9.

59. Le Bellec Y, Loy S, Touam C, et al. Surgical treatment for boutonniere deformity of the fingers: retrospective study of 47 patients. Chir Main 2001;20(5):362–7.

60. Hame SL, Melone CP. Boxer's knuckle in the professional athlete. Am J Sports Med 2000;28(6):879–82.

61. Melone CP Jr, Polatsch DB, Beldner S. Disabling hand injuries in boxing: boxer's knuckle and traumatic carpal boss. Clin Sports Med 2009;28(4):609–21.

62. Rayan GM, Murray D. Classification and treatment of closed sagittal band injuries. J Hand Surg Am 1994;19(4):590–4.

63. Rayan GM, Murray D, Chung KW, et al. The extensor retinacular system at the metacarpophalangeal joint. Anatomical and histological study. J Hand Surg 1997;22B:585–90.

64. Gonzalez MH, Papierski P, Hall RF Jr. Osteomyelitis of the hand after a human bite. J Hand Surg Am 1993;18:520–2.

65. Kang L, Carlson MG. Extensor tendon centralization at the metacarpophalangeal joint: surgical technique. J Hand Surg Am 2010;35(7):1194–7.

66. Saldana MJ, McGuire RA. Chronic painful subluxation of the metacarpal phalangeal joint extensor tendons. J Hand Surg Am 1986;11(3):420–3.

67. Pfirrmann CW, Theumann NH, Botte MJ, et al. MR imaging of the metacarpophalangeal joints of the fingers: part II. Detection of simulated injuries in cadavers. Radiology 2002;222(2):447–52.

68. Araki S, Ohtani T, Tanaka T. Acute dislocation of the extensor digitorum communis tendon at the metacarpophalangeal joint. A report of five cases. J Bone Joint Surg Am 1987;69:616–9.

69. Carroll C 4th, Moore JR, Weiland AJ. Posttraumatic ulnar subluxation of the extensor tendons: a reconstructive technique. J Hand Surg Am 1987;12:227–31.

70. Catalano LW III. Closed treatment of nonrheumatoid extensor tendon dislocations at the metacarpophalangeal joint. J Hand Surg Am 2006;31(2):242–5.

71. Nagaoka M. Extensor retinaculum graft for chronic boxer's knuckle. J Hand Surg Am 2006;31(6):947–51.

72. Patel MR, Lipson LB, Desai SS. Conservative treatment of mallet thumb. J Hand Surg 1986;11:45–7.

73. Fulcher SM, Kiefhaber TR, Stern PJ. Upper-extremity tendinitis and overuse syndromes in the athlete. Clin Sports Med 1998;17(3):433–48.

74. Rettig AC. Athletic injuries of the wrist and hand: part II: overuse injuries of the wrist and traumatic injuries to the hand. Am J Sports Med 2004;32:262–73.

75. Goubau JF, Goubau L, Van Tongel A, et al. The wrist hyperflexion and abduction of the thumb (WHAT) test: a more specific and sensitive test to diagnose de Quervain tenosynovitis than the Eichhoff's Test. J Hand Surg Eur Vol 2014;39(3): 286–92.

76. Finkelstein H. Stenosing tendovaginitis at the radial styloid process. J Bone Joint Surg Am 1930;12:509–40.

77. Brunelli G. Finkelstein's versus Brunelli's test in De Quervain tenosynovitis. Chir Main 2003;22:43–5 [in French].

78. Mardani-Kivi M, Karimi Mobarakeh M, Bahrami F, et al. Corticosteroid injection with or without thumb spica cast for de Quervain tenosynovitis. J Hand Surg Am 2014;39(1):37–41.

79. Weiss AP, Akelman E, Tabatabai M. Treatment of de Quervain's disease. J Hand Surg Am 1994;19(4):595–8.
80. Leslie BM, Ericson WB Jr, Morehead JR. Incidence of a septum within the first dorsal compartment of the wrist. J Hand Surg Am 1990;15(1):88–91.
81. Ta KT, Eidelman D, Thomson JG. Patient satisfaction and outcomes of surgery for de Quervain's tenosynovitis. J Hand Surg Am 1999;24:1071–7.
82. Witt J, Pess G, Gelberman RH. Treatment of deQuervain's tenosynovitis. J Bone Joint Surg Am 1991;73A:219–22.
83. Grundberg AB, Reagan DS. Pathologic anatomy of the forearm: intersection syndrome. J Hand Surg Am 1985;10:A299–302.
84. Howard N. Peritendinitis crepitans: a muscle-effort syndrome. J Bone Joint Surg Am 1937;19:447–59.
85. Wood M, Linscheid R. Abductor pollicis bursitis. Clin Orthop 1973;93:293–6.
86. Montalvan B, Parier J, Brasseur JL, et al. Extensor carpi ulnaris injuries in tennis players: a study of 28 cases. Br J Sports Med 2006;40:424–9.
87. Burkhart SS, Wood MB, Linscheid RL. Posttraumatic recurrent subluxation of the extensor carpi ulnaris tendon. J Hand Surg 1982;7:1–3.
88. Graham TJ. Pathologies of the extensor carpi ulnaris (ECU) tendon and its investments in the athlete. Hand Clin 2012;28:345–56.
89. Rowland SA. Acute traumatic subluxation of the extensor carpi ulnaris tendon at the wrist. J Hand Surg 1986;11A(6):809.
90. Inoue G, Tamura Y. Surgical treatment for recurrent dislocation of the extensor carpi ulnaris tendon. J Hand Surg Br 2001;26B:556–9.
91. MacLennan AJ, Nemechek NM, Waitayawinyu T, et al. Diagnosis and anatomic reconstruction of extensor carpi ulnaris subluxation. J Hand Surg 2008;33A:59–64.

Evaluation and Treatment of Flexor Tendon and Pulley Injuries in Athletes

Lauren M. Shapiro, MD[a], Robin N. Kamal, MD[b],*

KEYWORDS

- Flexor digitorum profundus • Flexor pulley system • Jersey finger • Pulley injuries

KEY POINTS

- A thorough understanding of the anatomy and mechanism of injury are critical for diagnosis, treatment, and postoperative management.
- Jersey finger injuries should be promptly diagnosed to allow timely surgical repair and prevention of complications.
- Meticulous suturing, tensioning, bony reduction, and fixation techniques are critical to postoperative tendon tracking and outcomes.
- It is important to understand the demands and treatment goals of injured athletes to allow them to make informed treatment decisions.

INTRODUCTION

Finger injuries make up more than a third of all upper extremity injuries presenting to emergency rooms in the United States.[1] Given its location and need for function, the finger is not only particularly vulnerable to athletic injuries but may result in significant functional consequences after injury. Although the exact incidence of athletic-related flexor tendon and flexor pulley injuries has not been described, they can be debilitating to the athletes. An understanding of the anatomy, mechanism, diagnosis, and treatment options of such injuries can ensure appropriate and efficient treatment.

Two injuries involving the flexor tendon-pulley system, namely avulsion injuries of the flexor digitorum profundus (FDP) tendon from its insertion onto the base of the distal phalanx (eg, jersey finger) and flexor pulley injuries are described given their high incidence within this patient population.

[a] Department of Orthopaedic Surgery, Stanford University, 300 Pasteur Drive, Room R144, Mail Code: 5341, Stanford, CA 94305, USA; [b] Department of Orthopaedic Surgery, Stanford University, Stanford, CA, USA
* Corresponding author. Department of Orthopaedic Surgery, Stanford University, 450 Broadway Street MC: 6342, Redwood City, CA 94603.
E-mail address: rnkamal@stanford.edu

Clin Sports Med 39 (2020) 279–297
https://doi.org/10.1016/j.csm.2019.12.004
0278-5919/20/© 2019 Elsevier Inc. All rights reserved.
sportsmed.theclinics.com

ANATOMY AND MECHANISM

An understanding of the anatomy of the digital flexor tendon and pulley system is critical to understanding the principles of injury, diagnosis, and treatment of FDP avulsion injuries and flexor pulley injuries. The extrinsic flexor muscles (FDP, flexor digitorum superficialis [FDS], and flexor pollicis longus) originate in the volar forearm and insert onto the volar base of the distal phalanx of the index through small fingers, the radial and ulnar aspect of the proximal half of the middle phalanx of these digits, and the volar base of the distal phalanx of the thumb, respectively. In these digits, the FDS tendon splits into 2 slips volar to the proximal phalanx through which the FDP passes (termed the Camper chiasm). At this level, the flexor tendons receive nutrition from both vascular perfusion (via the vincular system) and synovial diffusion (via the parietal paratenon). The vincular system, composed of short and long connections to the FDS and FDP, has implications for treatment of jersey finger injuries based on their disruption, as described in more detail later (**Fig. 1**). Given that the vincular system and synovial diffusion via the parietal paratenon are the predominant vascular supply to the tendons proximal to their insertion, the vascular supply at the bone-tendon interface has relevance for injuries at this interface. Leversedge and colleagues[2] evaluated the vascular anatomy of the FDP insertion and found a consistent and dense vascular supply to the palmar and dorsal regions from the distal phalanx and the vinculum brevis profundus (**Fig. 2**).

Five flexor tendon zones were described based on anatomy that help dictate treatment principles (**Fig. 3**).[3,4]An avulsion injury of the FDP off the distal phalanx occurs in zone 1, identified as the region in the finger that is distal to the FDS insertion. This injury, aptly termed jersey finger, describes an injury in which there is forced extension of the finger against flexion (eg, when a player, usually in rugby or football, grabs or gets a finger stuck in another player's jersey). The ring finger is especially susceptible to injury for a variety of proposed reasons: (1) the ring finger extends more prominently than the other digits during power grip,[2,5] (2) its biomechanical load to failure is significantly less than that of the long finger,[5–7] (3) it is anatomically restrained by the lumbrical muscles in the palm but shares a common muscle belly with the long and small fingers in the forearm.[8,9]

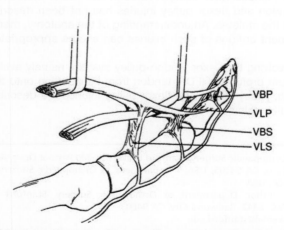

Fig. 1. Vincular blood supply to the flexor tendons. VBP, vinculum brevis profundus; VLP, vinculum longum to the profundus tendon; VBS, vinculum brevis superficialis; VLS, vinculum longum to the superficialis tendon.

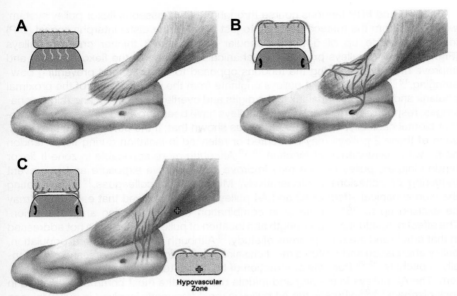

Fig. 2. Vascular anatomy of the FDP insertion. (*A*) Interosseous vessels from the phalanx penetrate the tendon at its insertion, (*B*) vessel leash from bony ostia penetrate the palmar tendon, (*C*) vascular network from the vincula penetrates the tendon substance. (*Adapted from* Leversedge FJ, Ditsios K, Goldfarb CA, et al. J Hand Surg 2002;27A:806-12; with permission.)

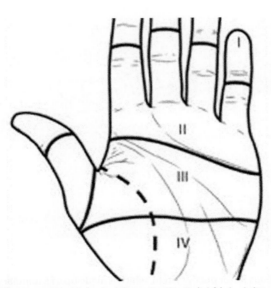

Fig. 3. Anatomic flexor zones. (*Adapted from* Dy CJ, Daluiski A. *J Am Acad Orthop Surg.* 2014;22:791-799; with permission.)

The FDS and FDP tendons course through the fibro-osseous flexor pulley system, which runs from the metacarpal neck to just distal to the distal interphalangeal (DIP) joint. It is made up of 5 thicker annular pulley and 3 thinner cruciate pulleys (**Fig. 4**).[10,11] The pulleys provide a mechanical advantage to the flexor tendons and improve motion by keeping the tendons opposed to the bone and preventing bow-stringing.[12,13] The A2 and A4 pulleys originate from the proximal third of the proximal phalanx and the middle phalanx in the digits and overlie the proximal and middle phalanges, respectively. Although these 2 pulleys have been shown to be the most important biomechanically,[14,15] further study has shown that, if the other pulleys are intact, each of these 2 pulleys may be vented or released in isolation during flexor tendon repair with maintenance of function.[16–18] Although more applicable in zone II flexor tendon injures, pulley release may improve intraoperative exposure and/or prevent triggering or adhesions postoperatively. Mitsionis and colleagues,[18] in evaluating the biomechanical effect of A2 and A4 pulley excision, showed that each pulley may be excised up to 25% alone or in combination without affecting angular rotation. The effect of residual pulley strength and location of pulley release were not addressed in that article and are current areas of study.[19] Although rare in the general population, pulley attenuation and ruptures most classically occur in rock climbers, and occasionally in pitchers,[20–22] from the contraction of the flexor tendons against the pulley system. The A2 pulleys in the ring and middle digits are the most commonly involved in rock climbers,[23–24] whereas the A4 pulley is most frequently involved in pulley injuries in baseball pitchers.[22] The crimp position, in which the proximal interphalangeal (PIP) joints are flexed 90° or more and the DIPs are slightly hyperextended, is common in rock climbing to allow maximum holding contact.[25] Pitchers with pulley ruptures have typically thrown fastballs in a similar mechanism that places an extension force on the DIP joint of a flexed digit.[22] In this position, the flexor tendons are contracting under high loads, which places a great amount of force on the pulley system. It is not clear why A4 pulley injuries may be more common in pitchers and A2 pulley injuries are

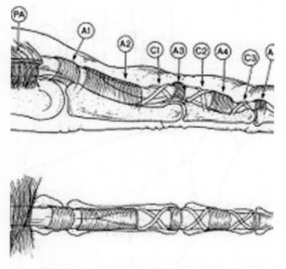

Fig. 4. The fibro-osseous flexor pulley system, which is made up of 5 annular pulleys and 3 cruciate pulleys. PA, palmar aponeurosis pulley. (*From* Strickland JW. Development of flexor tendon surgery: twenty-five years of progress. J Hand Surg Am 2000;25:214-35; with permission.)

more common climbers, but a biomechanical study of 19 fingers placed in the crimp position and loaded showed that, of those with isolated pulley ruptures, 82.4% failed at the A4 pulley, whereas the remaining digits (17.6%) failed at the A2 pulley.[25]

Zone 1 Flexor Digitorum Profundus Avulsions

Clinical evaluation and diagnosis

A thorough history and physical examination are critical for managing athletes. For example, recognizing concomitant or associated injuries may affect overall management, whereas an understanding of the chronicity of the injury may affect an athlete's treatment options. Patients may present with a painful and/or swollen digit that lacks isolated DIP joint flexion. Digital tenodesis shows relative extension of the involved distal phalanx (**Fig. 5**). Stabilizing the proximal and middle phalanxes and asking the patient to flex the finger isolates the FDP and allows evaluation of the tendon (**Fig. 6**). Critical to note is that an injured FDP may weakly flex the DIP via a bony avulsion trapped at the A5/A4 pulley or through an intact volar plate and distal vinculum (**Fig. 7**).[26,27] For this reason, some investigators advocate conducting this examination with resistance.[26,27] Palpation of the digit and palm is likely to elicit pain at the FDP insertion site (although patients with chronic injuries may be pain free) and may provide information as to the level of tendon retraction.

Although a diagnosis can typically be made based on history and physical examination alone, plain radiographs may help to identify an avulsion of a bony fragment, associated fractures, and/or dislocations. Advanced modalities such as ultrasonography and MRI may be useful adjuncts to help identify the level of retraction, especially in chronic injuries (**Fig. 8**).[28] Ultrasonography is a dynamic and inexpensive modality; however, it is operator dependent. MRI is less operator dependent but with an added expense.

Classification

Understanding the mechanism and nature of zone 1 flexor tendon injuries is important because it helps guide further work-up, prognosis, and treatment. The Leddy and Packer[7] classification schema, which was later augmented by Robins and Dobyns[29]

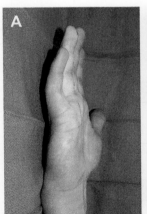
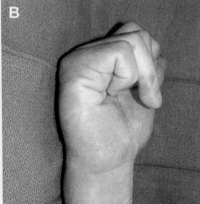

Fig. 5. Characteristic presentation of an FDP avulsion injury with loss of DIP tenodesis. (*A*) Fingers extended. (*B*) Fingers flexed demonstrate a lack of distal interphalangeal (DIP) joint flexion indicative of an FDP avulsion injury. (*From* Polfer EM, Sabino JM, Katz RD. J Hand Surg Am 2019;44:e1-164.e5; with permission.)

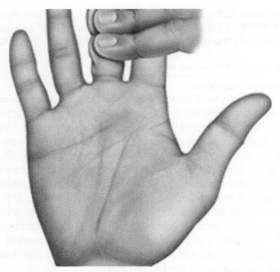

Fig. 6. Clinical examination technique that isolates the FDP tendon to evaluate for injury. (*From* Naumann JA, Leversedge FL. Sports Med Arthrosc Rev 2014;22:56-65; with permission.)

is frequently used and includes 4 primary injury types based on the level of tendon retraction[9,29–31] (**Table 1**).

In type I injuries, the FDP tendon retracts into the palm and the vincula are disrupted, thereby compromising the vascular supply. Type II injuries are the most common and occur when the tendon is retracted to the level of the PIP joint, leaving the long vinculum intact. It may be difficult to differentiate between type I and II injuries without advanced imaging. In addition, type II injuries may become type I injuries with continued activity.[32] Type III injuries occur when a large bony fragment has been

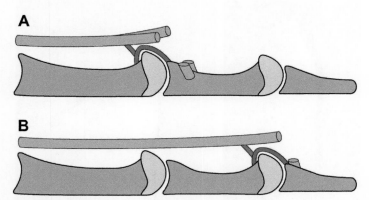

Fig. 7. An intact volar plate or distal vinculum (demonstrated in both *A* and *B*) that may lead to a clinical examination in which DIP flexion is feasible despite an FDP injury. (*From* Stewart DA, Smitham PJ, Gianoutsos MP, et al. Biomechanical influence of the vincula tendinum on digital motion after isolated flexor tendon injury: a cadaveric study. J Hand Surg Am 2007;32:1190–4; with permission.)

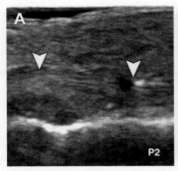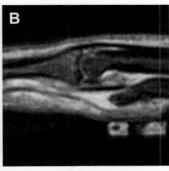

Fig. 8. Advanced imaging showing an FDP injury. (*A*) Ultrasonography image.; The arrowheads delineate the FDP tendon and the arrow indicates an avulsed fragment. (*B*) MRI. ([A] *From* Cockenpot E, Lefebvre G, Demondion X, Chantelot C, Cotton A. Imaging of sports-related hand and wrist injuries: sports imaging series. Radiology 2016;279:674-92; with permission; and [B] Image courtesy of Dr. Jeffrey Yao, Stanford Hospital and Clinics.)

avulsed that prevents retraction proximal to the distal aspect of the A4 pulley. In these scenarios, the vincula remain intact. Type IV is the least common type and includes both a fracture and an avulsion in which the FDP tendon has avulsed from the fracture fragment. In these injuries, the bony fragment retracts to the same level as that of a type III injury and the tendon retracts into the palm or to the PIP level.

Treatment
Type I Because the blood supply is disrupted in type I injuries, the prognosis is poor compared with that of type II and III injuries, and prompt (within 7 to 10 days) surgical treatment is recommended. A midlateral or Brunner-style incision is used to expose the distal flexor pulley system and the distal insertion of the FDP. The retracted portion of the tendon is retrieved through another incision made near or proximal to the A1 pulley. It may be necessary to extend this incision proximally or create transverse windows to identify and retrieve the reacted tendon. The retracted tendon may be "milked" distally within its sheath and held in place with a 25-gauge needle. Alternatively, a pediatric feeding tube may be used to help bring the tendon distal through the pulley system. The edges of the FDP tendon may need to be trimmed to healthy tendon. Although it is best to preserve the A4 pulley, it may be safely vented to prevent complications related to tendon gliding, as described earlier.[16–18] The bony insertion site of the tendon should be prepared and the tendon stump should be carefully debrided. Although various techniques exist to reinsert the FDP tendon to the distal phalanx, no one technique has proved to be superior.[33] A pullout suture sutured through the tendon and transosseous tunnels may be used. Sutures may be secured with or without a button on the nail plate dorsally (**Fig. 9**). The button and suture are

Table 1		
Classification of zone 1 flexor digitorum profundus avulsions		
Type	**Level of Retraction**	**Notes**
I	Palm	Vincula disrupted, prognosis poor
II	PIP joint	Vincula intact, prognosis fair
III	A5/A4 pulley	Vincula intact, prognosis good
IIIa/IV	Bone: A5/A4 pulley, Tendon: PIP joint or palm	Prognosis fair/poor

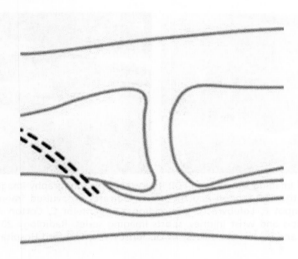

Fig. 9. One described technique for FDP repair. Pullout sutures are used in the FDP tendon and transosseous tunnels are used. Here, the sutures are secured with a button on the nail plate. (*From* Huq S, George S, Boyce DE. Zone 1 flexor tendon injuries: a review of the current options for acute treatment. *J Plast Reconstr Aesthet Surg.*2013;66:1023-1031; with permission.)

typically removed after 4 to 6 weeks. Alternatively, if the distal phalanx is large enough, miniature suture anchors may be used (**Fig. 10**). An all-inside repair using two 3-0 Ethibond sutures to attach to the distal FDP via a Massachusetts General Hospital (MGH)/ modified method to bone with 2 Keith needles, and a knot tied over the dorsal distal phalanx, has also been described (**Fig. 11**).[34] In each technique, it is critical to ensure the FDP tendon is well approximated to the bony footprint when the knot is tied. In order to minimize the risk of nail bed deformity when using the pullout or suture anchor technique is to ensure the needle (in the pullout suture and transosseous tunnel technique) and the tip of the suture anchor (in the suture anchor technique) do not exit through or penetrate the germinal or sterile matrices.

Matsuzaki and colleagues[35] compared the biomechanical properties of FDP to bone repairs using the pullout suture technique (with a dorsal button and Supramid suture) and the suture anchor technique (with 2 suture anchors and Supramid, Ethibond, or FiberWire suture). The investigators noted that the pullout technique had the greatest ultimate force to failure but had inferior stiffness compared with the anchor techniques. Although the FiberWire anchor technique had the best combination of mechanical properties, the investigators showed a positive correlation between bone mineral density and cortical thickness to ultimate load to failure, which may raise concerns in osteoporotic bone. Chu and colleagues[34] found no difference in tensile stiffness, ultimate load, or work to failure when comparing the all-inside technique with the pullout suture technique and the suture anchor technique.

McCallister and colleagues[36] compared the 1-year outcomes of the suture anchor technique with the pullout button technique in a nonrandomized manner. There were no differences in clinical outcomes between groups aside from a quicker return-to-work time in the suture anchor group. Tempelaere and colleagues[37] evaluated outcomes (via the Buck-Gramcko classification) of 16 patients undergoing surgical fixation of a type I jersey finger. Of the 15 patients with follow-up, 3 had an excellent

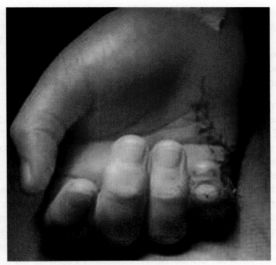

Fig. 10. Another described technique for FDP repair. When the fragment of bone is large enough, 1 or 2 miniature suture anchors may be used to secure the FDP tendon to the distal phalanx. (*From* McCallister WV, Ambrose HC, Katolik LI, Trumble TE. Comparison of pullout button versus suture anchor for zone 1 flexor tendon repair. J Han Surg Am 2006;31:246-51; with permission.)

outcome, 4 had a good outcome, 3 had a moderate outcome, and 5 had a poor outcome. The study did not report on comparisons between the surgical techniques.

Type II Given the lack of proximal retraction of the FDP tendon within the palm, the recommended time to surgery for type II is within 1 to 2 weeks, although delayed

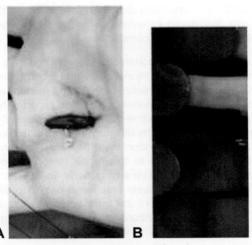

A   **B**

Fig. 11. (*A,B*) An all-inside repair technique using Ethibond sutures to attach the distal FDP to bone via an MGH/modified Becker method. (*From* Chu JY, Chen T, Awad HA, Elfar J, Hammert WC. Comparison of an all-inside suture technique with traditional pull-out suture and suture anchor repair techniques for flexor digitorum profundus attachment to bone. *J Hand Surg.* 2013;38:1084-1090; with permission.)

treatment (3–6 weeks) has been described. However, as noted earlier, these may become type I injuries so surgical delay should be avoided. These injuries are surgically managed similarly to type I injuries; however, typically only a finger incision is required, because retrieval of a proximally retracted tendon is not necessary. Tempelaere and colleagues[37] evaluated 4 patients with type II injuries and reported 1 good and 3 poor outcomes (via the Buck-Gramcko classification).

Type III Treatment of acute type III injuries is typically based on the amount of bony displacement. For displaced fractures (>2 mm), surgical treatment is recommended between 1 and 2 weeks, although repair can be completed from 3 to 6 weeks for type III injuries because the bony fragment prevents significant proximal retraction and the vincula are intact. The size of the avulsed bony fragment dictates surgical treatment. A small fragment, if extra-articular, may be excised and the FDP tendon may be sutured down to the bony footprint using the techniques described for type I injuries. In larger fragments, transosseous sutures or fracture reduction with miniscrews may be used to approximate the fracture and restore articular congruity if needed. Conservative management in the form of a finger-based splint with the DIP at 0° and close follow-up may be satisfactory for nondisplaced or minimally (<2 mm) displaced fractures. Conservative treatment depends on an accurate diagnosis (not missing a type IV injury) and close follow-up to ensure the fracture does not displace. Halát and colleagues[38] reviewed 29 patients with type III injuries with a mean follow-up of 7 years. Sixteen patients with nondisplaced to minimally displaced fractures treated with a splint reported no functional deficits at follow-up (mean of 0 on the Disabilities of the Arm, Shoulder, and Hand [DASH] score) and 95% tip pinch strength compared with the contralateral side. One patient had a 15° DIP extension deficit. In this same study, 13 patients treated operatively (with a variety of techniques and >2 mm of displacement preoperatively reported) had an average 9° extension deficit and 75% tip pinch strength compared with the contralateral side. The decrease in function as measured by DASH on follow-up was 1.6. These operative results are in line with other reports of operatively treated FDP avulsions (36 patients observed to have a 10°–15° extension deficit on follow-up).[7] Although it is possible that surgery itself may lead to an extension deficit, it is important to preoperatively counsel patients about this potential complication.

Type IV Although uncommon, it is important to recognize and treat type IV injuries early (within 7 to 10 days). Because type IV injuries represent a combination of a type I injury and a type III injury, they should be treated in the same manner as discussed earlier. Henry and colleagues,[39] in a literature review, detailed all reported type IV jersey fingers. Despite the surgical technique and outcomes varying substantially between these 19 cases, the investigators did reiterate the difficulty in surgical fixation of these injuries.

A wide-awake local anesthetic no tourniquet (WALANT) technique has been purported to have several advantages in the repair flexor tendon injuries.[40,41] The WALANT technique allows the avoidance of general anesthetic and/or sedation, in addition to the ability to intraoperatively test the repair to prevent repair gapping and/or bunching. Although the authors are transitioning to the use of the WALANT technique, we still commonly use monitored sedation for our surgically treated jersey fingers and pulley injuries.

Chronic injuries

Although there is no specific definition, the authors consider chronic injuries to be about 6 weeks or greater from the initial traumatic insult. Jersey fingers in athletes can present in a delayed fashion if they created limited dysfunction and the athlete preferred to simply tape the DIP joint to continue to play. It is important to obtain a detailed history and physical examination in these patients and tailor their care toward their functional goals. In patients who are pain free and functioning at their desired level, no treatment may be needed. In a review of 36 athletes with FDP avulsions, Leddy and Packer[7] reported on 13 late untreated injuries in athletes who were relatively asymptomatic. All of these athletes had full PIP range of motion and no DIP instability. Rarely, the retracted tendon stump interferes with tendon gliding and digit motion or causes pain, in which case the stump may be excised. DIP arthrodesis may be considered if the chronic injury has led to an unstable joint. In patients that show dysfunction from lack of active DIP flexion, and who can show reliability with therapy, a 2-stage reconstruction can be considered. The 2-stage reconstruction technique consists of an exploration to evaluate the injury and any other concomitant injuries, correction of any fixed flexion deformities with a capsulectomy as well as volar plate and accessory collateral ligament release, and placement of silicone tendon implant. Stage I starts with a Brunner or midaxial incision. The injured FDP tendon is transected proximally at the level of the lumbrical origin. Silicone implants are trialed to determine the appropriate size that allows for a smooth glide within the pulley system. The implant is first sutured to the distal phalanx. The proximal aspect of the implant is placed near the intended motor target for the graft. Postoperative treatment after stage I includes a posterior splint that holds the wrist in about 30° to 35° of flexion, the metacarpophalangeal (MP) joints in about 60° to 70°° of flexion, and the interphalangeal joints extended allowing for more proximal placement of the implant. Passive motion is started about 3 days after surgery with the goal of achieving full passive range of motion before stage II. Stage II is usually performed about 6 to 12 weeks after stage I (and when full passive range of motion is achieved). During this stage, incisions are made at the level of the distal phalanx and at the proximal extent of the injury. The pseudosheath is incised at these levels to identify the rod. The FDP tendon is typically used as the proximal motor. A tendon graft (eg, palmaris, plantaris) is sutured at the proximal end of the rod and fed through the pseudosheath before its fixation distally. Prior studies have shown good to fair results[42]; however, in athletes this can require extensive time away from sport (6–12 months).

In-season considerations
Diagnosing a jersey finger may be challenging for in-season athletes because timely surgical intervention is important to ensure an adequate repair. In activities in which grasp is not required or the patient may return without significant functional limitation, a fist-type immobilization (in which a loose and bulky dressing is placed around the hand/wrist to keep the hand in a loose flexed fist position for the purpose of protection) may be used. Ultimately, it is the clinician's job to present the treatment options, risks, and benefits and create a treatment plan with the athlete that aligns with the athlete's values and preferences.

Postoperative care and return to play
Postoperative care and return-to-play timing and precautions are similar for repair of all types of jersey fingers. A well-padded dorsal splint from the midforearm to the fingertips is applied to hold the wrist, MP, PIP, and DIP joints in slight flexion. Patients can begin a supervised early active motion protocol within 5 days after surgery with the goal of adding resistance and strength at around 8 weeks and full activity at around 10 to 12 weeks. A less bulky dorsal blocking splint may be fashioned by the hand therapist. Our protocols are similar to those of flexor tendon repair protocols, which have been a source of extensive research and debate. A systematic review of 9 intervention

studies of postoperative rehabilitation for flexor tendon repairs found that, despite there being significant variety in how investigators describe their protocols, a place-and-hold rehabilitation protocol results in better outcomes than passive flexion protocols.[43] Ultimately, the literature (and clinical practice) are moving toward earlier active motion and decreased wrist immobilization; however, robust intervention studies have yet to establish this as superior to place-and-hold protocols. Briefly, our hand therapists commence passive range of motion (recommended every 2 hours while the patient is awake) with place-and-hold flexion of all digits at a half fist with active extension to the dorsal blocking splint for the first 3 weeks (with the wrist extended 10°). Within this same period, active motion into a half fist is also encouraged with the guidance of hand therapists. The authors recommend no functional use of the hand and no participation in sports for the first 3 weeks. During weeks 3 to 6 postoperatively, we allow patients to advance digit flexion and tendon gliding exercises with the goal of achieving full digital extension without any forceful active flexion. During this period, we may consider allowing athletes to return to training without the use of their hands. Athletes who return may continue the use of the dorsal blocking splint or wrap the hand in a flexed/loose fist posture during play. Around 6 to 8 weeks after surgery, we discontinue the use of the dorsal blocking splint and encourage hand use for all functional activities. Athletes may initiate light upper body strengthening and training with the avoidance of forceful gripping. At 8 weeks, patients may begin strengthening exercises with a full release to sport at 12 weeks.

Flexor Pulley Injuries

Clinical evaluation and diagnosis

Patients typically present with pain and/or swelling on the volar aspect of the digit in the acute scenario with a history of an irregular or forceful movement during climbing. Occasionally, pain and swelling present a couple weeks before ultimate rupture.[44] Point tenderness over the injured pulley and pain or discomfort with gripping and resisted flexion of the affected digit are common. Decreased range of digital flexion secondary to swelling and/or flexor system inefficiency may be present, and bowstringing of the flexor tendons may be visualized with resisted digit flexion.

Although radiographs are frequently obtained to rule out other injuries, ultrasonography and/or MRI are frequently used for diagnostic confirmation.[45–49] Both may show increased tendon-to-bone distance in the axial or sagittal planes (**Fig. 12**). Although less expensive, ultrasonography is dynamic and the study may be conducted with resistance and throughout an arc of motion. MRI may additionally show injury to the pulley structure and/or surrounding edema.

Classification

A classification system for flexor pulley injuries was described and may help guide treatment.[50] Grade 1 represents a pulley strain. Grade 2 represents a complete A4 rupture or a partial A2 or A3 rupture. Grade 3 represents a complete A2 or A3 rupture. Grade 4 represents either multiple pulley ruptures or a single rupture with a concomitant injury (eg, collateral ligament or lumbrical injury).

Treatment

Grade 1 to 3 injuries are typically managed nonsurgically with a combination of rest, immobilization, antiinflammatories, and ice. Pulley support tape or rings are often used when the patient returns to climbing. Grade 1 injures do not require immobilization. Functional therapy and full sport-specific activities may resume based on comfort but can take 2 to 6 weeks. Grade 2 injuries are managed with about 10 days of immobilization (with the digit in a slightly flexed position) followed by

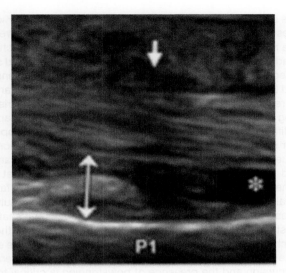

Fig. 12. Ultrasonography image of a patient with a flexor pulley injury. The single arrow represents the hypoechoic pulley that has been injured. The double-headed arrow shows the bowstringing or volar displacement of the tendon from the bone. The asterisk represents edema within the tendon sheath. (*From* Cockenpot E, Lefebvre G, Demondion X, Chantelot C, Cotton A. Imaging of sports-related hand and wrist injuries: sports imaging series. Radiology 2016;279:674-92; with permission.)

functional therapy and light sport-specific activity at 2 to 4 weeks, and return to full activity based on comfort thereafter. Grade 3 injuries are first treated with an external pulley ring splint. Functional therapy begins about 10 days postinjury, light sport-specific activity begins about 6 to 8 weeks postinjury, with full return to sport at about 3 months postinjury. If progression to sport seems hindered by the pulley ring or symptoms continue, we offer surgical reconstruction. Grade 4 injuries may warrant surgical repair or reconstruction if the patient is symptomatic. Surgical options vary and must account for (1) whether to repair the injury or reconstruct the pulley, (2) which repair or reconstruction technique to use, and (3) from where to obtain a graft if needed. The principles of either repair or reconstruction are to (1) place and maintain the flexor tendons near the centers of rotation of the DIP and PIP joints, and (2) obtain a repaired or reconstructed construct strong enough to allow for early mobilization given the risk of adhesions and loss of range of motion. As such, the patients should have near-full passive range of motion before considering surgery. Reconstruction involves using a graft to reconstitute the pulley by either connecting it to the remaining rims (nonencircling technique) or by wrapping the graft around the entire phalanx (encircling technique).

A volar Brunner incision is used to approach the pulley system. The decision to repair or reconstruct the pulley is made depending on the adequacy of the remaining tissue. Tissue adequacy is determined intraoperatively, both visually and by tactile feedback. The tissue is visualized and inspected to determine whether it is robust enough and sufficient for repair (eg, not scarred or attenuated), also allowing for normal gliding of the underlying flexor tendon after repair. Typically, if the tissue is inadequate for repair, a reconstruction is required. Scar tissue should be resected to prevent abnormal tendon gliding. Graft choices include the palmaris longus, the plantaris, a slip of FDS (ring finger), or a section of the dorsal wrist retinaculum.[51–53]

Several methods of pulley reconstruction have been described: the Kleinert and Bennett's[50] ever-present rim technique, in which a thin tendon graft is weaved back and forth through the rim of the pulley system; the Doyle and Blythe[54] technique, in which drill holes are made in the phalanx through which a graft is passed and sutured back to itself; the Lister technique,[55] in which a portion of the dorsal wrist extensor retinaculum is passed around the phalanx; the Karev technique,[56] in which the volar plate is slit and used for pulley reconstruction. The authors prefer to use a palmaris autograft in a looped encircling reconstructive manner (Okutsu technique).[57] In an in vitro study comparing 6 different reconstruction techniques, encircling looped techniques showed superior strength to failure compared with rim reconstruction techniques.[58] Lin and colleagues,[53] in a cadaveric study evaluating the biomechanical properties of tendon-based techniques for pulley reconstruction, showed that the triple-loop technique was the only studied technique able to withstand a load to failure equivalent to that of a natural pulley. When using the Okutsu technique, using multiple loops (2 to 3 loops) increases the width and more accurately reproduces the anatomy and function of the reconstructed pulley. Surgeons should take care to place the graft beneath the extensor mechanism at the A2 pulley level, place the graft over the extensor mechanism, and make 2 loops at the A4 pulley level (**Fig. 13**).[59] Intraoperative testing of flexor tendon excursion and the presence of bowstringing is critical to prevent overtensioning or undertensioning of the pulley. The authors advocate the use of WALANT in flexor pulley injury repair and reconstruction because it allows intraoperative tensioning and testing.

In a retrospective review of 56 patients who underwent an A2 or A4 pulley reconstruction (in which either palmaris longus or extensor retinaculum was sutured to the remnant pulley in a nonencircling technique), Arora and colleagues[60] noted that all nonclimbing patients were able to regain full digit dexterity in their previous occupations and that those who were rock climbers were able to return to their prior level of climbing at a mean of 48 months. Okutsu and colleagues[57] evaluated 6 patients who

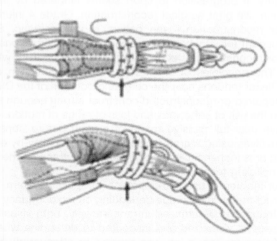

Fig. 13. The looped autograft tendon (*arrows*) for flexor pulley reconstruction. The graft is placed beneath the extensor mechanism and 3 loops are made at the A2 pulley level, while the graft is placed over the extensor mechanism and 2 loops are made at the A4 pulley level. (*From* Okutsu I, Ninomiya S, Hiraki S, et al. Three-loop technique for A2 pulley reconstruction. J Hand Surg Am 1987;12:790-4; with permission.)

had undergone a pulley reconstruction with the Okutsu technique with a mean follow-up of 21 months and found significant improvements in range of motion from preoperatively to postoperatively and reported satisfactory grip functions for all patients.

Chronic injuries
Although no exact definition of a chronic pulley exists, the authors consider 6 weeks or greater from injury to be chronic. Physician avoidance by the athlete or an unrecognized initial injury may result in a chronic injury. Again, it is critical to obtain a detailed history and physical examination in these patients and tailor their care toward their functional goals. Patients without injury or functional limitation may be managed without treatment. Chronic injury can make surgical treatment more challenging, and any preoperative joint stiffness (eg, interphalangeal joint contractures) should be addressed before surgery if possible and may need to be addressed intraoperatively.

In-season considerations
Athletes diagnosed with a pulley injury during the season or those who are unable to take time off from their athletic activities may be challenging. Return to sport before healing may lead to further injury and/or may make an acute injury more difficult to treat. However, this does not preclude early return to sport in those athletes who understand their options. In a review of overuse injuries, Rohrbough and colleagues[61] evaluated 42 elite climbers participating in competition and found that 26% of patients with physical examination findings consistent with pulley rupture were still participating at a high level despite bowstringing. Another report evaluating 21 rock climbers with pulley injuries (82% of which were type II and III injuries) treated conservatively found no difference with regard to finger strength between the injured and uninjured fingers at about 3.5 years from the date of injury.[62] In this same cohort, all patients returned to rock climbing within 1 year of injury, and follow-up ultrasonography showed no increase in bowstringing. Taping or ring splinting may be an option during the season until the athlete has the ability to undergo a period of immobilization or surgery and postoperative rehabilitation.

Postoperative care and return to play
Grade 1 to 3 pulley injury return-to-play timing consists of a graduated level of activity and may require 6 weeks to 3 months, based on injury grade and symptoms/demands for an athlete to return to the prior level of activity. Frequently taping and/or ring splinting may be used for weeks to months following an athlete's return because they may help to minimize stress on reconstructed pulleys. If an athlete has undergone repair or reconstruction, passive tendon gliding protocols with place-and-hold maneuvers are used immediately after surgery. The authors initially teach patients to conduct place-and-hold and action motion flexion exercises of all digits to a half fist with the pulley ring splint for the first 3 weeks after surgery. We do not allow functional use of the hand or participation in sports during the first 3 weeks after surgery. During postoperative week 3 to 4, we advance active digital flexion and initiate tendon gliding exercises. In this time period, we consider allowing athletes to return to sport without the use of their injured hands. During weeks 4 to 6, light resistive activity begins and we encourage the use of the hand for functional activities. Athletes may begin light upper body strengthening and training programs. At the 8-weel to 12-week point, strength training may begin, with a full release to sport around the 12-week mark.

SUMMARY

Flexor tendon injuries of competitive athletes present unique challenges to clinicians. The complex anatomy and treatment of the injury becomes more complicated when associated with delays in diagnoses, in-season considerations, and the athlete's eagerness to return to play as quickly as possible. Many athletes, with early recognition and appropriate treatment, may return to play without surgical intervention. Various treatment options exist for those requiring surgical treatment. Basic principles of meticulous surgical technique, open reduction and internal fixation of associated fractures when applicable, and tendon or graft tensioning remain. Wide-awake local anesthetic techniques with no tourniquet may be used for intraoperative evaluation of tensioning and tendon tracking. Adherence to postoperative therapy protocols is crucial to prevent complications. In addition, it is critical to maintain an open line of communication and understanding between clinician, patient, and any other involved parties (eg, coach, agent) regarding the diagnosis, treatment options, risks, and benefits, and create an environment in which the patient can come to an informed decision.

ACKNOWLEDGMENTS

The authors would like to acknowledge Wendy Moore, OTR/L, CHT for her assistance with this article.

DISCLOSURE

The authors, research organizations, or educational institutions received no payments or benefits related to the production of this work.

REFERENCES

1. Ootes D, Lambers KT, Ring DC. The epidemiology of upper extremity injuries presenting to the emergency department in the United States. Hand (N Y) 2012;7: 18–22.
2. Leversedge FJ, Ditsios K, Goldfarb CA, et al. Vascular anatomy of the human flexor digitorum profundus tendon insertion. J Hand Surg 2002;27A:806–12.
3. Kleinert H, Kutz J, Ashbell T, et al. Primary repair of lacerated flexor tendons in "no man's land." J Bone Joint Surg Am 1967;49:577.
4. Verdan CE. Half a century of flexor-tendon surgery: current status and changing philosophies. J Bone Joint Surg Am 1972;54:472–91.
5. Bynum DK Jr, Gilbert JA. Avulsion of the flexor digitorum profundus: anatomic and biomechanical considerations. J Hand Surg Am 1988;13:222–7.
6. Manske PR, Lesker PA. Avulsion of the ring finger flexor digitorum profundus tendon: an experimental study. Hand 1978;10:52–5.
7. Leddy JP, Packer JW. Avulsion of the profundus tendon insertion in athletes. J Hand Surg Am 1977;2:66–9.
8. Lunn PG, Lamb DW. "Rugby finger"—avulsion of profundus of ring finger. J Hand Surg Br 1984;9:69–71.
9. Leddy JP. Avulsions of the flexor digitorum profundus. Hand Clin 1985;1:77–83.
10. Doyle JR, Blythe WF. Anatomy of the flexor tendon sheath and pulleys of the thumb. J Hand Surg Am 1977;2:149–51.
11. Cohen MJ, Kaplan L. Histology and ultrastructure of the human flexor tendon sheath. J Hand Surg Am 1987;12:25–9.

12. Idler RS. Anatomy and biomechanics of the digital flexor tendons. Hand Clin 1985;1:3–11.
13. Amadio PC, Lin GT, An KN. Anatomy and pathomechanics of the flexor pulley system. J Hand Ther 1989;2:138–41.
14. Lin GT, Amadio PC, An KN, et al. Functional anatomy of the human digital flexor pulley system. J Hand Surg 1989;14:949–56.
15. Peterson WW, Manske PR, Bollinger BA, et al. Effect of pulley excision on flexor tendon biomechanics. J Orthop Res 1986;4:96–101.
16. Kwai Ben I, Elliot D. "Venting" or partial lateral release of the A2 and A4 pulleys after repair of zone 2 flexor tendon injuries. J Hand Surg Br 1998;23B:649–54.
17. Tang JB. Indications, methods, postoperative motion and outcome evaluation of primary flexor tendon repairs in zone 2. J Hand Surg Eur Vol 2007;32:118–29.
18. Mitsionis G, Bastidas JA, Grewal R, et al. Feasibility of partial A2 and A4 pulley excision: effect on finger flexor tendon biomechanics. J Hand Surg Am 1999;24:310–4.
19. Chow JC, Sensinger J, McNeal D, et al. Importance of proximal A2 and A4 pulleys to maintaining kinematics in the hand: a biomechanical study. Hand (N Y) 2014;9:105–11.
20. Bollen SR. Injury to the A-2 pulley in rock climbers. J Hand Surg Br 1990;15:268–70.
21. Merritt AL, Huang JL. Hand injuries in rock climbing. J Hand Surg Am 2011;36:1859–61.
22. Lourie GM, Hamby Z, Raasch WG, et al. Annular flexor pulley injuries in professional baseball pitchers: a case series. Am J Sports Med 2011;39:421–4.
23. Zafonte B, Rendulic D, Szabo R. Flexor pulley system: anatomy, injury, and management. J Hand Surg Am 2014;39:2525–32.
24. Moutet F, Forli A, Voulliaume D. Pulley rupture and reconstruction in rock climbers. Tech Hand Up Extrem Surg 2004;8:149–55.
25. Marco RAW, Sharkey NA, Smith TS, et al. Pathomechanics of closed rupture of the flexor tendon pulleys in rock climbers. J Bone Joint Surg Am 1998;80(7):1012–9.
26. Stewart DA, Smitham PJ, Gianoutsos MP, et al. Biomechanical influence of the vincula tendinum on digital motion after isolated flexor tendon injury: a cadaveric study. J Hand Surg Am 2007;32:1190–4.
27. Sasaki Y, Nomura S. An unusual role of the vinculum after complete laceration of the flexor tendons. J Hand Surg 1987;12B:105–8.
28. Cockenpot E, Lefebvre G, Demondion X, et al. Imaging of sports-related hand and wrist injuries: sports imaging series. Radiology 2016;279:674–92.
29. Robins PR, Dobyns JH. Avulsion of the insertion of the flexor digitorum profundus tendon associated with fracture of the distal phalanx. A brief review. American Academy of Orthopaedic Surgeons Symposium on Tendon Surgery in the Hand. St Louis (MO): CV Mosby; 1975.
30. Trumble TE, Vedder NE, Benirschke SK. Misleading fractures after profundus tendon avulsions: a report of 6 cases. J Hand Surg Am 1992;17:902–6.
31. Smith JH. Avulsion of the profundus tendon with simultaneous intra-articular fracture of the distal phalanx: case report. J Hand Surg 1981;6:600.
32. Stamos BD, Leddy JP. Closed flexor tendon disruption in athletes. Hand Clin 2000;16:359–65.
33. Huq S, George S, Boyce DE. Zone 1 flexor tendon injuries: a review of the current treatment options for acute injuries. J Plast Reconstr Aesthet Surg 2013;66:1023–31.

34. Chu JY, Chen T, Awad HA, et al. Comparison of all-inside suture technique with traditional pull-out suture and suture anchor repair techniques for flexor digitorum profundus attachment to bone. J Hand Surg Am 2013;38:1084–90.

35. Matsuzaki H, Zaegel MA, Gelberman RH, et al. Effect of suture material and bone quality on the mechanical properties of zone 1 flexor tendon-bone reattachment with bone anchors. J Hand Surg Am 2008;33:709–17.

36. McCallister WV, Ambrose HC, Katolik LI, et al. Comparison of pullout button versus suture anchor for zone 1 flexor tendon repair. J Hand Surg Am 2006;31: 246–51.

37. Tempelaere C, Brun M, Doursounian L, et al. Traumatic avulsion of the flexor digitorum profundus tendon. Jersey finger, a 29 cases report. Hand Surg Rehabil 2017;36:368–72.

38. Halát G, Negrin L, Erhart J, et al. Treatment options and outcome after bony avulsion of the flexor digitorum profundus tendon: a review of 29 case. Arch Orthop Trauma Surg 2017;137:285–92.

39. Henry SL, Katz MA, Green DP. Type IV FDP avulsion: lessons learned clinically and through review of the literature. HAND 2009;4:357–61.

40. Lalonde D, Higgins A. Wide awake flexor tendon repair in the finger. Plast Reconstr Surg Glob Open 2016;4:e797.

41. Lalonde D. Decreasing tendon rupture and tenolysis with wide awake surgery. BMC Proc 2015;9:A66.

42. Amadio PC, Wood MB, Cooner WP 3rd, et al. Staged flexor tendon reconstruction in the fingers and hand. J Hand Surg Am 1988;13:559–62.

43. Neiduski RL, Powell RK. Flexor tendon rehabilitation in the 21st century: a systematic review. J Hand Ther 2019;32(2):165–74.

44. Bodner G, Rudisch A, Gabl M, et al. Diagnosis of digital flexor tendon annular pulley disruption: comparison of high frequency ultrasound and MRI. Ultraschall Med 1999;20:131–6.

45. Hauger O, Chung CB, Lektrakul N, et al. Pulley system in the fingers: normal anatomy and simulated lesions in cadavers at MR imaging, CT, and US with and without contrast material distention of the tendon sheath. Radiology 2000;217: 201–12.

46. Martinoli C, Bianchi S, Nebiolo M, et al. Sonographic evaluation of digital annular pulley tears. Skeletal Radiol 2000;29:387–91.

47. Martinoli C, Bianchi S, Cotton A. Imaging of rock climbing injuries. Semin Musculoskelet Radiol 2005;9:334–45.

48. Guntern D, Goncalves-Matoso V, Gray A, et al. Finger A2 pulley lesions in rock climbers: detection and characterization with magnetic resonance imaging at 3 Tesla—initial results. Invest Radiol 2007;42:435–41.

49. Schoffl V, Hochholzer T, Winkelmann HP, et al. Pulley injuries in rock climbers. Wilderness Environ Med 2003;14:94e100.

50. Kleinert HE, Bennett JB. Digital pulley reconstruction employing the always present rim of the previous pulley. J Hand Surg Am 1978;3:297–8.

51. Karev A, Stahl S, Taran A. The mechanical efficiency of the pulley system in normal digits compared with a reconstructed system using the "belt loop" technique. J Hand Surg Am 1987;12:596–601.

52. Mehta V, Phillips CS. Flexor tendon pulley reconstruction. Hand Clin 2005;21: 245–51.

53. Lin GT, Amadio PC, An KN, et al. Biomechanical analysis of finger flexor pulley reconstruction. J Hand Surg Br 1989;14:278–82.

54. Doyle JR, Blythe WF. Anatomy of the flexor tendon sheath and pulleys of the tendon sheath and pulleys of the thumb. J Hand Surg Am 1977;2:149–51.
55. Lister GD. Reconstruction of pulleys employing extensor retinaculum. J Hand Surg Am 1979;4:461–4.
56. Karev A. The "belt loop" technique for the reconstruction of pulleys in the first stage of flexor tendon grafting. J Hand Surg Am 1984;9:923–4.
57. Okutsu I, Ninomiya S, Hiraki S, et al. Three-loop technique for A2 pulley reconstruction. J Hand Surg Am 1987;12:790–4.
58. Widstrom CJ, Doyle JF, Johnson G, et al. A mechanical study of six digital pulley reconstruction techniques: part II. Strength of individual reconstructions. J Hand Surg 1989;14:826–9.
59. Inkellis E, Altman E, Wolfe SW. Management of flexor pulley injuries with proximal interphalangeal joint contracture. Hand Clin 2018;34:251–66.
60. Arora R, Fritz D, Zimmermann R, et al. Reconstruction of the digital flexor pulley system: a retrospective comparison of two methods of treatment. J Hand Surg Eur Vol 2007;32:60–6.
61. Rohrbough JT, Mudge MK, Schilling RC. Overuse injuries in the elite rock climber. Med Sci Sports Exerc 2000;32:1369–72.
62. Schoffl VR, Einwag F, Strecker W, et al. Strength measurement and clinical outcome after pulley ruptures in climbers. Med Sci Sports Excerc 2006;38(4):637–43.

Distal Radius Fractures in the Athlete

Andrew D. Sobel, MD, Ryan P. Calfee, MD, MSc*

KEYWORDS

- Distal radius fracture • Athletic injury • Wrist • Sports • Surgery

KEY POINTS

- Athletes have specialized needs surrounding the diagnosis and treatment of distal radius fractures.
- Return to play is a point of emphasis for athletes, especially those at high levels of sport.
- Early return involves frank conversation with the treating surgeon to ensure an understanding of the risks by the patient.
- Prompt and proper rehabilitation is critical to achieving the best outcome.

INTRODUCTION

Distal radius fractures are common injuries that are seen in younger and older populations.[1] Although treatment options of distal radius fractures vary depending on many factors including age, bone quality, functional demand, and fracture characteristics, there are unique subsets of patients that require specialized approaches and care to attain the best possible outcomes.

Athletes are motivated and healthy individuals who engage in activities that often directly require the use of their hands and wrists or place them at higher risk for sustaining wrist injuries. These patients are usually focused on the most expeditious return to function and competition. Treating surgeons must keep this need in mind and consider the level of competition when balancing the risks and benefits of timing the athletes' return to play. Conventional surgical and nonsurgical options are often appropriate, but there are instances where this may not be the case. This article discusses the presentation and treatment of distal radius fractures in athletes.

EPIDEMIOLOGY

Distal radius fractures are the most common upper extremity fracture in the United States, accounting for nearly 25% of all upper extremity fractures.[1] Distal radius fractures are becoming more frequent over the past five decades.[2,3] Patients younger than

Department of Orthopedic Surgery, Washington University in St. Louis, Campus Box 8233, 660 South Euclid Avenue, St. Louis, MO 63108, USA
* Corresponding author.
E-mail address: calfeer@wustl.edu

Clin Sports Med 39 (2020) 299–311
https://doi.org/10.1016/j.csm.2019.10.005
0278-5919/20/© 2019 Elsevier Inc. All rights reserved.

sportsmed.theclinics.com

the age of 18 and older than 50 years are the most affected,[1] although the reasons for sustaining distal radius fractures in these populations are quite disparate.[4-7] Younger patients typically sustain distal radius fractures during sports or play and older patients typically have lower-energy mechanisms, such as ground-level falls resulting in fragility fractures. Distal radius fractures account for 23% and 17% of all sport-related fractures in adolescents and adults, respectively.[8] Athletes with distal radius fractures are often younger and healthier than the general population with the same injury[9] because, like the younger population in general, they have higher bone density and fracture their distal radii only through higher energy mechanisms.[10-14]

The risk of an athlete suffering a distal radius fracture varies by sport. Eighty-seven percent of all sport-related fractures result from athletes participating in only 10 sports, with 31 other sports resulting in the remaining 13% of the fractures.[9] Distal radius fractures are more common with in-line skating, badminton, gymnastics, ice-skating, snowboarding, football, and horseback riding[9] and in less-competitive athletic activities, such as riding hoverboards.[15] The relative risks of fracture by sport likely varies across populations because studies have reported soccer contributing from 20%[16] to 50%[13] of distal radius fractures sustained during sport. Despite the high energy collisions, only 5% of all injuries in professional football players are distal radius fractures, making it only the seventh most common upper extremity injury from the elbow to hand in this sport.[17]

The complexity of the type of distal radius fracture can vary based on the sport involved. Skiing and horseback riding often result in more complex fractures given falls at higher speeds and from larger heights, whereas fractures from soccer and rugby are typically extra-articular.[13] Even within the same sport, fracture patterns can differ in subgroups of athletes. Experienced snowboarders sustained more intra-articular fractures than beginners, which was likely related to the expert snowboarders performing more jumps.[14]

PREVENTION

Wrist guards have been shown to decrease the strain at the distal radius during impact by sharing load and absorbing energy.[18] Biomechanically, this can translate into different patterns of and potential less severe wrist injuries.[19,20] Clinically, the use of wrist guards reduced the incidence of distal radius fracture during snowboarding by 85%[21] and resulted in an approximately 10-times lower risk of wrist injury in in-line skaters.[22] However, not all sports permit or can accommodate the use of personal protective equipment and younger athletes typically discard this equipment because it is cumbersome or unfashionable. In these instances, focusing on education and building skill is protective against sustaining a distal radius fracture based on the protective effect of heightened athletic prowess.[23]

DISTAL RADIUS ANATOMY

The distal radius articulates with the distal ulna, lunate, and scaphoid, but given its morphology, affords limited bony constraint to these structures. Forearm pronosupination and load transmission[24] occurs through the sigmoid notch of the radius as part of the distal radioulnar joint. Appropriate congruity and contact between the radius and ulna is imperative for painless motion. The lunate and scaphoid articulate with the lunate and scaphoid fossae on the radius, which are often involved in intra-articular fractures of the distal radius. Normal anatomic alignment of the distal radius involves assessment of standard radiographic parameters, such as height, inclination, tilt, and length. Radius height refers to the proximodistal distance from the ulnar portion of the lunate facet to the tip of the radial styloid (normal 12 mm). Radial incli-nation is the angulation of a line from the ulnar portion of the lunate facet to the tip of the radial styloid in relation to a line perpendicular to the longitudinal axis of the radial metaphysis starting at the ulnar portion of the lunate facet (normal 22°) (**Fig. 1**). Volar tilt is the angulation on the lateral radiograph of the articular surface of the distal radius in relation to a line perpendicular to the axis of the radial shaft (normal is about 11° volar) (**Fig. 2**). Radius length is the variance in proximodistal distance between the radial-most portion of the ulnar head and the ulnar most portion of the lunate facet (neutral is typically normal) (**Fig. 3**).[25] These average normal values may not perfectly describe each individual, so comparison with the contralateral wrist is helpful to detect subtle fracture displacement. Re-establishment and maintenance of these radio-graphic parameters and joint congruity is a principal goal of distal radius fracture treatment.

Besides the osseous architecture, stability and function of the wrist is conferred by stout ligamentous and other soft tissue structures. Carpal stability is afforded by volar radiocarpal ligaments (radioscaphocapitate, radiolunate), which originate across and obscure the volar margin of the distal radius articular lip and insert onto the scaphoid, capitate, and lunate and dorsal radiocarpal ligaments that origi-nate on the dorsal rim of the radius and insert into the dorsal lunate and triquetrum. Assessment of the volar lip of the distal radius is critical because there may be a separate fracture fragment encompassing this small, but important component of the bone (**Fig. 4**). Displacement of this volar bony support produces changes in the "teardrop angle," carpal translation, lunate subsidence, and length of the volar lip fragment.[26] Although these fragments are small, specialized plates or fixation constructs should be used because standard locking plates placed distal and volar past the "watershed" line risk flexor tendon irritation and possible rupture.[27] Distal radioulnar joint stability is afforded by the triangulofibrocartilage complex (TFCC) and associated radioulnar ligaments. These stabilizing structures are frequently

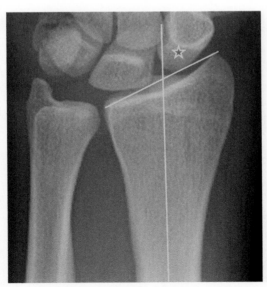

Fig. 1. Posteroanterior radiograph of a normal distal radius indicating the angle of radius inclination relative to the long axis of the radius. The *star* marks the normal 22° angle.

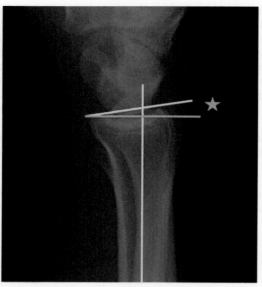

Fig. 2. Lateral radiograph of normal distal radius indicating the volar tilt of the distal radius with normal 11° angle indicated by the *star*.

injured in distal radius fractures and careful consideration to their treatment may improve patient outcomes.[28]

The radial and ulnar arteries give main contributions to the deep and superficial palmar arches, respectively, but there are numerous anastomoses between the two

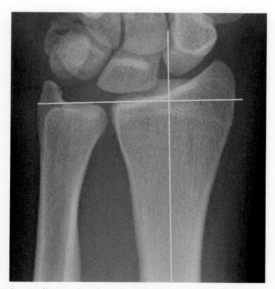

Fig. 3. Posteroanterior radiograph of a normal distal radius demonstrating neutral ulnar variance as ulnar length equal to ulnar corner of distal radius articular surface.

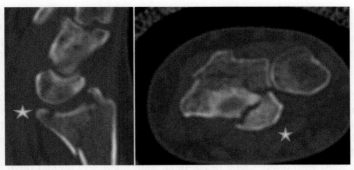

Fig. 4. Sagittal and axial computed tomography images with volar lunate facet fracture marked with *stars*.

systems along the course of the hand. The median nerve runs between the flexor digitorum profundus and flexor digitorum superficialis in the forearm and becomes more superficial as it runs distally to pass into the carpal tunnel in a volar and radial position. Before entry, the palmar cutaneous nerve branches off 5 cm proximal to the wrist flexion crease and this branch typically becomes superficial, piercing through the antebrachial fascia, between the palmaris longus and flexor carpi radialis tendons. The palmar cutaneous nerve often makes its way into a separate fascial tunnel superficial to the carpal tunnel as it passes to the palm. These relationships are important because fractures of the distal radius can increase carpal canal pressure, leading to compression on the median nerve and acute carpal tunnel syndrome[29] and the flexor carpi radialis approach to the radius can injure the palmar cutaneous nerve, which at times courses within the flexor carpi radialis sheath.[30]

PATIENT EVALUATION

Depending on the acuity and nature of the injury, a formal trauma evaluation may need to be performed on the patient. For example, a fall from a large height in a skateboarder or motocross racer requires an on-field primary survey, which involves an assessment of airway, breathing, circulation, and neurologic status, whereas a badminton player with wrist pain after diving for a shuttlecock may require a more focused examination. Once the patient is stabilized, the wrist is assessed noting skin integrity, deformity, tenderness, and neurovascular status. After ruling out acute compartment syndrome or carpal tunnel syndrome in high-energy injury mechanisms, one can proceed with a semielective approach to treatment with ultimate choices made depending on fracture and patient characteristics.

Orthogonal radiographs are necessary to determine the personality of the fracture. The previously discussed radiographic parameters are used as guides defining acceptable reductions, which ultimately impacts the choice of operative versus nonoperative treatment. Intra-articular incongruity may be readily apparent on radiographs, but is clarified by computed tomography scan when necessary. Intra-articular displacement is typically surgically corrected because of its association with post-traumatic arthritis.[31] Dorsal tilt more than 10° from neutral can lead to loss of wrist flexion in addition to adaptive midcarpal instability and pain. Radial shortening can result in ulnar-positive variance and ulnocarpal impaction.

Ligamentous wrist injuries frequently occur in the setting of a distal radius fracture. Mehta and colleagues[32] determined that the prevalence of ligamentous injury is 69% in the setting of distal radius fractures. Provocative wrist testing is often difficult to perform because pain from the fracture can preclude wrist motion or confound feedback from palpation. If there is concern for scapholunate ligament injury, an MRI is helpful to confirm the presence of this injury, although intraoperative fluoroscopy or arthroscopy are alternatives. TFCC injuries are more common, comprising 61% of the soft tissue injuries in the athlete presenting with distal radius fractures.[33] Despite the high incidence of concomitant carpal soft tissue injuries, it does not seem necessary to treat most of these.[34,35] However, we believe that the athlete with associated completed scapholunate ligament rupture or TFCC tear associated with gross distal radial-ulnar joint instability should have those injuries treated surgically.

Finally, talking with the athlete and determining their goals for recovery is the final step before making any recommendation for treatment. There are many additional considerations when treating athletes, such as their current level of play, commitment to advancing to or staying at the highest level of play, contract negotiations, time left in-season, available time for recovery, and risk of secondary surgeries or complications with early return to play. All of these must be discussed frankly and openly to set expectations and achieve the desired outcome.

TREATMENT OPTIONS
Nonoperative Treatment

Most athletes are younger, active patients that have a desire to return to sport quickly without permanent dysfunction. Nondisplaced fractures are typically indicated for nonoperative management in all patients and in the athlete, this is generally true as well. However, displaced fractures with excellent postreduction alignment present a unique decision point. Questions to ask are:

- Is the athlete able to maintain a cast for 4 to 6 weeks and potentially longer weight-bearing restrictions?
- Will the time immobilized and the associated muscular atrophy result in significant rehabilitation and delay in returning to sport?
- Does the athlete's sport allow return to play in a cast?
- Is the athlete able to have weekly follow-up radiographs to determine if the fracture has maintained its alignment?

After reduction and splinting, initial treatment should involve weekly radiographs for 3 weeks to assess fracture alignment. Splints are transitioned to casts after fracture stability is confirmed and removable orthoses may be initiated after 6 weeks. Nondisplaced fractures may be transitioned to a removable brace at 4 weeks. These guidelines are general, with decreasing pain and tenderness and radiographic signs of osseous bridging assisting the decision making. Strengthening is delayed until there is no tenderness at the fracture site and radiographs demonstrate fracture line resolution.

It is not advisable for athletes to attempt nonoperative management with displaced distal radius fractures in the hopes of having "off season surgery." Unless the season is ending within a week or 2 and surgery can be delayed until then, a longer postponement is not recommended because fracture malunion repair would require an osteotomy. Compared with primary fracture surgery, malunion correction is associated with outcomes that are less predictable and more modest.[36]

Operative Treatment

Open reduction with internal fixation of all other distal radius fractures is the mainstay in adult athletes. The timing of this procedure is similar to nonathletes; it is ideally performed within 2 weeks after the injury. If the patient is comfortable and has no neurovascular compromise, it is possible to delay surgical intervention by placing the athlete in a cast in order for them to return to sport before their operative procedure. This is usually only considered in patients at the highest level of sport and follows an honest discussion of the risks of play. Although returning to sports that do not require wrist involvement rarely risks substantial reinjury, repeat falls or unintended collisions could risk more extensive injury.

The choice of the ideal internal fixation construct is generally based on fracture morphology. Most fractures are fixed with volar locking plates (**Fig. 5**). Although many studies show no difference in results at 1 to 2 years between methods of fixation,[37,38] there is evidence that volar plating has fewer complications and improved functional outcomes when compared with external and dorsal plate fixation.[39–42] Intra-articular fractures with depressed fragments are best accessed via a dorsal approach because the surgeon can visualize the articular surface directly (**Fig. 6**). Volar rim fractures must be addressed to provide stability to the carpus and these fractures often require specialized fixation distal, such as hook plates placed distal to the watershed line to capture the osteoligamentous fragments. Occasionally, a combination of fixation strategies is indicated to achieve stable reduction (**Fig. 7**). Finally, severely comminuted fractures may require spanning fixation for indirect reduction purposes.

Although many athletes are young, skeletally mature individuals, there are unique populations of athletes that do not fit this description and treatment should be tailored accordingly. Skeletally immature athletes with distal radius fractures is a rapidly growing cohort.[43] These young athletes are rarely in such high-level competition that their sport should supersede standard care for their injury. Most pediatric distal radius fractures can be treated nonoperatively given robust healing of fractures and remodeling of postreduction deformity if growth from the physis is still possible. However, the young athlete and their family may not want to risk the 39% loss of reduction after closed treatment and subsequent time taken to remodel and instead take the 38% risk of pin-related complications with Kirschner wire fixation (**Fig. 8**A, B).[44] Alternatively, some metadiaphyseal fractures in the child are well stabilized with small plates that spare the physis (**Fig. 9**A, B). The slightly older, but still growing, adolescent athlete who has already secured an athletic scholarship may have less motivation to

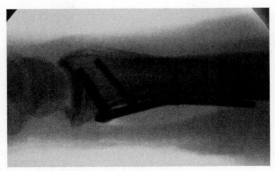

Fig. 5. Lateral radiograph of a well-placed volar locking plate tightly applied to the bone and proximal to the volar lip of the distal radius.

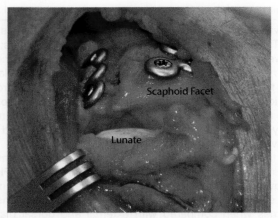

Fig. 6. Dorsal intraoperative view of intra-articular fracture reduced now with volar plates. Advantage here of dorsal approach is that fracture lines through the dorsal lunate facet and between the lunate and scaphoid facets reduced under direct vision.

expedite return to play. The contrary is expected in those yet to obtain a scholarship and who are under the watchful eye of scouts.

Older athletes are becoming more common as the population continues to live longer. Athletes older than age 60 have lower bone density and should be assumed to have osteoporosis and treated as such. The benefit of operative treatment of distal radius fractures in the high-functioning geriatric population is debated because those with malunion do not differ in functional outcomes compared with those with well-aligned fractures. If operative management is selected based on the patient's risk

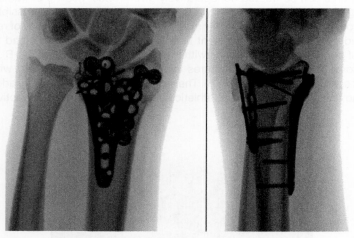

Fig. 7. Anteroposterior and lateral radiographs of a 42-year-old mountain biker with a complex, intra-articular distal radius fracture. Volar lunate facet rim fracture is hooked with a rim plate and a more proximal volar fracture plane is fixated with a volar locking plate. Dorsally, the articular surface of the distal radius was directly evaluated and a depressed, central articular fragment was reduced. The dorsal cortical and articular components were fixed with low-profile locking plates.

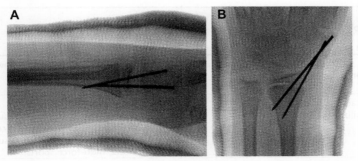

Fig. 8. Lateral (*A*) and anteroposterior (*B*) radiographs of a skeletally immature dirt bike rider who was treated with percutaneous Kirschner wire fixation for a displaced Salter-Harris type II distal radius fracture now well aligned.

tolerance and preference, often with consideration of the need for earlier return and utility of the affected extremity in their sport, standard approaches used for all adult patients should be selected.

Return to Sport

There is no consensus approach to return to sport after distal radius fracture. Some take a regimented approach in permitting return to sport when the fracture has healed and the range of motion and grip strength of the affected extremity is 80% of the contralateral.[45] Alternatively, we have typically made more personalized decisions based on sport demands and the risk-tolerance of the patient. **Table 1** comprises many situations that could be witnessed by the treating surgeon.

REHABILITATION

Regardless of the type of intervention, finger, forearm, elbow, and shoulder motion is initiated immediately and emphasized throughout healing. This prevents atrophy and stiffness of the unaffected muscles and joints and limits tendinous adhesions. In

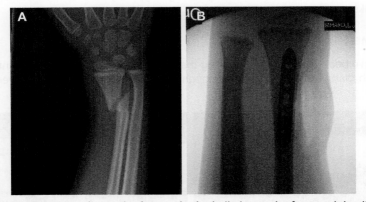

Fig. 9. Anteroposterior radiograph of young basketball player who fractured the distal one-third of his radius for the second time in 5 months (*A*) prompting fixation with a short 2.4-mm plate remaining proximal to the physis (*B*).

Table 1
Return to sport situations

Situation	Approximate Time to Return
Athlete's sport permits casts/immobilization and patient is accepting of risk	Immediately after casting as definitive treatment. As soon as skin healed following surgery.
Athlete cannot return until all immobilization is discontinued	4 wk (nonoperative, nondisplaced), 6 wk (nonoperative, displaced/reduced). 2–4 wk following surgery for noncontact, low-force sports. 6 wk following surgery for contact, high-force sports.
Athlete requires full, painless motion and strength	6–8 wk (operative), 8–12 wk (nonoperative).
Athlete participates in contact sport and cast is permitted	Follow chosen protocol and then add about 6 wk in a playing cast (only during sport).
Pediatric athletes	As early as 4 wk (either nonoperative or nonoperative if not requiring full, painless motion and strength), 6–8 wk (all others).

addition, muscle contractions and elevation can reduce edema, helping to limit pain and speed recovery. Postoperative splint removal occurs at 10 to 14 days and a removable orthosis is fashioned for stability and comfort, whereas motion exercises are initiated if the operative construct is considered rigid enough to support this motion (**Fig. 10**A, B). Otherwise, a period of casting for about 2 to 4 weeks follows. Motion after fractures managed nonoperatively begins after about 6 weeks of immobilization. Although one study had shown therapist-guided rehabilitation programs did not result in a difference in functional outcomes after volar plate fixation of distal radius fractures,[46] the high-level athlete was not separately studied. For most athletes treated surgically for distal radius fractures, we begin motion of the wrist and forearm within the first 2 weeks after surgery. Our intent is to achieve functional arcs of motion by the time of fracture union at which point a return to contact sports is considered for most nonprofessional athletes. Strengthening is typically initiated after fracture union at 6 weeks.

OUTCOMES

There have been few studies evaluating the specific outcomes after treatment of athletes with distal radius fractures. Although it may be assumed that achievement of

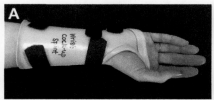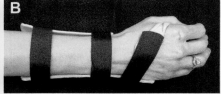

Fig. 10. Volar (*A*) and dorsal (*B*) view of a routine wrist orthosis fashioned by a hand therapist for early postoperative support after distal radius fracture allowing full finger motion.

functional outcomes would parallel the general population, these patients are healthy, highly motivated, and often unencumbered by pain. In a small subset of their overall cohort of rugby players sustaining fractures, Robertson and colleagues[47] showed that 90% of athletes with distal radius fractures were able to return to sport at their pre-injury level and all did so within 3 months. In soccer players sustaining distal radius fractures, Robertson and colleagues[16] showed 77% were able to return to the same level of play at a mean of 8.9 weeks and 100% of professional athletes achieved this outcome. Finally, Lawson and colleagues[13] determined that 73% of athletes, most of whom played soccer, skied, danced, or played rugby, returned to their original sport after treatment. Overall, these studies support a high rate of return, especially in high-level athletes and those in sports where the wrist is not a predominate component of function.

SUMMARY

Athletes commonly sustain distal radius fractures and although the fractures themselves may look similar to patients in the general population, there are numerous additional considerations in the decision-making process, treatment, and recovery of these patients. Efficient and speedy recovery is maximized by understanding the athlete's specific needs related to their sport and outcomes are generally good in this healthy, often young, population.

DISCLOSURE

R.P. Calfee reports research support from Medartis outside of the submitted work.

REFERENCES

1. Karl JW, Olson PR, Rosenwasser MP. The epidemiology of upper extremity fractures in the United States, 2009. J Orthop Trauma 2015;29(8):e242-4.
2. Bengner U, Johnell O. Increasing incidence of forearm fractures. A comparison of epidemiologic patterns 25 years apart. Acta Orthop Scand 1985;56(2):158-60.
3. Nellans KW, Kowalski E, Chung KC. The epidemiology of distal radius fractures. Hand Clin 2012;28(2):113-25.
4. Curtis EM, van der Velde R, Moon RJ, et al. Epidemiology of fractures in the United Kingdom 1988-2012: variation with age, sex, geography, ethnicity and socioeconomic status. Bone 2016;87:19-26.
5. Ismail AA, Pye SR, Cockerill WC, et al. Incidence of limb fracture across Europe: results from the European Prospective Osteoporosis Study (EPOS). Osteoporos Int 2002;13(7):565-71.
6. Sakai A, Oshige T, Zenke Y, et al. Association of bone mineral density with deformity of the distal radius in low-energy Colles' fractures in Japanese women above 50 years of age. J Hand Surg Am 2008;33(6):820-6.
7. Louer CR, Boone SL, Guthrie AK, et al. Postural stability in older adults with a distal radial fracture. J Bone Joint Surg Am 2016;98(14):1176-82.
8. Wood AM, Robertson GA, Rennie L, et al. The epidemiology of sports-related fractures in adolescents. Injury 2010;41(8):834-8.
9. Court-Brown CM, Wood AM, Aitken S. The epidemiology of acute sports-related fractures in adults. Injury 2008;39(12):1365-72.
10. Schipilow JD, Macdonald HM, Liphardt AM, et al. Bone micro-architecture, estimated bone strength, and the muscle-bone interaction in elite athletes: an HR-pQCT study. Bone 2013;56(2):281-9.

11. Sherk VD, Bemben MG, Bemben DA. Comparisons of bone mineral density and bone quality in adult rock climbers, resistance-trained men, and untrained men. J Strength Cond Res 2010;24(9):2468–74.

12. Tenforde AS, Fredericson M. Influence of sports participation on bone health in the young athlete: a review of the literature. PM R 2011;3(9):861–7.

13. Lawson GM, Hajducka C, McQueen MM. Sports fractures of the distal radius: epidemiology and outcome. Injury 1995;26(1):33–6.

14. Matsumoto K, Sumi H, Sumi Y, et al. Wrist fractures from snowboarding: a prospective study for 3 seasons from 1998 to 2001. Clin J Sport Med 2004;14(2): 64–71.

15. Sobel AD, Reid DB, Blood TD, et al. Pediatric orthopedic hoverboard injuries: a prospectively enrolled cohort. J Pediatr 2017;190:271–4.

16. Robertson GA, Wood AM, Bakker-Dyos J, et al. The epidemiology, morbidity, and outcome of soccer-related fractures in a standard population. Am J Sports Med 2012;40(8):1851–7.

17. Carlisle JC, Goldfarb CA, Mall N, et al. Upper extremity injuries in the National Football League: part II: elbow, forearm, and wrist injuries. Am J Sports Med 2008;36(10):1945–52.

18. Staebler MP, Moore DC, Akelman E, et al. The effect of wrist guards on bone strain in the distal forearm. Am J Sports Med 1999;27(4):500–6.

19. Moore MS, Popovic NA, Daniel JN, et al. The effect of a wrist brace on injury patterns in experimentally produced distal radial fractures in a cadaveric model. Am J Sports Med 1997;25(3):394–401.

20. Lewis LM, West OC, Standeven J, et al. Do wrist guards protect against fractures? Ann Emerg Med 1997;29(6):766–9.

21. Hagel B, Pless IB, Goulet C. The effect of wrist guard use on upper-extremity injuries in snowboarders. Am J Epidemiol 2005;162(2):149–56.

22. Schieber RA, Branche-Dorsey CM, Ryan GW, et al. Risk factors for injuries from in-line skating and the effectiveness of safety gear. N Engl J Med 1996;335(22): 1630–5.

23. Machold W, Kwasny O, Eisenhardt P, et al. Reduction of severe wrist injuries in snowboarding by an optimized wrist protection device: a prospective randomized trial. J Trauma 2002;52(3):517–20.

24. Shaaban H, Giakas G, Bolton M, et al. The distal radioulnar joint as a load-bearing mechanism: a biomechanical study. J Hand Surg Am 2004;29(1):85–95.

25. Fernandez DL, Wolfe S. Distal radius fractures. 5th edition. Philadelphia: Elsevier; 2005.

26. Beck JD, Harness NG, Spencer HT. Volar plate fixation failure for volar shearing distal radius fractures with small lunate facet fragments. J Hand Surg Am 2014; 39(4):670–8.

27. Soong M, Earp BE, Bishop G, et al. Volar locking plate implant prominence and flexor tendon rupture. J Bone Joint Surg Am 2011;93(4):328–35.

28. Ruch DS, Yang CC, Smith BP. Results of acute arthroscopically repaired triangular fibrocartilage complex injuries associated with intra-articular distal radius fractures. Arthroscopy 2003;19(5):511–6.

29. Gelberman RH, Szabo RM, Mortensen WW. Carpal tunnel pressures and wrist position in patients with Colles' fractures. J Trauma 1984;24(8):747–9.

30. Jones C, Beredjiklian P, Matzon JL, et al. Incidence of an anomalous course of the palmar cutaneous branch of the median nerve during volar plate fixation of distal radius fractures. J Hand Surg Am 2016;41(8):841–4.

31. Knirk JL, Jupiter JB. Intra-articular fractures of the distal end of the radius in young adults. J Bone Joint Surg Am 1986;68(5):647–59.
32. Mehta JA, Bain GI, Heptinstall RJ. Anatomical reduction of intra-articular fractures of the distal radius. An arthroscopically-assisted approach. J Bone Joint Surg Br 2000;82(1):79–86.
33. Hanker GJ. Radius fractures in the athlete. Clin Sports Med 2001;20(1):189–201.
34. Mrkonjic A, Geijer M, Lindau T, et al. The natural course of traumatic triangular fibrocartilage complex tears in distal radial fractures: a 13-15 year follow-up of arthroscopically diagnosed but untreated injuries. J Hand Surg Am 2012;37(8): 1555–60.
35. Mrkonjic A, Lindau T, Geijer M, et al. Arthroscopically diagnosed scapholunate ligament injuries associated with distal radial fractures: a 13- to 15-year follow-up. J Hand Surg Am 2015;40(6):1077–82.
36. Lozano-Calderon SA, Brouwer KM, Doornberg JN, et al. Long-term outcomes of corrective osteotomy for the treatment of distal radius malunion. J Hand Surg Eur Vol 2010;35(5):370–80.
37. Gartland JJ Jr, Werley CW. Evaluation of healed Colles' fractures. J Bone Joint Surg Am 1951;33-A(4):895–907.
38. Karnezis IA, Fragkiadakis EG. Association between objective clinical variables and patient-rated disability of the wrist. J Bone Joint Surg Br 2002;84(7):967–70.
39. Chappuis J, Boute P, Putz P. Dorsally displaced extra-articular distal radius fractures fixation: dorsal IM nailing versus volar plating. A randomized controlled trial. Orthop Traumatol Surg Res 2011;97(5):471–8.
40. Grewal R, Perey B, Wilmink M, et al. A randomized prospective study on the treatment of intra-articular distal radius fractures: open reduction and internal fixation with dorsal plating versus mini open reduction, percutaneous fixation, and external fixation. J Hand Surg Am 2005;30(4):764–72.
41. Ruch DS, Papadonikolakis A. Volar versus dorsal plating in the management of intra-articular distal radius fractures. J Hand Surg Am 2006;31(1):9–16.
42. Wei DH, Poolman RW, Bhandari M, et al. External fixation versus internal fixation for unstable distal radius fractures: a systematic review and meta-analysis of comparative clinical trials. J Orthop Trauma 2012;26(7):386–94.
43. de Putter CE, van Beeck EF, Looman CW, et al. Trends in wrist fractures in children and adolescents, 1997-2009. J Hand Surg Am 2011;36(11):1810–5.e2.
44. Miller BS, Taylor B, Widmann RF, et al. Cast immobilization versus percutaneous pin fixation of displaced distal radius fractures in children: a prospective, randomized study. J Pediatr Orthop 2005;25(4):490–4.
45. Henn CM, Wolfe SW. Distal radius fractures in athletes: approaches and treatment considerations. Sports Med Arthrosc Rev 2014;22(1):29–38.
46. Souer JS, Buijze G, Ring D. A prospective randomized controlled trial comparing occupational therapy with independent exercises after volar plate fixation of a fracture of the distal part of the radius. J Bone Joint Surg Am 2011;93(19):1761–6.
47. Robertson GA, Wood AM, Heil K, et al. The epidemiology, morbidity and outcome of fractures in rugby union from a standard population. Injury 2014; 45(4):677–83.

Surgical Techniques for the Treatment of Acute Carpal Ligament Injuries in the Athlete

Jacob D. Gire, MD, Jeffrey Yao, MD*

KEYWORDS

- Wrist pain • Carpal ligament injury • Wrist instability • Wrist arthroscopy
- Intercarpal ligament repair • Scapholunate ligament • Lunotriquetral ligament

KEY POINTS

- The treatment of carpal ligament injuries in athletes is highly individualized, sport specific, and requires an open discussion between the athlete, family, coaches, trainers, and the physician.
- Early recognition and treatment of carpal ligament injuries is essential to ensure optimal outcomes.
- A short trial of immobilization for occult injuries often improves symptoms, followed by early surgical treatment if symptoms persist.
- Acute dynamic and static injuries should be treated early for the most predictable outcome, even if this requires forfeiting the current season.

INTRODUCTION

The normal wrist involves a complex, balanced synchrony between the carpal bones and rows. These bones are stabilized by intrinsic and extrinsic carpal ligaments.[1–3] Disruption of these ligaments can result in pain, instability, and loss of function. Untreated, or inadequately treated, these injuries can lead to progressive degenerative change that may be career threatening.[4] With athletes, our initial goals remain to make a timely and accurate diagnosis, provide options, and create an environment for shared decision making. Restoring their unique skill set can be challenging. An appreciation of the nuances of patient wishes, risk tolerance, and demands of the sport allows an individualized treatment strategy to be provided.

Athletes of any discipline involving violent contact with the ground or other players are prone to carpal ligament injury.[5,6] This injury is often related to a fall or impact resulting in forced hyperextension of the wrist.[7] Patients often present with dorsal wrist pain and swelling and may complain of decreased motion, grip strength, and the

Robert A. Chase Hand and Upper Limb Center, Department of Orthopaedic Surgery, Stanford University Medical Center, 450 Broadway Street, MC 6342, Redwood City, CA 94063, USA
* Corresponding author.
E-mail address: jyao@stanford.edu

Clin Sports Med 39 (2020) 313–337
https://doi.org/10.1016/j.csm.2019.12.001
0278-5919/20/© 2019 Elsevier Inc. All rights reserved.

feeling of sudden shifts or clunks. The most commonly injured carpal ligaments are the scapholunate interosseous ligament (SLIL) and the lunotriquetral interosseous ligament (LTIL) (**Fig. 1**), with SLIL injury occurring at a rate of about 6 times that of LTIL injuries.[5] Injuries to the carpal ligaments occurs on a spectrum and can range from partial tear with occult instability to complete tear with injury to associated secondary ligamentous stabilizers. Without treatment, these injuries often progress to arthrosis.[4] These injuries may be ignored by athletes for weeks or years, which creates a treatment dilemma, as outcomes of operative treatment for chronic injuries are less predictable. In this article, we focus on surgical treatment of carpal ligament injuries in athletes who are identified in the acute phase.

PHYSICAL EXAMINATION

For any athlete presenting with acute wrist pain, a comprehensive physical examination is performed. Specific clinical findings that may suggest an SLIL injury include tenderness over the carpus, particularly dorsal and radial, prominence of the scaphoid proximal pole, and in some cases, an enlarged gap between the scaphoid and lunate. Dorsal wrist pain that seems out of proportion or is not responsive to a brief course of immobilization should raise suspicion for a carpal ligament injury. Specific provocative maneuvers may be limited initially owing to pain and swelling, but may be more appreciable upon repeat examination. The scapholunate ligament injury is tested with Watson's test. With the wrist in ulnar deviation, the scaphoid is stabilized in extension with the examiners thumb on its tubercle and index finger on the dorsal proximal pole. As the wrist is radially deviated, the scaphoid's natural tendency is to flex. This action is limited by the surgeon's thumb on the tubercle. If the SLIL is incompetent, the patient may experience pain or a painful dorsal clunk as the scaphoid is displaced dorsally. Additionally, pain with resisted index and long finger extension with the wrist partially flexed is a sensitive finding for injury or insufficiency of the dorsal SL ligament.[8] The SLIL may also be tested with the scaphoid lift test. With the elbow on the table and the forearm fully pronated, the lunate is stabilized in one hand and the scaphoid tubercle is pushed upward in an attempt to extend the scaphoid in relation to the lunate,

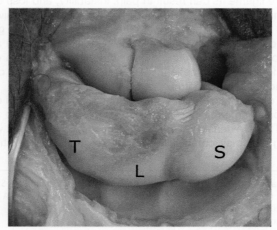

Fig. 1. Proximal row of the carpus demonstrating the scapholunate ligament between the scaphoid (S) and lunate (L) and the lunotriquetral ligament between the lunate (L) and triquetrum (T).

with pain indicating the test is positive.[9] LT ligament injury and instability can be evaluated with the shuck, ballottement, and shear tests, with the shear test being most specific.[10] The shuck test is performed by stabilizing the lunate to the radius and attempting to translate the triquetrum in a volar and dorsal direction in relation to the lunate. A test is positive when pain or increased laxity is noted.[11] With the ballottement test, the examiner uses his or her thumb to push the medial body of the triquetrum radially against the lunate in a rocking or balloting manner.[10] For the shear test, the examiner steadies and supports the dorsal body of the lunate while a firm load is applied on the LT joint through compressing the pisiform against the triquetrum.[12] A positive finding for the ballottement and shear tests is the presence of pain.

IMAGING

Standard posteroanterior, lateral, and oblique radiographs are obtained routinely with contralateral views for comparison. These radiographs are scrutinized for incongruity of arcs, intercarpal distance abnormalities, and the intercarpal angles are measured using standard techniques.[13] When static instability is absent but SLIL injury is suspected, a clenched pencil grip view provides the best method to evaluate for dynamic instability (**Fig. 2**).[14] Additional stress views of the carpus such as an axial loading view, ulnar deviation view, and distraction view may help to identify malalignment. Static findings such as SL diastasis, a positive ring sign, and dorsal scaphoid translation should raise suspicion for more significant ligamentous injury (**Fig. 3**). Fluoroscopy, computed tomography scans, and MRIs can all provide useful information to supplement the clinical examination. We rely primarily on MRI to evaluate for intercarpal ligament injuries, with a 3 T magnet preferred because this has been shown to be superior to 1.5 T magnets (**Fig. 4**).[15,16] The sensitivity and specificity of 3-T MR for SLIL tears has been reported between 70% to 90% and 94% to 100%, respectively. For LTIL tears, the sensitivity is lower from 50% to 82%, and specificity is comparable from 94% to 100%.[17,18]

GENERAL MANAGEMENT

In the absence of radiographic abnormalities, many intercarpal ligament injuries improve with a brief period of immobilization,[7,19] whereas athletes with radiographic

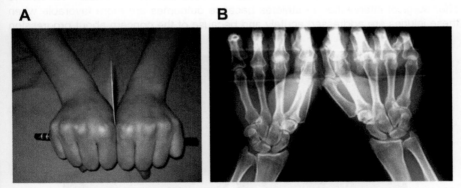

A   **B**

Fig. 2. Pencil grip view demonstrating (*A*) proper patient position and (*B*) the radiographic image demonstrating scapholunate interval widening on the right. (*From* Lee SK, Desai H, Silver B, Dhaliwal G, Paksima N. Comparison of radiographic stress views for scapholunate dynamic instability in a cadaver model. J Hand Surg 2011;36A:1149–1157; with permission.)

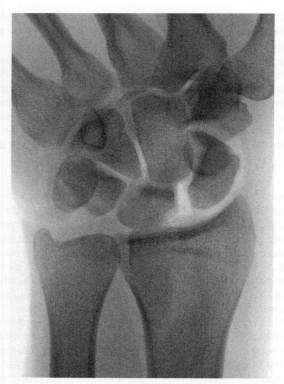

Fig. 3. Posteroanterior view of the left wrist demonstrating SL widening and a signet ring sign suggesting SL injury with rotatory subluxation.

evidence of acute carpal ligament injury with static or dynamic change are indicated for early surgery. Significant ligament injuries may still be present even in the absence of static or dynamic instability on the initial plain radiograph. A high clinical suspicion is necessary to ensure timely diagnosis because the window of opportunity for repair is limited and early intervention is preferable to ensure optimal outcomes.[20] We tend to offer surgical intervention in athletes because outcomes are more favorable when these injuries are addressed acutely and because of the concern about progression

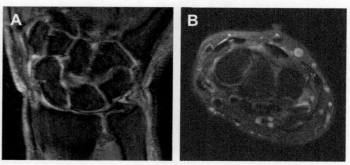

Fig. 4. MRI of the wrist with (A) coronal and (B) axial T2-weighted images demonstrating increased signal intensity in the SL and LT ligaments suggestive of partial tear.

to scapholunate advanced collapse arthritis. It should be noted, however, that the true natural history of intercarpal ligament injuries is unknown; many acute injuries go undetected and are often written off as a sprain. Additionally, it has been observed in a small cohort of patients that partial ligament injuries may not in fact progress to static gap, dorsal intercalated segment instability deformity, or arthritis, although all of these patients reported some level of pain, decreased grip strength, and decreased range of motion after nonoperative treatment.[19] Athletes with clinically suspected carpal ligament injuries but normal radiographs are immobilized and reevaluated at 1 and 3 weeks after injury. This schedule provides the opportunity to repeat provocative testing maneuvers once pain and swelling subside, as well as to confirm improvement in symptoms. Often elite athletes present with or request high-resolution MRIs, which can be helpful in evaluating the anatomic structures of the carpus and facilitate early injury identification, assuming adequate imaging protocol, radiologist experience, and sufficiently strong magnet.[15,16] However, this cannot supplant clinical evaluation because there is a high rate of asymptomatic tears found on MRI.[21,22] If the MRI is equivocal and a patient remains symptomatic after 4 weeks of immobilization, and suspicion for carpal ligament injury remains high, wrist arthroscopy for diagnostic and therapeutic purposes is indicated. Diagnostic arthroscopy provides the best means of assessing the intrinsic and extrinsic ligaments of the wrist. The Geissler classification is used to classify the degree of injury noted to the SL and LT interosseous ligaments (**Table 1**)[23] and the European Wrist Arthroscopy Society classification has also been described for the SL ligament.[24] Garcia-Elias and colleagues[25] proposed 5 questions to help guide treatment: (1) Is the dorsal SL Ligament intact and functional? (2) Does the ligament have sufficient tissue and healing potential? (3) Is the scaphoid aligned normally? (4) Is any carpal malalignment easily reducible? and (5) Is the articular cartilage normal? These questions help stratify stages of scapholunate injury and have been used to create stage-oriented algorithms for treatment.[25,26] In general, attempts at restoring bony relationships with a soft tissue repair or reconstruction is attempted when a wrist is without fixed bony deformity, as is often the case with acute carpal ligament injury. However, in the presence of fixed bony deformity, which occurs with chronic or neglected injury, this strategy is likely to fail and as such salvage surgical procedures are favored, such as a partial wrist fusion.

Table 1	
Geissler arthroscopic classification of interosseous ligament injury	
Grade	**Description**
I	Attenuation/hemorrhage of the interosseous ligament viewed from the radiocarpal space without midcarpal malalignment.
II	Attenuation/hemorrhage of the interosseous ligament viewed from the radiocarpal space with incongruency/step-off of carpal alignment. May have a gap less than the width of a probe.
III	Incongruency/step-off of carpal alignment viewed from the radiocarpal and midcarpal space and a probe can be passed through a gap between the carpal bones.
IV	Incongruency/step-off of carpal alignment viewed from the radiocarpal and midcarpal space with gross instability and a 2.7 mm arthroscope may be passed through the gap between the carpal bones.

From Geissler WB, Freeland AE, Savoie FH, McIntyre LW, Whipple TL. Intracarpal soft-tissue lesions associated with an intra-articular fracture of the distal end of the radius. *JBJS*. 1996;78(3):357-365; with permission.

For athletes with acute carpal ligament injuries, we generally treat partial SL liga-ment tears (Geissler grades I–III) with arthroscopic debridement and capsular shrinkage and temporary pinning of the SL joint depending on the amount of instability (Geissler grade III). We immobilize the patient for 6 weeks after surgery and then initiate hand therapy with return to play allowed when athletes can tolerate the activ-ities of their sport and when grip strength is at least 50% of the contralateral side, often at 12 weeks. In those with complete tears (Geissler grade IV), an open dorsal approach is made and the ligament is repaired primarily or acutely reconstructed if insufficient tissue is present. When rotatory instability of the scaphoid is also observed, a dorsal capsulodesis is also performed to address the sagittal plane instability. After ligament repair with or without capsulodesis, the wrist is immobilized in a short arm cast for 6 to 8 weeks. Pins are then removed and the athlete is transitioned to a removable splint for 4 additional weeks and dart thrower's range of motion exercises are begun. Return to play is typically allowed at 4 to 6 months postoperatively after these parameters are met. For those who present in the chronic phase, reconstruction is considered in the off season with an understanding that results are less predictable and salvage pro-cedures may be necessary at the end of an athlete's career. Operative treatment of LT ligament tears is less well-studied, but largely mirrors SL treatment algorithms and is detailed elsewhere in this article.

SURGICAL TECHNIQUES
Diagnostic Arthroscopy

Wrist arthroscopy remains the gold standard for the diagnosis of carpal ligament injury. Both the radiocarpal and midcarpal joints are evaluated using standard tech-niques. The 3-4, 6R, and midcarpal portals are marked. The radiocarpal joint is insuf-flated with saline through the 3-4 interval. Distension of the midcarpal joint may be palpated during injection of the radiocarpal joint in the presence of interosseous liga-ment injuries.[27] The skin is sharply incised and a small curved hemostat is used to bluntly spread down to and then enter capsule. The blunt trocar with arthroscopic can-nula followed by the arthroscope is inserted through the 3-4 portal. The 6R portal is then made under direct vision. The radiocarpal joint is evaluated in a systematic fashion noting the presence of synovitis and the quality of the articular surface and intrinsic and extrinsic ligaments. A shaver and/or thermal probe is used to address sy-novitis and remove debris to improve visualization. The SLIL, LTIL, and triangular fibro-cartilage complex are probed for structural integrity. The 3-4 portal provides the best view of the SLIL, where it should have a concave appearance (**Fig. 5**). The arthroscope is then transitioned to the 6R portal, where the LT ligament is better visualized. The normal ligament should also be concave in appearance between the lunate and trique-tral articular surfaces (**Fig. 6**). From the 6R portal, the camera is then directed dorsally to evaluate for dorsal capsular injury. Typically, communicating fibers of the dorsal intercarpal ligament insert onto the SLIL and a dorsal bow of the capsule will be observed. When injured, this arch or septum will be absent and when probed no resis-tance will be felt as the probe moves dorsally toward the midcarpal joint (**Fig. 7**).

The midcarpal–radial and midcarpal–ulnar portals are then created, located approx-imately 1 cm distal to the 3-4 and 4-5 portals. When there is an SLIL injury, we typically create the ulnar midcarpal portal first given the displacement of the scaphoid, which can make the radial midcarpal portal more challenging to create. A volar radial portal may be added to better visualize the volar SL and the dorsoradiocarpal (DRC) ligaments. The midcarpal radial portal is used to evaluate the scapholunate interval, followed by the midcarpal ulnar portal for the LT interval, and presence of instability is noted and graded

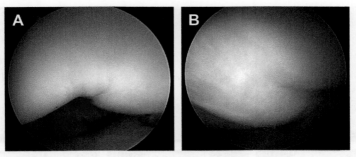

Fig. 5. SLIL viewed through the 3-4 portal with (*A*) normal appearance and (*B*) abnormal appearance with loss of concavity and laxity observed.

as described by Geissler.[23] The arthroscope is usually started in the midcarpal radial portal, except in smaller wrists where the midcarpal ulnar portal may be easier to enter or if the patient is suspected to have a large SLIL tear with scaphoid displacement. Individuals with a normal interval will have tight apposition of the scaphoid and lunate, without step off or the ability to get a probe between the bones (**Fig. 8**). As level of injury worsens, coronal plane instability is first observed with gapping between the carpal bones, followed by sagittal plane instability in the presence of associated extrinsic ligament injury, with articular step-off observed in the midcarpal joint as the lunate flexes or extends in relation to the scaphoid and triquetrum.

Scapholunate Interosseous Ligament Injuries

Occult instability

Partial SL ligament tears may result in occult instability and often improve with a brief course of immobilization followed by dedicated therapy. Strengthening the flexor carpi radialis, abductor pollicis longus, and extensor carpi radialis longus after cast removal may improve scaphoid stability and gradual return to play is allowed if the activities required for their sport are tolerable and grip strength is at least 50% of the contralateral side.[28–30] Specific rehabilitation protocols for partial SL ligament tears, which

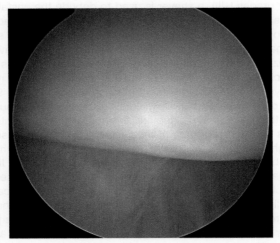

Fig. 6. Normal concave appearance of the lunotriquetral joint viewed through the 6R portal.

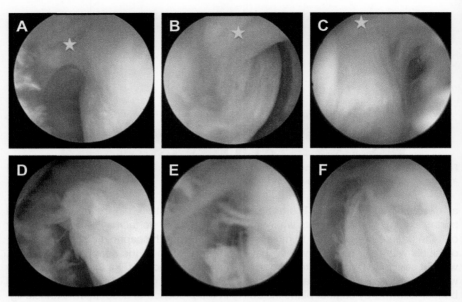

Fig. 7. Arthroscopic view of the (*A–C*) normal dorsal capsuloscapholunate septum (*stars*) in 3 patients and (*D–F*) a torn dorsal capsuloscapholunate septum in 3 patients viewed from the 6R portal. (*From* Binder AC, Kerfant N, Wahegaonkar AL, et al. Dorsal Wrist Capsular Tears in Association with Scapholunate Instability: Results of an Arthroscopic Dorsal Capsuloplasty. J Wrist Surg 2013;2:160-167; with permission.)

include dart-throwers motion and/or proprioception training have been described with promising early outcomes.[31–33] In those patients who remain symptomatic, or in skill position athletes such as quarterbacks and basketball and baseball players who require wrist motion to perform, we favor early surgical treatment with arthroscopy, debridement, and thermal shrinkage. After arthroscopic confirmation of stable partial SL tear (Geissler grades I–III), a shaver is used to debride the unstable tissue flaps, preserving the healthy intact fibers. A monopolar or bipolar radiofrequency probe is then inserted into the midcarpal joint and used to perform thermal shrinkage of the distal volar SL ligament and the dorsal SLIL as needed. This maneuver is performed using the cauterization setting and the ligament and volar capsule is spot welded at the palmar junction of the scaphoid and lunate until a color change is noted from pearl white to golden yellow/light brown without ablating the tissue (**Fig. 9**). The probe is applied in bursts of a few seconds while maintaining adequate fluid outflow and irrigation to decrease the risk of heat buildup and thermal injury. If present, redundancy of the membranous and dorsal portion of the ligament is also addressed with thermal shrinkage through the radiocarpal portal. After thermal shrinkage, the scapholunate joint is again probed to confirm stability. In Geissler grades I and II ligament injuries we immobilize the wrist for 6 weeks but do not transfix the joint, whereas in Geissler grade III injuries, two 0.045-inch K-wires are used to transfix the scapholunate joint and protect the ligament for 6 weeks, after which the short arm thumb spica cast and K-wires are removed. Therapy with motion in the dart throwers plane is started immediately after discontinuation of immobilization and activity is advanced to full active range of motion as tolerated thereafter. Full return to activity is allowed at 12 weeks.

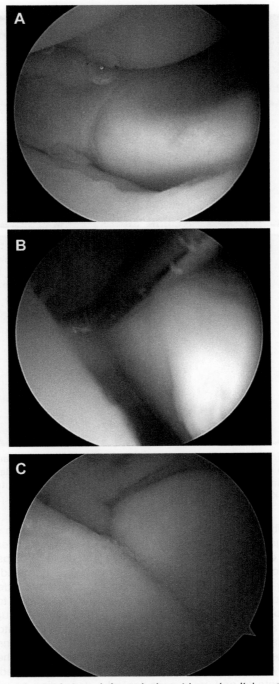

Fig. 8. Scapholunate interval viewed through the midcarpal radial portal demonstrating (*A*) abnormal widening suggestive of SL injury determined to be (*B*) Geissler grade III on probing. (*C*) Normal SL interval for comparison with tight apposition of the scaphoid and lunate.

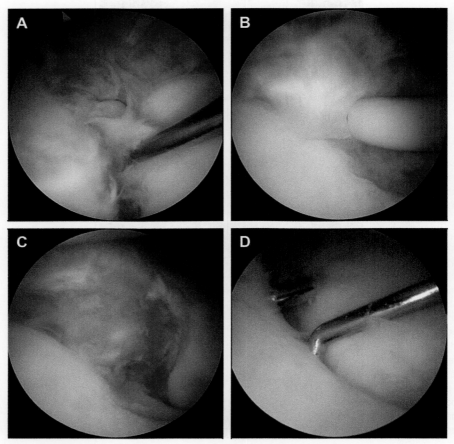

Fig. 9. Arthroscopic view of the scapholunate interval through the midcarpal radial portal demonstrating (A) Geissler grade III SL injury, (B) volar SLIL and capsule before thermal shrinkage, (C) golden yellow/tan color change, and (D) improvement in interval stability after shrinkage and K-wire fixation.

Occult instability of the scapholunate has also been described to occur with dorsal intercarpal ligament injuries, without associated SL ligament tear.[34,35] Loss of the normal arch of the dorsal capsuloscapholunate septum is observed through the radiocarpal joint and minimal to no resistance is encountered as a probe is passed from the radiocarpal to the midcarpal joint. Often abundant synovitis is encountered. Repair of the dorsal capsuloscapholunate septum to the SLIL has been described by using a needle to pass a 3-0 PDS suture through the capsule at the 3-4 portal, advancing it through the capsule and dorsal SL into the midcarpal joint and tying this down over dorsal capsule with the wrist in extension.[34,35] When we have encountered this pathology in practice, we have used either debridement alone followed by immobilization or a single suture anchor placed on the dorsal aspect of the lunate to perform a capsuloplasty, depending on whether the patient's complaints were pain or instability. Postoperatively the patient is placed in a short arm cast for 4 weeks, followed by therapy and return to full activity at 12 weeks.

Isolated injury of the DRCL without associated SLIL tear has also been observed to result in occult and dynamic instability. The ligament is visualized through the volar radial portal. This is created through a 2-cm longitudinal incision at the proximal wrist crease over the flexor carpi radialis tendon. The sheath is incised and the tendon is retracted ulnar after which a 22-gauge needle, followed by blunt trocar and cannula are introduced through the floor of the flexor carpi radialis sheath into the radiocarpal joint. The ligament is captured using an outside in technique with a horizontal mattress stitch passed through the ligament using the 3-4 and 4-5 portals. The tails are then passed under the extensor tendons and tied over the capsule at either the 3-4 or 4-5 portal.[36]

Outcomes Outcomes data after arthroscopic treatment of occult SL instability are limited to case series and expert opinion, typically involving chronic injuries with normal carpal alignment after failure of nonoperative measures. Ruch and Poehling[37] performed debridement alone of membranous SL tears in patients with at least 6 months of mechanical symptoms with satisfactory improvement and no progression to instability in all 7 of their patients with at least 2 years of follow-up. Weiss and colleagues[38] reported on debridement of partial tears in patients with symptoms refractory to a minimum of 6 weeks of nonoperative treatment, with satisfactory improvement in 11 of 13 patients at a mean follow-up of 27 months. Debridement is thought to address any mechanical symptoms and associated synovitis related to unstable tissue flaps.

Early results for arthroscopic debridement and thermal shrinkage for partial tears with normal carpal alignment have also been favorable. Darlis and colleagues[39] reported improvement in pain in 14 of 16 patients with a minimum of 3 months of symptoms, with complete resolution of symptoms in 8 of 16, without evidence of instability at a mean of 19 months. Lee and colleagues[40] reported on 16 wrists with isolated partial SL or LT tear and a minimum of 3 months of symptoms, with significant improvement in pain at rest and with activity, as well as excellent functional scores in 13 of 16, and good in 3 of 16 at a mean of 53 months of follow-up. No radiographic instability or arthritic change was noted in their follow-up period. Battistella and Taverna[41] similarly reported improvement in patients with Geissler grade I injury treated with debridement and thermal shrinkage alone, and in those with grades II and III change treated with arthroscopic reduction, k-wire fixation, and thermal shrinkage. Thermal shrinkage is thought to improve symptoms of instability by tightening the ligaments through heating and denaturing of collagen, which is followed by tissue repair with vascular invasion and fibroblastic activity.[39,42–44] Additionally, pain symptoms may be alleviated through ligament denervation.[45]

Patients may benefit from arthroscopic reduction and K-wire fixation, without thermal shrinkage. In a series of 40 patients with less than 3 months of symptoms and 3 mm or less of side-to-side difference in the scapholunate interval, 83% had maintenance of reduction and symptom relief. Stability was observed to be maintained for 2 to 7 years of follow-up.[46] Arthroscopic dorsal capsuloplasty for isolated dorsal capsuloscapholunate septum tear as performed by Binder and colleagues[34] had significant improvement in wrist range of motion, grip strength, functional scores, and pain scores in 10 patients with a history of at least 7 months of chronic dorsal wrist pair that was refractory to nonoperative measures, with a mean follow-up of 16 months.

Complications Heat-related complications including collagen necrosis and chondrolysis are concerns with thermal shrinkage.[47] Although these complications have not been reported with wrist arthroscopy, issues with thermal capsulorrhaphy of the glenohumeral joint including recurrent instability, deficient anterior capsule, and chondrolysis have decreased its frequency of use.[48,49] Strict attention to maintaining adequate outflow and using the probe in a pulsed manner for no longer than a few seconds at a time help to ensure adequate heat dissipation and may decrease the risk of heat-related complications.[50,51]

Complete scapholunate interosseous ligament tear amenable to repair

Complete disruption of the SLIL alone results in dynamic instability and is only apparent on stress examination. With additional injury of the scaphotrapezial and dorsal intercarpal ligaments, static SL interval diastasis can occur. When this includes scaphotrapezial trapezoid injury, the scaphoid will flex and rotatory subluxation will occur. When this is observed, it is important that surgical repair or reconstruction stabilizes the carpus in both coronal and sagittal planes to ensure optimal outcome.[26] Arthroscopy will demonstrate instability of the scapholunate interval with step off in the radiocarpal and midcarpal joints (Geissler grades III and IV). In the acute (<1 week) and subacute phases (<6–8 weeks), repair is preferable if tissue quality is of adequate quality. Arthroscopic reduction and fixation may be adequate in Geissler III injuries, and techniques to reduce and repair a complete SLIL tear (Geissler grade IV) with dorsal capsulodesis have been described.[52] Our preference for athletes is to perform an open reduction and dorsal ligament repair and K-wire fixation, with or without capsulodesis when the injury is sustained within 8 weeks of presentation.

A dorsal approach to the carpus with a radially based ligament-sparing capsulotomy is performed.[53] The capsulotomy runs from the radial styloid along the dorsal rim of the radius to the center of the lunate fossa, extending in line with the dorsal radiotriquetral ligament to its insertion, and then from the triquetrum to the scaphotrapezial trapezoid joint in line with the fibers of the dorsal intercarpal ligament (**Fig. 10**). Two 0.062-inch K-wires are inserted into the lunate and scaphoid as joysticks to assist with reduction at the planned insertion site of a suture anchor. The carpus is stabilized with two 0.045-inch K-wires through the scapholunate and scaphocapitate joints[54] and then a dorsal ligament repair is performed using suture anchors (**Fig. 11**). Most commonly, the ligament has avulsed off of the scaphoid, followed by a tear in the midsubstance, and then the lunate.[26] The suture from the anchor is left intact and half of the dorsal intercarpal ligament, which was maintained on the distal scaphoid, is

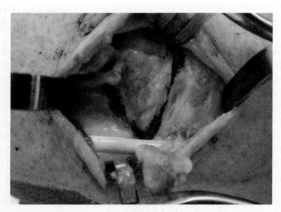

Fig. 10. Dorsal ligament-sparing capsulotomy with the dorsal intercarpal and dorsal radiocarpal ligaments outlined. (*From* Paci GM, Yao J. Surgical Techniques for the Treatment of Carpal Ligament Injury in the Athlete. Clin Sports Med 2015;34:11-35; with permission.)

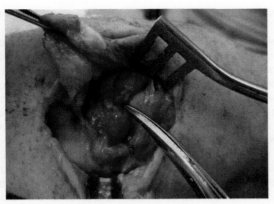

Fig. 11. Repair of the scapholunate ligament back to the lunate using suture anchors. (*From* Paci GM, Yao J. Surgical Techniques for the Treatment of Carpal Ligament Injury in the Athlete. Clin Sports Med 2015;34:11-35; with permission.)

brought over and attached to the dorsal scaphoid and lunate reinforcing the SL repair and completing the capsulodesis (**Fig. 12**). The capsulotomy is then closed to the dorsal radiotriquetral ligament, the pins are cut beneath the skin and the wrist is immobilized in a short arm cast for 6 to 8 weeks. Pins are then removed and the athlete is transitioned to a removable splint for 4 additional weeks and dart thrower's range of

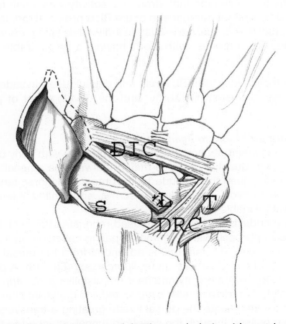

Fig. 12. The modified dorsal intercarpal (DIC) capsulodesis with a strip of the DIC maintained on the scaphoid (S) and transferred from the triquetrum (T) to the dorsal lunate (L). DRC, dorsoradiocarpal. (*From* Manuel J & Moran SL. The diagnosis of treatment of scapholunate instability. Hand Clinic 2010; 26: 129-144; used with permission of Mayo Foundation for Medical Education and Research, all rights reserved.)

motion exercises are begun. Return to play is allowed at 4 to 6 months postoperatively.

An alternative technique to stabilize the scapholunate interval that affords early motion involves placement of a headed 3.0-mm screw across the scapholunate interval instead of Kirschner wires. After the scapholunate joint is reduced, a screw is placed through the 1-2 portal starting midlateral at the waist of the scaphoid and advance through the scapholunate joint and into the proximomedial corner of the lunate.[55] The athlete is transitioned into a removable brace at 1 to 2 weeks and therapy is initiated. The screw is retained for a minimum of 3 months to protect the repair and removal is planned thereafter.[56]

For those with sagittal plane instability, the dorsal capsulodesis is an important component of SL ligament repair. Various capsulodesis techniques have been described, including all arthroscopic techniques,[34] a proximal radius based flap,[57] a radial-based dorsal intercarpal capsulodesis,[58] and an ulnar-based dorsal intercarpal ligamentoplasty[59,60] fixed to the scaphoid or lunate.

Outcomes In general, pain and symptoms improve with treatment; however, there is often some slight loss of grip strength and motion. Early operative treatment of the scapholunate ligament (<6 weeks) improves the chances of a successful outcome.[20] Melone and colleagues[61] treated 25 professional basketball players with acute ligament repair and capsulodesis, resulting in considerable improvement in symptoms and all returning to full participation, and no need for further surgery at an average of 5 years of follow-up. Three patients in this cohort had evidence of carpal malalignment and arthritis present 7 or more years after surgery, which is in line with another study that observed that strenuous activity was a risk factor for deterioration over time.[62] A direct comparison of the Blatt proximal radius-based flap to the distal ulnar dorsal intercarpal based flap in individuals with chronic tears did not show a difference in outcome, with both having a comparable loss of wrist flexion.[58,63]

Complications Complications after SL repair and capsulodesis include pin site infections, wrist stiffness, persistent instability, and the development of post-traumatic arthritis.

Complete injury not amenable to ligament repair

After injury, the SL ligament degenerates quickly and even with early operative intervention the quality and quantity of tissue may not always be amenable to repair. In these situations, techniques that include tendon reconstructions, tenodesis, bone–tendon–bone reconstruction, scapholunate screw, and limited intercarpal fusions have been used with variable results.[64–74]

The triligament tenodesis is a commonly used reconstruction technique.[25] In this procedure, a dorsal approach with a ligament-sparing capsulotomy is performed. A guidewire for a cannulated 3.2-mm drill is advanced from the dorsal SLIL origin to the palmar distal scaphoid tuberosity under fluoroscopy (**Fig. 13**). A palmar incision is made over the scaphoid tuberosity and an 8-cm distally based strip of flexor carpi radialis approximately 3 mm in diameter is harvested and drawn into the wound. A rongeur is then used to decorticate the dorsal lunate creating a transverse trough. The tendon strip is then passed through the scaphoid tunnel, attached to the lunate with a suture anchor, and then tensioned around the radiotriquetral ligament and secured to itself (**Fig. 14**). The scapholunate and scaphocapitate joints are then transfixed with two 0.045-inch K-wires to protect the reconstruction, the capsulotomy is closed, and the wrist is immobilized in a short arm thumb spica. After 6 weeks the pins are

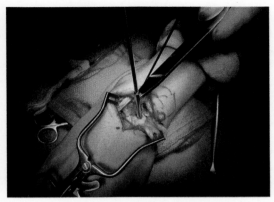

Fig. 13. A cannulated 3.2-mm drill is used to create a bone tunnel from the dorsal SL insertion to the scaphoid tuberosity along the central axis in preparation for ligament reconstruction. (*From* Paci GM, Yao J. Surgical Techniques for the Treatment of Carpal Ligament Injury in the Athlete. Clin Sports Med 2015;34:11-35; with permission.)

removed and the athlete is transitioned to a removable brace. Return to play is allowed 6 to 9 months after surgery.

Our preference for SL reconstruction is the scapholunate axis method using a palmaris or a half strip flexor carpi radialis graft.[75] The scapholunate articulation must remain easily reducible with 0.062-inch K-wires without bending them, and have carpal bones of sufficient size to support a tendon graft and tenodesis screw. A standard dorsal approach and a separate radial approach over the anatomic snuffbox is used (**Fig. 15**). A dorsal and radial capsulotomy is performed. The scapholunate interval is manually reduced with a volar directed force on the capitate or using K-wires as joy sticks. A transverse incision is made just ulnar to the radiotriquetral ligament and the tip of a c-shaped drill guide is placed on the proximal ulnar aspect of the lunate midpoint in the anteroposterior plane. The cannulated sleeve is placed midlateral on the scaphoid and a guidewire is passed through the central axis of the scaphoid

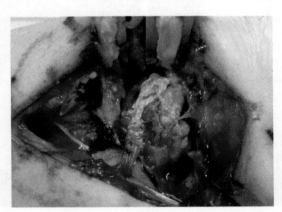

Fig. 14. The tendon graft is tensioned and attached to the lunate with a suture anchor and then passed through the radiotriquetral ligament and secured to itself. (*From* Paci GM, Yao J. Surgical Techniques for the Treatment of Carpal Ligament Injury in the Athlete. Clin Sports Med 2015;34:11-35; with permission.)

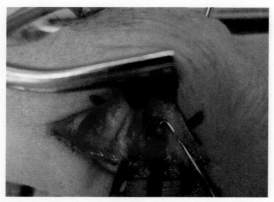

Fig. 15. The radial approach through the anatomic snuffbox for the scapholunate axis method exposing the starting point midlateral on the right of the scaphoid as indicated by the probe. (*From* Paci GM, Yao J. Surgical Techniques for the Treatment of Carpal Ligament Injury in the Athlete. Clin Sports Med 2015;34:11-35; with permission.)

and lunate and a second wire is passed just distal through the guide (**Fig. 16**). Acceptable reduction and wire placement is confirmed and then a step drill is used to prepare the bone tunnels (**Fig. 17**). A palmaris or partial flexor carpi radialis free tendon graft is harvested, passed, and secured to the lunate with a bullet anchor (**Fig. 18**). The graft is then tensioned and an interference screw is placed (**Fig. 19**), after which the remaining graft is sutured to the remnant dorsal SLIL and then secured to the dorsal radiocarpal ligament (**Fig. 20**).

Outcomes Most ligament reconstruction techniques achieve pain relief and satisfactory functional outcomes, but incomplete return of grip strength, loss of motion, and difficulty with long-term maintenance of alignment remains common.[25,58,76] Williams

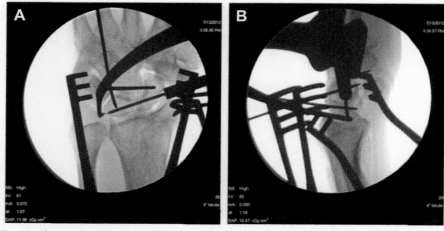

Fig. 16. The guidewire is placed along the central axis of the scaphoid and lunate as visualized on the posteroanterior (*A*) and lateral (*B*) radiographs, respectively, ending at the proximoulnar corner of the lunate (*A*). (*From* Paci GM, Yao J. Surgical Techniques for the Treatment of Carpal Ligament Injury in the Athlete. Clin Sports Med 2015;34:11-35; with permission.)

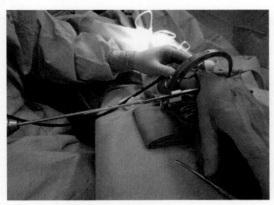

Fig. 17. A cannulated step drill (2.9 leading, 3.8 trailing) is used to create the graft tunnel over the central guidewire. (*From* Paci GM, Yao J. Surgical Techniques for the Treatment of Carpal Ligament Injury in the Athlete. Clin Sports Med 2015;34:11-35; with permission.)

and colleagues[77] described their experience with a modified Brunelli SLIL reconstruction in 14 athletes with 79% returning to play after 4 months but notably, only 64% of their cohort were able to return to their pre-injury level of competition.

Complications Carpal fracture and osteonecrosis of the scaphoid or the lunate are the most significant complications that can occur secondary to bone tunnel creation.[76,78,79] Meticulous guidewire placement ensuring central bone tunnel placement can decrease the risk of fracture; however, osteonecrosis is speculated to be

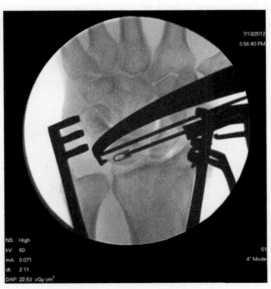

Fig. 18. The tendon graft is threaded through the bullet anchor and placed in the proximoulnar corner of the lunate. (*From* Paci GM, Yao J. Surgical Techniques for the Treatment of Carpal Ligament Injury in the Athlete. Clin Sports Med 2015;34:11-35; with permission.)

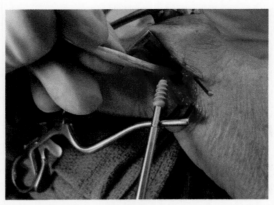

Fig. 19. The tendon graft is tensioned and secured with a 4-mm interference screw into the scaphoid. (*From* Paci GM, Yao J. Surgical Techniques for the Treatment of Carpal Ligament Injury in the Athlete. Clin Sports Med 2015;34:11-35; with permission.)

secondary to loss of intraosseous blood supply and may be harder to prevent. Incomplete return of function and ongoing pain can be problematic after reconstruction. Long-term recurrent instability and loss of carpal alignment leading to arthrosis has also been observed.[25,58,76]

Lunotriquetral Interosseous Ligament Injuries

Occult instability
Isolated LT injuries are less well-studied than those to the SLIL and as such indications for operative treatment are largely extrapolated from SLIL injuries. Often, nonoperative treatment of acute partial injuries with immobilization followed by dedicated therapy provides adequate healing and symptom relief. In those where nonoperative measures fail, arthroscopic debridement with or without thermal shrinkage and K-wire fixation may be used in a similar fashion to partial SLIL injuries as described elsewhere in this article.

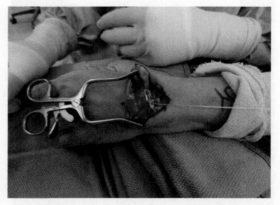

Fig. 20. The remaining graft is passed dorsal to the scaphoid and then secured to the lunate and the dorsal radiocarpal ligament. (*From* Paci GM, Yao J. Surgical Techniques for the Treatment of Carpal Ligament Injury in the Athlete. Clin Sports Med 2015;34:11-35; with permission.)

Outcomes Arthroscopic debridement of partial tears was demonstrated to provide pain relief in 13 of 14 patients without progressive instability at 34 months.[37] Lee and colleagues[40] also observed symptomatic pain relief and function improvements without the development of instability in 10 wrists with Geissler grades I and II injuries after debridement and thermal shrinkage with an average of 4.5 years of follow-up.

Acute complete injury with repairable lunotriquetral interosseous ligament
Dorsal or palmar tears of the LTIL may result in synovitis, dynamic volar intercalated segmental instability, and abnormal carpal motion. When tears are associated with extrinsic ligament injury to the dorsal radiocarpal ligament and ulnocapitate ligament, static volar intercalated segmental instability deformity may arise. In these situations, an open dorsal approach to the radiocarpal and ulnocarpal articulation is used. A ligament-sparing capsulotomy is performed and the LTIL is inspected. The joint is manually reduced with the use of K-wires as joysticks, followed by placement of two or three 0.045-inch K-wires or a temporary screw to transfix the LT joint. Most commonly, the ligament is avulsed off of the triquetrum and is repaired with the use of suture anchors into the dorsal lunate and triquetrum. Similar to scapholunate ligament injuries, if there is sagittal plane instability a capsulodesis is performed by attaching the dorsal radiotriquetral ligament to the dorsal lunate after LT repair and an additional wire traversing the triquetrohamate joint is placed.[80] The pins are cut beneath the skin and the arm is immobilized in a long arm splint or cast for 6 weeks, followed by a short arm cast for an additional 4 to 6 weeks. K-wires are removed at 10 to 12 weeks postoperatively and range of motion exercises and extensor carpi ulnaris strengthening are initiated. Return to play is at 6 to 9 months after repair.[81,82]

Outcomes The described results of LT ligament repair primarily are in patients with subacute or chronic injury which limits their applicability to athletes undergoing acute repair. Reagan reported satisfactory results and pain resolution in 6 of 7 patients with an average of 42 months of follow-up.[11] Favero and colleagues[83] reported 90% patient satisfaction with only one case of failure in 21 wrists. Shin and colleagues[84] observed short-term improvement in pain in function; however, they observed a complication rate of 40% in their series with a mean of 6.5 years of follow-up. Debridement alone has been described for complete tears, with satisfactory results in 7 of 9 patients at a mean of 27 months follow-up.[38]

Complete injury with irreparable ligament
In situations where the ligament is not amenable to primary repair, reconstruction is an acceptable alternative.[82,85] After standard dorsal exposure, the remaining LTIL is debrided and a 0.045-inch K-wire is passed from the dorsal ulnar aspect of the triquetrum toward the volar radial corner, exiting within the LT joint. A second wire is then passed from the dorsal radial to the volar ulnar lunate. A 3.2-mm cannulated drill or a series of awls is then used to create bone tunnels. A transverse incision approximately 6 cm proximal to the ulnar styloid is then made and a 3 mm width distally based strip of extensor carpi ulnaris is harvested from the radial aspect of the tendon. The extensor carpi ulnaris subsheath is opened dorsally at the level of the carpometacarpal joint and a wire loop or suture lasso is used to shuttle the tendon graft distally and then it is passed ulnar to radial through the previously made bone tunnels. The LT joint is then anatomically reduced and the tendon graft is tensioned and secured to itself. Two 0.045-inch K-wires are passed percutaneously and buried and a long arm cast is applied. This is maintained for 6 to 8 weeks, after which the point pins are removed

and a removable brace is provided and motion is started. Return to play is allowed at 6 to 9 months after reconstruction.

One alternative to repair or reconstruction is an ulnar shortening osteotomy, with the goal of tightening the distal triangular fibrocartilage complex extension and ulnar extrinsic ligaments which stabilize the LT joint.[86] A 2.5-mm ulnar shortening osteotomy is performed regardless of ulnar variance.[87] This procedure is not selected, however, in patients with incompetent radiotriquetral and ulnolunate ligaments, or dynamic or static volar intercalated segmental instability deformity.

For those who fail reconstruction or develop early arthrosis, LT arthrodesis is considered as a salvage option. The LT joint is approached through the fifth extensor compartment taking care to protect the dorsal radiotriquetral ligament. The joint surface is prepared and grafted with distal radius bone graft and then reduced and maintained with 1 or 2 headless compression screws. The wrist is immobilized for 8 to 12 weeks until union has been confirmed radiographically and then therapy is initiated.[88,89]

Outcomes Case series for LT ligament reconstruction also focus on chronic injuries and demonstrated comparable pain and function improvement to repair. Reconstruction seems to be more durable than LT repair or arthrodesis, with a 5-year reoperation rate of 31% in comparison with 77% and 78%, respectively.[84] LT arthrodesis has unpredictable results with a high rate of nonunion ($\leq$57%).[88,90] Even if union is achieved, patients can continue to complain of ulnar wrist pain. Ulnar shortening osteotomy demonstrated significant symptom improvement in 53 patients over a mean of 10 months. In their cohort, 83% reported excellent or good outcomes scores with a lower complication rate than other intercarpal procedures, however, almost all patients required reoperation for elective implant removal.[86]

DISCLOSURE

J.D. Gire: Research support: Acumed, LLC. J. Yao: IP Royalties: Arthrex; Paid presenter or speaker: Arthrex, Trimed; Stock or Stock Options: McGinley Orthopedics, Elevate Braces, 3D Systems; Financial or material support: Saunders/Mosby-Elsevier, Springer; Publishing royalties: Saunders/Mosby-Elsevier, Springer; Editorial or governing board: Saunders/Mosby-Elsevier; Board or committee member: American Association for Hand Surgery; American Society for Surgery of the Hand; Arthroscopy Association of North America.

REFERENCES

1. Ruby LK, Conney WP, An KN, et al. Relative motion of selected carpal bones: a kinematic analysis of the normal wrist. J Hand Surg Am 1988;13(1):1–10.

2. Berger RA, Crowninshield RD, Flatt AE. The three-dimensional rotational behaviors of the carpal bones. Clin Orthop Relat Res 1982;167:303–10.

3. De Lange A, Kauer JMG, Huiskes R. Kinematic behavior of the human wrist joint: a roentgen-stereophotogrammetric analysis. J Orthop Res 1985;3(1):56–64.

4. Watson HK, Ballet FL. The SLAC wrist: scapholunate advanced collapse pattern of degenerative arthritis. J Hand Surg Am 1984;9(3):358–65.

5. Slade JF, Milewski MD. Management of carpal instability in athletes. Hand Clin 2009;25(3):395–408.

6. Tosti R, Shin E. Wrist Arthroscopy for Athletic Injuries. Hand Clin 2017;33(1): 107–17.

7. Geissler WB, Burkett JL. Ligamentous sports injuries of the hand and wrist. Sports Med Arthrosc Rev 2014;22(1):39–44.
8. Watson HK, Ashmead D, Makhlouf MV. Examination of the scaphoid. J Hand Surg Am 1988;13(5):657–60.
9. Young D, Papp S, Giachino A. Physical examination of the wrist. Orthop Clin North Am 2007;38(2):149–65.
10. Kleinman WB. Physical examination of the wrist: useful provocative maneuvers. J Hand Surg Am 2015;40(7):1486–500.
11. Reagan DS, Linscheid RL, Dobyns JH. Lunotriquetral sprains. J Hand Surg Am 1984;9(4):502–14.
12. Kleinman WB. Diagnostic exams for ligamentous injuries. Am Soc Surg Hand, Corresp Club Newsl 1985;51.
13. Larsen CF, Stigsby B, Lindequist S, et al. Observer variability in measurements of carpal bone angles on lateral wrist radiographs. J Hand Surg Am 1991;16(5): 893–8.
14. Lee SK, Desai H, Silver B, et al. Comparison of radiographic stress views for scapholunate dynamic instability in a cadaver model. J Hand Surg Am 2011;1149–57.
15. Saupe N, Prüssmann KP, Luechinger R, et al. MR imaging of the wrist: comparison between 1.5-and 3-T MR imaging—preliminary experience. Radiology 2005;234(1):256–64.
16. Ringler MD. MRI of wrist ligaments. J Hand Surg Am 2013;38(10):2034–46.
17. Magee T. Comparison of 3-T MRI and arthroscopy of intrinsic wrist ligament and TFCC tears. Am J Roentgenol 2009;192(1):80–5.
18. Anderson ML, Skinner JA, Felmlee JP, et al. Diagnostic comparison of 1.5 Tesla and 3.0 Tesla preoperative MRI of the wrist in patients with ulnar-sided wrist pain. J Hand Surg Am 2008;33(7):1153–9.
19. O'Meeghan CJ, Stuart W, Mamo V, et al. The natural history of an untreated isolated scapholunate interosseus ligament injury. J Hand Surg Am 2003;28(4): 307–10.
20. Rohman EM, Agel J, Putnam MD, et al. Scapholunate interosseous ligament injuries: a retrospective review of treatment and outcomes in 82 wrists. J Hand Surg Am 2014;39(10):2020–6.
21. Couzens G, Daunt N, Crawford R, et al. Positive magnetic resonance imaging findings in the asymptomatic wrist. ANZ J Surg 2014;84(7–8):528–32.
22. Linkous MD, Pierce SD, Gilula LA. Scapholunate ligamentous communicating defects in symptomatic and asymptomatic wrists: characteristics. Radiology 2000; 216(3):846–50.
23. Geissler WB, Freeland AE, Savoie FH, et al. Intracarpal soft-tissue lesions associated with an intra-articular fracture of the distal end of the radius. J Bone Joint Surg Am 1996;78(3):357–65.
24. Fairplay T, Mathoulin C, Messina J, et al. The EWAS classification of scapholunate tears: an anatomical arthroscopic study. J Wrist Surg 2013;02(02):105–9.
25. Garcia-Elias M, Lluch AL, Stanley JK. Three-ligament tenodesis for the treatment of scapholunate dissociation: indications and surgical technique. J Hand Surg Am 2006;31(1):125–34.
26. Kitay A, Wolfe SW. Scapholunate instability: current concepts in diagnosis and management. J Hand Surg Am 2012;37(10):2175–96.
27. Master DL, Yao J. The wrist insufflation test: a confirmatory test for detecting intercarpal ligament and triangular fibrocartilage complex tears. Arthroscopy 2014; 30(4):451–5.

28. Salva-Coll G, Garcia-Elias M, Hagert E. Scapholunate instability: proprioception and neuromuscular control. J Wrist Surg 2013;2(2):136.

29. Salva-Coll G, Garcia-Elias M, Leon-Lopez MT, et al. Effects of forearm muscles on carpal stability. J Hand Surg Eur Vol 2011;36(7):553–9.

30. Hagert E. Proprioception of the wrist joint: a review of current concepts and possible implications on the rehabilitation of the wrist. J Hand Ther 2010; 23(1):2–17.

31. Anderson H, Hoy G. Orthotic intervention incorporating the dart-thrower's motion as part of conservative management guidelines for treatment of scapholunate injury. J Hand Ther 2016;29(2):199–204.

32. Holmes MK, Taylor S, Miller C, et al. Early outcomes of 'The Birmingham Wrist Instability Programme': a pragmatic intervention for stage one scapholunate instability. Hand Ther 2017;22(3):90–100.

33. Hagert E, Lluch A, Rein S. The role of proprioception and neuromuscular stability in carpal instabilities. J Hand Surg Eur Vol 2016;41(1):94–101.

34. Binder AC, Kerfant N, Wahegaonkar AL, et al. Dorsal wrist capsular tears in association with scapholunate instability: results of an arthroscopic dorsal capsuloplasty. J Wrist Surg 2013;2(2):160.

35. Van Overstraeten L, Camus EJ, Wahegaonkar A, et al. Anatomical description of the dorsal capsulo-scapholunate septum (DCSS)—arthroscopic staging of scapholunate instability after DCSS sectioning. J Wrist Surg 2013;2(2):149.

36. Slutsky DJ. Arthroscopic dorsal radiocarpal ligament repair. Arthroscopy 2005; 21(12):1486.

37. Ruch DS, Poehling GG. Arthroscopic management of partial scapholunate and lunotriquetral injuries of the wrist. J Hand Surg Am 1996;21(3):412–7.

38. Weiss A-PC, Sachar K, Glowacki KA. Arthroscopic debridement alone for intercarpal ligament tears. J Hand Surg Am 1997;22(2):344–9.

39. Darlis NA, Weiser RW, Sotereanos DG. Partial scapholunate ligament injuries treated with arthroscopic debridement and thermal shrinkage. J Hand Surg Am 2005;30(5):908–14.

40. Lee JI, Nha KW, Lee GY, et al. Long-term outcomes of arthroscopic debridement and thermal shrinkage for isolated partial intercarpal ligament tears. Orthopedics 2012;35(8):e1204–9.

41. Battistella F, Taverna E. Arthroscopic Thermal Shrinkage for Scapholunate Ligament Injuries (SS-63). Arthroscopy 2007;23(6):e32.

42. Wallace AL, Hollinshead RM, Frank CB. The scientific basis of thermal capsular shrinkage. J Shoulder Elbow Surg 2000;9(4):354–60.

43. Hayashi K, Markel MD. Thermal capsulorrhaphy treatment of shoulder instability: basic science. Clin Orthop Relat Res 2001;390:59–72.

44. Medvecky MJ, Ong BC, Rokito AS, et al. Thermal capsular shrinkage: basic science and clinical applications. Arthroscopy 2001;17(6):624–35.

45. Pirolo JM, Le W, Yao J. Effect of electrothermal treatment on nerve tissue within the triangular fibrocartilage complex, scapholunate, and lunotriquetral interosseous ligaments. Arthroscopy 2016;32(5):773–8.

46. Whipple TL. The role of arthroscopy in the treatment of scapholunate instability. Hand Clin 1995;11(1):37–40.

47. Manuel J, Moran SL. The diagnosis and treatment of scapholunate instability. Orthop Clin North Am 2007;38(2):261–77.

48. Toth AP, Warren RF, Petrigliano FA, et al. Thermal shrinkage for shoulder instability. HSS J 2011;7(2):108–14.

49. Good CR, Shindle MK, Kelly BT, et al. Glenohumeral chondrolysis after shoulder arthroscopy with thermal capsulorrhaphy. Arthroscopy 2007;23(7):797.e1-5.
50. Sotereanos DG, Darlis NA, Kokkalis ZT, et al. Effects of radiofrequency probe application on irrigation fluid temperature in the wrist joint. J Hand Surg Am 2009;34(10):1832-7.
51. Huber M, Eder C, Mueller M, et al. Temperature profile of radiofrequency probe application in wrist arthroscopy: monopolar versus bipolar. Arthroscopy 2013; 29(4):645-52.
52. Carratalá V, Lucas FJ, Miranda I, et al. Arthroscopic scapholunate capsuloligamentous repair: suture with dorsal capsular reinforcement for scapholunate ligament lesion. Arthrosc Tech 2017;6(1):e113-20.
53. Berger RA, Bishop AT, Bettinger PC. New dorsal capsulotomy for the surgical exposure of the wrist. Ann Plast Surg 1995;35(1):54-9.
54. Jakubietz MG, Zahn R, Gruenert JG, et al. Kirschner wire fixations for scapholunate dissociation: a cadaveric, biomechanical study. J Orthop Surg 2012;20(2): 224-9.
55. Aviles AJ, Lee SK, Hausman MR. Arthroscopic Reduction-Association of the Scapholunate. Arthroscopy 2007;23(1):105.e1-5.
56. Souer JS, Rutgers M, Andermahr J, et al. Perilunate fracture–dislocations of the wrist: comparison of temporary screw versus k-wire fixation. J Hand Surg Am 2007;32(3):318-25.
57. Blatt G. Capsulodesis in reconstructive hand surgery. Dorsal capsulodesis for the unstable scaphoid and volar capsulodesis following excision of the distal ulna. Hand Clin 1987;3(1):81-102.
58. Moran SL, Cooney WP, Berger RA, et al. Capsulodesis for the treatment of chronic scapholunate instability. J Hand Surg Am 2005;30(1):16-23.
59. Slater RR, Szabo RM, Bay BK, et al. Dorsal intercarpal ligament capsulodesis for scapholunate dissociation: biomechanical analysis in a cadaver model. J Hand Surg Am 1999;24:232-9.
60. Szabo RM. Scapholunate ligament repair with capsulodesis reinforcement. J Hand Surg Am 2008;33(9):1645-54.
61. Melone CP, Polatsch DB, Flink G, et al. Scapholunate interosseous ligament disruption in professional basketball players: treatment by direct repair and dorsal ligamentoplasty. Hand Clin 2012;28(3):253-60.
62. Pomerance J. Outcome after repair of the scapholunate interosseous ligament and dorsal capsulodesis for dynamic scapholunate instability due to trauma. J Hand Surg Am 2006;31(8):1380-6.
63. Gajendran VK, Peterson B, Slater RR Jr, et al. Long-term outcomes of dorsal intercarpal ligament capsulodesis for chronic scapholunate dissociation. J Hand Surg Am 2007;32(9):1323-33.
64. Linscheid RL, Dobyns JH. Treatment of scapholunate dissociation. Rotatory subluxation of the scaphoid. Hand Clin 1992;8(4):645-52.
65. Brunelli GA, Brunelli GR. A new technique to correct carpal instability with scaphoid rotary subluxation: a preliminary report. J Hand Surg Am 1995;20(3): S82-5.
66. Rosenwasser MP, Miyasajsa KC, Strauch RJ. The RASL procedure: reduction and association of the scaphoid and lunate using the Herbert screw. Tech Hand Up Extrem Surg 1997;1(4):263-72.
67. Weiss A-PC. Scapholunate ligament reconstruction using a bone-retinaculum-bone autograft. J Hand Surg Am 1998;23(2):205-15.

68. Svoboda SJ, Eglseder WA Jr, Belkoff SM. Autografts from the foot for reconstruction of the scapholunate interosseous ligament. J Hand Surg Am 1995;20(6): 980–5.

69. Hofstede DJ, Ritt MJPF, Bos KE. Tarsal autografts for reconstruction of the scapholunate interosseous ligament: a biomechanical study. J Hand Surg Am 1999;24(5):968–76.

70. Harvey EJ, Berger RA, Osterman AL, et al. Bone–tissue–bone repairs for scapholunate dissociation. J Hand Surg Am 2007;32(2):256–64.

71. Lipton CB, Ugwonali OF, Sarwahi V, et al. Reduction and association of the scaphoid and lunate for scapholunate ligament injuries (RASL). Atlas Hand Clin 2003;8(2):249–60.

72. Watson HK, Belniak R, Garcia-Elias M. Treatment of scapholunate dissociation: preferred treatment-STT fusion vs other methods. Orthopedics 1991;14(3): 365–70.

73. Kleinman WB, Carroll C. Scapho-trapezio-trapezoid arthrodesis for treatment of chronic static and dynamic scapho-lunate instability: a 10-year perspective on pitfalls and complications. J Hand Surg Am 1990;15(3):408–14.

74. Horn S, Ruby LK. Attempted scapholunate arthrodesis for chronic scapholunate dissociation. J Hand Surg Am 1991;16(2):334–9.

75. Yao J, Zlotolow DA, Lee SK. ScaphoLunate axis method. J Wrist Surg 2016; 5(1):59.

76. Sousa M, Aido R, Freitas D, et al. Scapholunate ligament reconstruction using a flexor carpi radialis tendon graft. J Hand Surg Am 2014;39(8):1512–6.

77. Williams A, Ng CY, Hayton MJ. When can a professional athlete return to play following scapholunate ligament delayed reconstruction? Br J Sports Med 2013;47(17):1071–4.

78. Chan K, Engasser W, Jebson PJL. Avascular Necrosis of the Lunate Following Reconstruction of the Scapholunate Ligament Using the Scapholunate Axis Method (SLAM). J Hand Surg Am 2019;44(10):904.e1-4.

79. De Smet L, Sciot R, Degreef I. Avascular necrosis of the scaphoid after three-ligament tenodesis for scapholunate dissociation: case report. J Hand Surg Am 2011;36(4):587–90.

80. Omokawa S, Fujitani R, Inada Y. Dorsal radiocarpal ligament capsulodesis for chronic dynamic lunotriquetral instability. J Hand Surg Am 2009;34(2):237–43.

81. Paci GM, Yao J. Surgical techniques for the treatment of carpal ligament injury in the athlete. Clin Sports Med 2015;34(1):11–35.

82. Shin AY, Bishop AT. Treatment options for lunotriquetral dissociation. Tech Hand Up Extrem Surg 1998;2(1):2–17.

83. Favero KJ, Bishop AT, Linscheid RL. Lunotriquetral ligament disruption: a comparative study of treatment methods. In: 46th Annual Meeting of the American Society for Surgery of the Hand. Orlando, Florida, October 2-5, 1991.

84. Shin AY, Weinstein LP, Berger RA, et al. Treatment of isolated injuries of the lunotriquetral ligament: a comparison of arthrodesis, ligament reconstruction and ligament repair. J Bone Joint Surg Br 2001;83(7):1023–8.

85. Hoxie SC, Shin AY. Lunotriquetral ligament repair and augmentation. In: Operative techniques in hand, wrist, and forearm surgery. Wolters Kluwer Health Adis (ESP); 2012.

86. Mirza A, Mirza JB, Shin AY, et al. Isolated lunotriquetral ligament tears treated with ulnar shortening osteotomy. J Hand Surg Am 2013;38(8):1492–7.

87. Rayhack JM, Gasser SI, Latta LL, et al. Precision oblique osteotomy for shortening of the ulna. J Hand Surg Am 1993;18(5):908–18.

88. Van de Grift TC, Ritt M. Management of lunotriquetral instability: a review of the literature. J Hand Surg Eur Vol 2016;41(1):72–85.
89. Pin PG, Young VL, Gilula LA, et al. Management of chronic lunotriquetral ligament tears. J Hand Surg Am 1989;14(1):77–83.
90. Larsen CF, Jacoby RA, McCabe SJ. Nonunion rates of limited carpal arthrodesis: a meta-analysis of the literature. J Hand Surg Am 1997;22(1):66–73.

Acute Scaphoid Waist Fracture in the Athlete

Thomas B. Hughes, MD

KEYWORDS

- Scaphoid waist fractures • Scaphoid fractures • Athlete • Sports
- Scaphoid nonunion

KEY POINTS

- A high index of suspicion for a scaphoid fracture is required in athletes with a wrist sprain.
- Nonoperative options, and the complications seen with surgery, should be discussed in detail with the athlete when choosing a treatment regimen.
- Operative fixation of scaphoid waist fractures in athletes may lead to a shorter time out of sport and a quicker return to function.

INTRODUCTION

Scaphoid fractures are the most common carpal injury and provide a significant challenge in management (**Figs. 1–6**). In the athlete, specifically, scaphoid fractures lead to 2 significant challenges: (1) the difficulty of making an accurate, early diagnosis and (2) the need for early return to play.

Diagnosis of scaphoid fractures is a challenge in the general public, with no true gold standard test to confirm a diagnosis. In an athlete, it is even more complicated by the athlete's approach to injury. Scaphoid fractures can be associated with lower-energy injuries that do not seem significant to many athletes. The level of posttraumatic symptomatology can seem minimal, with nagging wrist pain that is not completely disabling. The athlete's mentality frequently ignores these symptoms and assumes that these will resolve spontaneously, as so many other trivial injuries have in the past. This can lead to a delayed or missed diagnosis.

The second challenge occurs when scaphoid fractures are identified. Management that minimizes immobilization and allows early return to sport is necessary to maximize an athlete's career. Athletes' careers, whether professional, collegiate, or high school, are brief, and management of their injuries requires an understanding of the specific time table under which their lives are managed. Shared decision making is necessary to optimize the outcome for an individual athlete.

University of Pittsburgh School of Medicine, UPMC, 9104 Babcock Boulevard, Pittsburgh, PA 15237, USA
E-mail address: Thughes424@aol.com

Clin Sports Med 39 (2020) 339–351
https://doi.org/10.1016/j.csm.2019.12.007
0278-5919/20/© 2020 Elsevier Inc. All rights reserved.

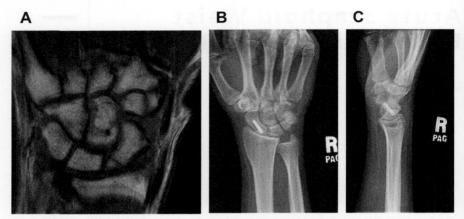

Fig. 1. A 20-year-old college hockey player was checked into the boards and hyperextended his wrist. He complained of snuffbox tenderness and decreased range of motion. Initial radiographs showed no evidence of fracture, but, due to clinical suspicion, MRI was obtained. (A) T1 MRI coronal sequence demonstrates a nondisplaced fracture of the proximal pole. A (B) 6-week postoperative anteroposterior radiograph and (C) lateral radiograph show no displacement of the fracture or avascular necrosis. The patient returned to play at 6 weeks.

EPIDEMIOLOGY

Scaphoid fractures account for 10.6% of all hand fractures (including finger and metacarpal)[1] and account for approximately 66% of all carpal fractures.[2] The rate of scaphoid fracture is approximately 12 per 100,00 in the population as a whole. In collegiate football players, however, the rate of scaphoid fractures may approach 1:100.[3] They have been reported to be nearly 8 times more common in male athletes than in female athletes[2] but, more recently, rates of injury were much closer in men and women, with a ratio of only 2:1. It was hypothesized by the authors that the relative increase in female scaphoid fractures may be due to a higher level of participation in sports.[4]

HISTORY AND EXAMINATION

A fall on an outstretched hand, especially with the hand in a pronated and ulnarly deviated position, is the mechanism most commonly described for a scaphoid fracture. In high-energy injuries, there is significant pain and swelling. In lower-energy injuries, however, the outward signs of trauma may be subtle. It is in these subtle injuries that early diagnosis is most critical. These are likely to be the nondisplaced injuries that may be managed nonoperatively if they are identified early. Delay in diagnosis can lead to fracture displacement and nonunion. Therefore, all patients with radial wrist pain, snuffbox tenderness, or scaphoid tubercle tenderness should be treated with immobilization until the scaphoid is definitively determined to be intact.

ANATOMY

The scaphoid is a cashew nut–shaped bone that is thinnest in its central portion, with slightly more bulbous ends. It creates a linkage between the proximal and distal rows of the carpus, neutralizing forces of extension and flexion on the midcarpal joint. As a

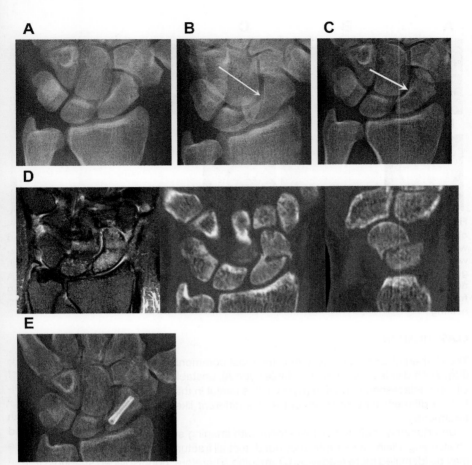

Fig. 2. A 30-year-old man suffered a fall and complained of knee and wrist pain. He had a history of chronic pain, so his wrist symptoms were minimized. (*A*) The initial anteroposterior radiograph was normal, but a subtle cortical disruption (*arrow*) is appreciated on (*B*) the initial lateral. He presented to orthopedics 2 months later with a subtle cystic (*arrow*) change on the (*C*) anteroposterior radiograph. (*D*) MRI shows a nonunion as well as the CT scan, which demonstrates a cystic nonunion. (*E*) Screw fixation with cancellous bone graft led to union.

result, there are significant forces across the scaphoid from its articulation with the trapezium and trapezoid. After injury, these forces contribute to a higher rate of nonunion than other carpal bones.

The scaphoid is covered almost entirely in articular cartilage and, therefore, bathed in synovial fluid. This fluid potentially can wash out valuable hematoma after scaphoid fractures. The cartilage also limits the potential entry points for vascularity (Fig. 1 from Gelberman[5] 1980 [Fig. 4]). The dorsal oblique ridge is a nonarticular portion of the scaphoid through which the vessel enters and supplies the proximal pole of the scaphoid. The volar vessel contributes the blood supply to the distal third of the scaphoid. This retrograde blood flow explains the particular difficulty in treating more proximal fractures, because these injuries disrupt the blood supply to the proximal pole.

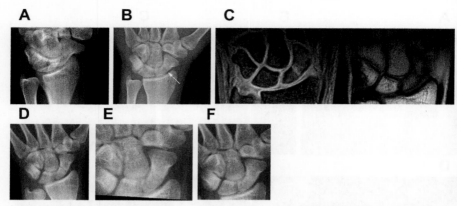

Fig. 3. A 16-year-old football player sustained a fall on his extended wrist. (*A*) Radiographs obtained the day after the injury demonstrate no obvious fracture line. He was diagnosed with a wrist sprain and allowed to return to football. One month later, he re-injured his wrist (although he admits he had persistent symptoms since the initial injury), and radiographs obtained 1 month later showed a clear fracture line (*arrow*). (*B, C*) An MRI was ordered that confirmed the diagnosis (T1 and T2 images show non-displaced scaphoid waist fracture). Serial radiographs, at (*D*) 2 months, (*E*) 3 months, and (*F*) months, show sequential healing.

CLASSIFICATION

The Herbert classification system is the most commonly used system in the literature (**Fig. 7**).[6] It divides fractures into stable (type A), unstable (type B), delayed union (type C), and established nonunion (type D). It is useful in that each of these types suggest both a different type of treatment and a different likelihood of success with these treatments.

Unfortunately, defining displacement with imaging studies of the scaphoid can be challenging. Plain radiographs may not detect all fracture displacement. Displacement may be identified more readily by CT imaging. Therefore, nondisplaced scaphoid fractures on radiography may miss displacement noted on CT scans and, therefore, may characterize fracture stability poorly.[7] Gilley and colleagues[7] showed that 26% to 34% of radiographically nondisplaced scaphoid fractures were displaced on CT scan imaging. Davis[8] has shown no difference in union rate between displaced and nondisplaced fractures when assessed with plain radiographs. When these injuries are assessed using CT scans, however, there is greater predictability. In 59 patients, 42 of 43 (98%) nondisplaced fractures went on to union with casting, whereas 5 of 16 (31%) displaced fractures went on to nonunion with casting. Therefore, in radiographically nondisplaced fractures, CT scans along the axis of the scaphoid should be used to confirm that the fractures are truly nondisplaced. In those that are found to be nondisplaced on CT imaging, there is evidence to show a significantly higher rate of union than for displaced fractures and, therefore, displaced fractures are considered unstable and surgical treatment typically is offered.

Although there is consensus in the differences between treatment and outcomes of stable and unstable injuries, it is unclear that this determination of stability can be performed with imaging alone. Buijze and colleagues[9] reported on a series of scaphoid fractures evaluated with arthroscopy and noted that in 58 patients, 38 were found unstable at the time of arthroscopic evaluation. Only 27 of the radiographs, however, showed displacement resulting, with 11 of the unstable fractures considered

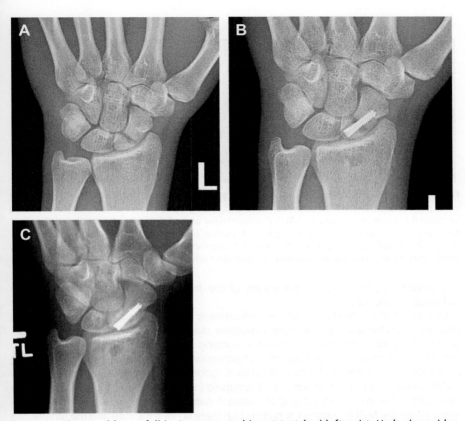

Fig. 4. An 18-year-old man fell in August onto his outstretched left wrist. He had consider-ations to continue football in college, so he did not report his injury until after the season. He had presented to the office in mid-December with (*A*) an established nonunion. The pa-tient also had college aspirations for track as a sprinter and hurdler, the season starting in March. A long discussion was undertaken with the patient and family regarding the timing of surgery as it related to his 2 sports. A decision was made to proceed with surgery imme-diately, with the plan to allow him to train but not compete prior to early healing of the fracture. (*B*) Screw fixation and bone-grafting were performed. (*C*) The fracture proceeded to union while the patient entertains opportunities at a Division III football program and Division I track program.

nondisplaced. So, although a fracture may be minimally displaced, it is not necessarily stable. This information brings into question determining stability of a fracture BASED on plain radiographs and the treatment recommendations that ensue.

IMAGING

Initial imaging for all patients with radial-sided wrist pain should include posteroante-rior and lateral radiographs as well as a dedicated scaphoid view. When these studies demonstrate a fracture, more advanced imaging typically is indicated. When the radio-graphs are negative, there are 2 ways for a clinician to proceed. In many cases, a period of immobilization, typically 10 days to 14 days, is followed by repeat radiographs. By this time, most scaphoid fractures have become more evident on

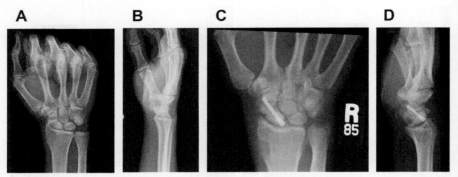

Fig. 5. A 26-year-old professional soccer player presented 4 years after a fall with persistent wrist pain and decreased motion. He never had radiographs after the initial injury because he thought it was only a sprain. (*A*) Anteroposterior and (*B*) lateral radiographs of the wrist demonstrating scaphoid nonunion. Ulnar deviation (*C*) anteroposterior and (*D*) lateral radiographs showing healed fracture after 1,2 intercompartmental supraretinacular artery vascularized bone graft and headless compression screw fixation.

radiographs, as the bone at the edges of the fracture resorbs, leading to greater radiographic lucency.

In many athletes, the period of immobilization is not ideal, because it interferes with their sport or training, and a more expedient diagnosis is desired. In these cases, advanced imaging (magnetic resonance imaging [MRI]/computed tomography [CT]) should be obtained to either diagnose a fracture or rule one out. Although CT imaging approaches the ability of MRI to accurately diagnose scaphoid fractures, MRI is nearly 100% sensitive and specific for occult scaphoid injury. Therefore, the author typically uses MRI as the advanced imaging of choice in patients with suspected scaphoid fractures. When the MRI is negative, it is likely that there is not a fracture and the athlete can

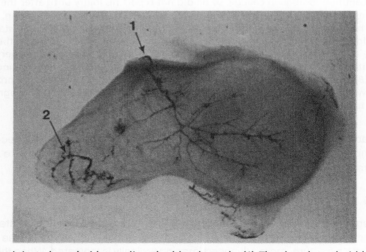

Fig. 6. An injected scaphoid revealing the blood supply. (1) The dorsal scaphoid branch of the radial artery enters on the dorsal ridge of the scaphoid and supplies the proximal two-thirds of the scaphoid. (2) The volar scaphoid branch of the radial artery supplies the distal one-third of the scaphoid.

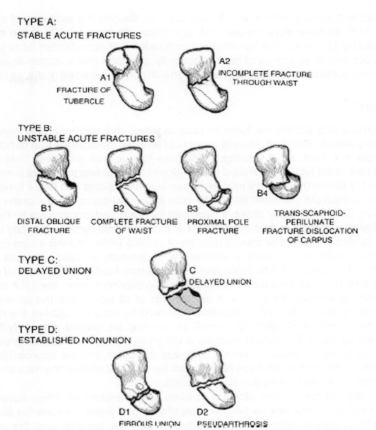

TYPE A:
STABLE ACUTE FRACTURES

A1
FRACTURE OF
TUBERCLE

A2
INCOMPLETE FRACTURE
THROUGH WAIST

TYPE B:
UNSTABLE ACUTE FRACTURES

B1
DISTAL OBLIQUE
FRACTURE

B2
COMPLETE FRACTURE
OF WAIST

B3
PROXIMAL POLE
FRACTURE

B4
TRANS-SCAPHOID-
PERILUNATE
FRACTURE DISLOCATION
OF CARPUS

TYPE C:
DELAYED UNION

C
DELAYED UNION

TYPE D:
ESTABLISHED NONUNION

D1
FIBROUS UNION

D2
PSEUDARTHROSIS

Fig. 7. The Herbert classification system of scaphoid fractures. This system divides fractures into stable injuries (type A) and unstable injuries (type B). Typically, type A fractures are more amenable to nonoperative management whereas type B injuries require surgery.[6] Type C injuries are delayed union, where surgical intervention may require less of a need for bone grafting. Type D injuries are the most difficult to treat and require operative fixation in association with bone grafting. (*From* Herbert TJ. The Fractured scaphoid. Thieme NY. 1990; with permission.)

play as tolerated. The athlete should be followed after playing to ensure that an undiagnosed injury does not manifest, for example, an occult scapholunate ligament injury.

Advanced imaging also is used for purposes other than diagnosis. As discussed previously, in fractures diagnosed with radiography, CT scans can make a more accurate assessment of displacement, they can better define the fracture morphology, and they can help to plan a surgical approach when needed. CT imaging also has been helpful in diagnosing avascular necrosis of the proximal pole of a scaphoid fracture.[10] MRI is the more typical imaging study used to assess vascularity of the proximal pole, although many surgeons feel that the best way to diagnose vascularity is to intraoperatively assess the blood flow of the proximal pole.[11]

Although proximal pole viability has long been considered an important factor for scaphoid healing, there are some data that healing can occur in the face of proximal pole ischemia.[12] Rancy and colleagues[12] looked at 35 nonunions (23 proximal pole nonunions) and identified avascularity using MRI (39.1%), intraoperative bleeding (84.8%), and intraoperative histopathologic analysis (54.5%). Despite the evidence of avascularity on MRI, intraoperative assessment, and histopathology, 94.3% of the fracture had healed by 12 weeks. The investigators concluded that vascularized bone grafting likely is not needed regardless of bone vascularity, provided that scaphoid anatomy is restored and stabilized with rigid internal fixation with nonvascularized grafts, as needed.

TREATMENT

The treatment of scaphoid fractures in athletes takes on a different tone than in the general population. There are several aspects of athletes' avocations that direct treatment decisions. First, most athletes participate in seasonal activities. That is, the timing of their sport typically is limited to a portion of the year and treatment is modified based on the timing of the injury relative to that season. Injuries that occur toward the end of the season are managed differently from those that occur 1 to 2 months before the season. Secondly, many athletes' windows for sport participation are limited to a reasonably short period of their overall life. For a recreational cyclist, who may ride for another 40 years, the loss of several months of cycling while wearing a cast may not lead to considering more invasive treatments. In contrast, a college football player may have only 1 season left to determine if football may lead to a professional career and may wish to consider a treatment that leads to playing sooner, even if it is associated with higher risks. Finally, there are athletes of all types, and the potential for young athletes to develop into professionals should be weighed against the risks of invasive treatment. A 12-year-old football player may be treated differently from a 12-year-old gymnast. The former typically is too young to have any serious prospects for scholarship or professional sports, whereas the latter may be approaching the peak of an athletic career. All these issues must be weighed against the risks and benefits of each treatment method in consideration.

Additionally, treating most athletes involves consideration of other associated stake-holders in an athlete's career. In cases of young athletes, they are the athlete's parents. In collegiate athletes, that group includes the parents and the college coaches. In professional athletes, there are frequently coaches, agents, and team leadership. Although the physician may need to communicate with many individuals about the treatment plans chosen, the needs of the patient always should remain the primary focus of the treating physician.

For all patients, the decision to proceed with operative management typically resolves around fracture stability. Those fractures that are deemed stable typically can be treated in a nonoperative fashion. Therefore, all fractures that are displaced or those that are of the proximal pole typically are treated surgically. It is less clear how to proceed with treatment in the minimally displaced waist fracture, where nonoperative treatment has been shown to lead to union in many cases.

Nonoperative Treatment

For stable fractures, nonoperative treatment can lead to a high rate of union and should be considered for nondisplaced scaphoid waist fractures. The time to union of scaphoid fractures treated with casting is affected by the fracture location.[13,14] Distal fractures heal rapidly, typically in approximately 6 weeks. Waist fractures heal more slowly, going on to union in 8 weeks to 12 weeks, on average. Proximal pole injuries can take 12 weeks to 24 weeks to heal with immobilization, which is difficult for almost any athlete to tolerate.

If nonoperative treatment is chosen, the type of cast or splint that is best is still unclear. Historically, long arm thumb spica casts have been used to provide the least motion at the wrist of the scaphoid. Comparative studies have not demonstrated a difference in union rates or outcomes with long arm cast immobilization; therefore, fewer physicians choose this method.[15,16] More recent studies have shown faster healing with the use of a short arm cast without thumb immobilization and equal final union rates[17]; Buijze et al looked at 62 patients with minimally displaced scaphoid fractures that were treated in short arm casts. They were randomized into 2 groups, those in a thumb spica cast compared with short arm casts with the thumb free. CT scans were performed after 10 weeks of casting. The percentage of the fracture line that had bridging bone across it was recorded and compared. There was a significantly higher percentage of healing (85% vs 70%) for the group without thumb immobilization. The overall union rate was 98%, with the only nonunion in a patient who did not tolerate casting and had surgical intervention.

Grewal and colleagues[16] investigated the effectiveness and speed of union for nonoperative treatment of nondisplaced scaphoid fractures; 172 patients were treated in a short arm thumb spica cast, leading to a union rate of 99.4% (1 nonunion). In patients without diabetes or cysts, the time to union averaged 49 days, as diagnosed by CT scan. This is shorter than most prior studies had suggested for union after nonoperative treatment. The investigators suggested that use of CT scans to assess union may lead to a shorter period of immobilization.

Another series of studies published in 2013[8] examined fracture types that can be treated successfully with cast immobilization. Davis found that fractures determined to be nondisplaced on CT scans or MRI would reliably go on to heal in 4 to 8 weeks with casting. Radiographic determination of displacement was inadequate, however, to predict reliable healing. Patients had CT scans performed after 4 weeks of casting. Many nondisplaced fractures already had signs of healing and then were removed from their cast all but 1 went on to complete union.

The author typically recommends 4 weeks of below-elbow thumb spica cast immobilization followed by additional short arm removable immobilization for 2 weeks. A CT scan is obtained at 6 weeks for in-season athletes. If greater than 50% of the fracture demonstrates bridging bone, the patient is released to activities as tolerated. For out-of-season athletes, the CT scan is delayed until 8 weeks to increase the likelihood that 50% bridging bone has formed.

Operative Treatment

All fractures that have been determined to be unstable require surgical treatment. The operative treatment of scaphoid fractures typically involves screw fixation, although Kirschner (K)-wires and plates also are used at times. The screw can be placed antegrade (from a dorsal approach) or retrograde (from a volar approach). It can be placed in an open fashion or percutaneously or arthroscopically assisted.[18] The difference in management is based on fracture location, fracture displacement, and surgeon preference and experience.

For displaced fractures, a reduction is required to restore normal anatomy. This typically is done most simply with open reduction. It also can be affected with percutaneously placed K-wires used as joy sticks. This percutaneous reduction can be assessed fluoroscopically and/or arthroscopically.

Once the reduction has been achieved, the screw is placed. Typically, a headless compression screw is used. More distal fractures are addressed more easily using a volar approach, whereas more proximal fractures are addressed dorsally. Percutaneous fixation is possible from either approach[19–22] (Fig. 8). Dorsally placed screws tend to be placed more centrally within the scaphoid, because the trapezium can lead to a slight obliquity to the path of the compression screw.[23,24] When the presence

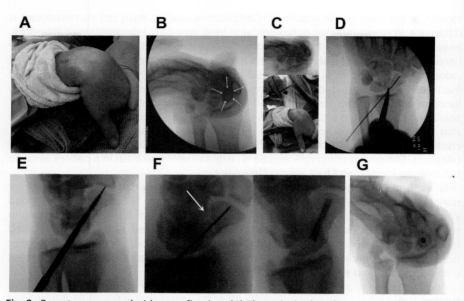

Fig. 8. Percutaneous scaphoid screw fixation. (*A*) The wrist is placed on a stack of towels and hyperflexed so that the scaphoid can be imaged down its long axis. (*B*) The scaphoid is then visualized as a circle (*arrows surround scaphoid*). The thumb is positioned slightly radial, so that it does not interfere with the imaging. (*C1*) A guide wire for a cannulated screw is in the center of the circle. (*C2*) Intraoperatively, this is placed slightly distal and ulnar to Lister's Tubercle. (*D*) The guide wire is then advanced, placing it in the center of the scaphoid down its long axis. A small incision is made and blunt dissection is performed to the scaphoid. To be certain a path is cleared through the soft tissues in the correct direction, an image with the tip of the scissors (*D*) in contact with the scaphoid can confirm the location of the soft tissue pathway. The wire then is measured to select the correct screw size. (*E*) The wire then is advanced through the subchondral bone to prevent it from being removed with the cannulated drill. The screw is placed over the guide wire. (*F*) Note the central placement of the guide wire (*F1*) and screw (*F2*) perpendicular to the fracture line (*arrow*). (*G*) The central position of the screw can be confirmed after removing the guide wire and placing the hand back into the hyperflexed position.

of the trapezium precludes appropriate screw positioning relative to the fracture, a transtrapezial approach has been shown effective without significant long-term problems at the scaphotrapeziotrapezoid (STT) joint.[25–28]

Treatment of Nondisplaced Scaphoid Waist Fractures

The greatest debate in the treatment of acute scaphoid fractures centers around the operative treatment of nondisplaced waist fractures. Early studies investigating the surgical treatment of these injuries were promising.[29] Many more studies comparing operative and nonoperative treatment of stable scaphoid waist fractures have since been performed, leading to an evolution on the treatment of these scaphoid fractures. Although operative treatment of these injuries commonly is performed for athletes at every level, the physician and patient should have an understanding of the data so that they can have appropriate expectations of outcomes.

Dias and colleagues[30] reported a randomized controlled comparison of these 2 treatment options. The motion, grip, and Patient Evaluation Measure all were better in the operative group at 8 weeks (the time of cast removal). At 12 weeks, however, only grip strength was better in surgical patients. Additionally, 10 of the 44 surgical patients had not healed at 12 weeks. Minor complications occurred in 13 of the operative group. These results lead Dias and colleagues to recommend nonoperative treatment of these patients due to the similar functional results and the higher complication rates in the surgical group. Clementson and colleagues[31] showed a slightly quicker return of function at 6 weeks and 10 weeks, but long-term follow-up showed less motion in the surgical group with high rates of STT arthritis.

Other studies, however, have seen some benefit to operative treatment of nondisplaced fractures. McQueen and colleagues[32] demonstrated a quicker time to union (9.2 weeks compared with 13.9 weeks for casting). These patients had a faster return to sport (6.4 weeks compared with 15.5 weeks for casting) as well as full-duty work (3.8 weeks compared with 11.4 weeks for casting), with few complications.

RETURN TO SPORT

Specific data on return to sport are sparse, so typically a long discussion with the patient about expectations for healing as well as expectations for the ability to perform guide a final return to sport. Rettig and Kollias[33] reported on 12 in-season athletes treated with screw fixation for waist fractures. In each patient, the sport precluded the use of a cast. Return to sport averaged 5.8 weeks; however, there was 1 nonunion.

Another study of 20 patients treated with screw fixation of a scaphoid waist fracture included 6 collegiate or professional athletes.[34] Five of the 6 returned to the previous level of play, although no explanation was given for the 1 athlete who could not.

A randomized study compared cast immobilization with screw fixation of nondisplaced fracture in 58 patients, including 6 athletes.[35] The study did not demonstrate a difference in union rates or time to union but did show earlier return of motion. The 2 athletes treated surgically returned to the sport, soccer, 6 weeks after surgery. The other 3 athletes (a swimmer, squash player, and soccer player) returned to sport at 12 weeks.

A meta-analysis of the 11 studies looked at rates of return to sport and return-to-sport times.[36] For nonoperative management, return rates of 90% at 9.6 weeks were obtained. This group had union rates of 85% at a mean time of 14.0 weeks. For operative fixation of the scaphoid, a return-to-sport rate of 98% was obtained. The return time averaged 7.3 weeks. Union rates of 97% at 9.8 weeks were noted.

SUMMARY

Scaphoid waist fractures are a common injury among athletes, and their treatment requires special understanding of multiple variables, including the type of injury and the type of athlete. For displaced fractures, early surgical reduction and stabilization can lead to a successful outcome and return to sport. For nondisplaced fractures, the literature demonstrates higher complication rates with surgical treatment. Surgery may lead to faster return of motion, function, and return to sport. Therefore, the key to treatment of an athlete is a detailed discussion regarding these risks as they relate to the athlete's goals and motivations revolving around the sport.

DISCLOSURE

The authors have nothing to disclose.

REFERENCES

1. Hove LM. Fractures of the hand. Distribution and relative incidence. Scand J Plast Reconstr Surg Hand Surg 1993;27(4):317–9.
2. Hey HW, Dennis HH, Chong AK, et al. Prevalence of carpal fracture in Singapore. J Hand Surg Am 2011;36(2):278–83.
3. Geissler WB. Arthroscopic management of scaphoid fractures in athletes. Hand Clin 2009;25(3):359–69.
4. Wolf JM, Dawson L, Mountcastle SB, et al. The incidence of scaphoid fracture in a military population. Injury 2009;40(12):1316–9.
5. Gelberman RH, Menon J. The vascularity of the scaphoid bone. J Hand Surg Am 1980;5(5):508–13.
6. Ten Berg PW, Drijkoningen T, Strackee SD, et al. Classifications of acute scaphoid fractures: a systematic literature review. J Wrist Surg 2016;5(2):152–9.
7. Gilley E, Puri SK, Hearns KA, et al. Importance of computed tomography in determining displacement in scaphoid fractures. J Wrist Surg 2018;7(1):38–42.
8. Davis TR. Prediction of outcome of non-operative treatment of acute scaphoid waist fracture. Ann R Coll Surg Engl 2013;95(3):171–6.
9. Buijze GA, Jørgsholm P, Thomsen NO, et al. Factors associated with arthroscopically determined scaphoid fracture displacement and instability. J Hand Surg Am 2012;37(7):1405–10.
10. Smith ML, Bain GI, Chabrel N, et al. Using computed tomography to assist with diagnosis of avascular necrosis complicating chronic scaphoid nonunion. J Hand Surg Am 2009;34(6):1037–43.
11. Günal I, Ozçelik A, Göktürk E, et al. Correlation of magnetic resonance imaging and intraoperative punctate bleeding to assess the vascularity of scaphoid nonunion. Arch Orthop Trauma Surg 1999;119(5–6):285–7.
12. Rancy SK, Swanstrom MM, DiCarlo EF, et al. Success of scaphoid nonunion surgery is independent of proximal pole vascularity. J Hand Surg Eur Vol 2018;43(1):32–40.
13. Buijze GA, Ochtman L, Ring D. Management of scaphoid nonunion. J Hand Surg Am 2012;37(5):1095–100 [quiz 1101].
14. Cooney WP, Dobyns JH, Linscheid RL. Nonunion of the scaphoid: analysis of the results from bone grafting. J Hand Surg Am 1980;5(4):343–54.
15. Clay NR, Dias JJ, Costigan PS, et al. Need the thumb be immobilised in scaphoid fractures? A randomised prospective trial. J Bone Joint Surg Br 1991;73(5):828–32.
16. Grewal R, Suh N, MacDermid JC. Is casting for non-displaced simple scaphoid waist fracture effective? A CT based assessment of union. Open Orthop J 2016;10:431–8.
17. Buijze GA, Goslings JC, Rhemrev SJ, et al. Cast immobilization with and without immobilization of the thumb for nondisplaced and minimally displaced scaphoid waist fractures: a multicenter, randomized, controlled trial. J Hand Surg Am 2014;39(4):621–7.
18. Slade JF, Gillon T. Retrospective review of 234 scaphoid fractures and nonunions treated with arthroscopy for union and complications. Scand J Surg 2008;97(4):280–9.
19. Slade JF, Grauer JN, Mahoney JD. Arthroscopic reduction and percutaneous fixation of scaphoid fractures with a novel dorsal technique. Orthop Clin North Am 2001;32(2):247–61.

20. Taras JS, Sweet S, Shum W, et al. Percutaneous and arthroscopic screw fixation of scaphoid fractures in the athlete. Hand Clin 1999;15(3):467–73.
21. Wozasek GE, Moser KD. Percutaneous screw fixation for fractures of the scaphoid. J Bone Joint Surg Br 1991;73(1):138–42.
22. Haddad FS, Goddard NJ. Acute percutaneous scaphoid fixation. A pilot study. J Bone Joint Surg Br 1998;80(1):95–9.
23. Chan KW, McAdams TR. Central screw placement in percutaneous screw scaphoid fixation: a cadaveric comparison of proximal and distal techniques. J Hand Surg Am 2004;29(1):74–9.
24. Jeon IH, Micic ID, Oh CW, et al. Percutaneous screw fixation for scaphoid fracture: a comparison between the dorsal and the volar approaches. J Hand Surg Am 2009;34(2):228–36.e1.
25. Geurts G, van Riet R, Meermans G, et al. Incidence of scaphotrapezial arthritis following volar percutaneous fixation of nondisplaced scaphoid waist fractures using a transtrapezial approach. J Hand Surg Am 2011;36(11):1753–8.
26. Meermans G, Verstreken F. Percutaneous transtrapezial fixation of acute scaphoid fractures. J Hand Surg Eur Vol 2008;33(6):791–6.
27. Meermans G, Van Glabbeek F, Braem MJ, et al. Comparison of two percutaneous volar approaches for screw fixation of scaphoid waist fractures: radiographic and biomechanical study of an osteotomy-simulated model. J Bone Joint Surg Am 2014;96(16):1369–76.
28. Verstreken F, Meermans G. Transtrapezial approach for fixation of acute scaphoid fractures. JBJS Essent Surg Tech 2015;5(4):e29.
29. Bond CD, Shin AY, McBride MT, et al. Percutaneous screw fixation or cast immobilization for nondisplaced scaphoid fractures. J Bone Joint Surg Am 2001; 83-A(4):483–8.
30. Dias JJ, Wildin CJ, Bhowal B, et al. Should acute scaphoid fractures be fixed? A randomized controlled trial. J Bone Joint Surg Am 2005;87(10):2160–8.
31. Clementson M, Jørgsholm P, Besjakov J, et al. Conservative treatment versus arthroscopic-assisted screw fixation of scaphoid waist fractures–a randomized trial with minimum 4-year follow-up. J Hand Surg Am 2015;40(7):1341–8.
32. McQueen MM, Gelbke MK, Wakefield A, et al. Percutaneous screw fixation versus conservative treatment for fractures of the waist of the scaphoid: a prospective randomised study. J Bone Joint Surg Br 2008;90(1):66–71.
33. Rettig AC, Kollias SC. Internal fixation of acute stable scaphoid fractures in the athlete. Am J Sports Med 1996;24(2):182–6.
34. Bedi A, Jebson PJ, Hayden RJ, et al. Internal fixation of acute, nondisplaced scaphoid waist fractures via a limited dorsal approach: an assessment of radiographic and functional outcomes. J Hand Surg Am 2007;32(3):326–33.
35. Adolfsson L, Lindau T, Arner M. Acutrak screw fixation versus cast immobilisation for undisplaced scaphoid waist fractures. J Hand Surg Br 2001;26(3):192–5.
36. Goffin JS, Liao Q, Robertson GA. Return to sport following scaphoid fractures: a systematic review and meta-analysis. World J Orthop 2019;10(2):101–14.

Carpal Fractures Other than Scaphoid in the Athlete

Bilal Mahmood, MD[a], Steve K. Lee, MD[b],*

KEYWORDS

• Carpal fractures • Athlete • Triquetrum • Trapezium • Trapezoid • Lunate
• Capitate • Hamate

KEY POINTS

- Approximately 15% to 41% carpal fractures occur in nonscaphoid carpal bones, and often occur as an avulsion, as part of a peri-lunate pattern of injury, or a direct blow/axial load.
- Triquetral fractures are the most common nonscaphoid carpal fractures, accounting for 4% to 29% of all carpal fractures.
- In treating athletes, the hand surgeon must determine whether further injury is risked or if early return can be accomplished safely.

Carpal fractures other than scaphoid occur at lower rates compared with scaphoid fractures.[1] Larsen and colleagues[2] estimated the annual incidence of nonscaphoid carpal fractures to be 36 fractures per 100,000 people in Odense, Denmark. The ratio of nonscaphoid to scaphoid fractures varies. Garcia-Elias reviewed 10,400 consecutive wrist injuries over 10 years and noted 249 carpal fractures. Out of these, 153, or 61% of carpal fractures involved the scaphoid, and 26% involved the triquetrum.[3] Others have noted a similar ratio of scaphoid to nonscaphoid fractures with 59% to 85% being a scaphoid fracture and the remaining 15% to 41% being various other carpal injuries.[3]

It is helpful to think of carpal fractures as belonging to 1 of 3 categories. They may be a result of an avulsion injury, usually a ligamentous avulsion. A second possibility is the occurrence of a perilunate pattern, where greater arc injuries may result in scaphoid, capitate triquetrum, and/or radial styloid fractures. Thirdly, a direct blow or an axial load can cause significant soft tissue injury along with unstable fracture patterns. In these cases, the direction of the force can be variable, resulting in a myriad of injury patterns.

[a] Department of Orthopaedic Surgery, University of Rochester, 601 Elmwood Avenue, Box 665, Rochester, NY 14642, USA; [b] Hospital for Special Surgery, 523 East 72nd Street, 4th Floor, New York, NY 10021, USA
* Corresponding author.
E-mail address: lees@hss.edu

Clin Sports Med 39 (2020) 353–371
https://doi.org/10.1016/j.csm.2019.12.006
0278-5919/20/© 2020 Elsevier Inc. All rights reserved.

sportsmed.theclinics.com

The high functional demands of an athlete place them in a category where suspicion for carpal fractures should be high. Carpal fractures, especially those other than the scaphoid are frequently missed on initial presentations.[3] Furthermore, the small size of carpal bones complicates surgery and there is the need for awareness of the vascular supply to each bone. Ligamentous injuries are often an important component of the overall injury, as well as secondary injuries to nerves or tendons.

When dealing specifically with athletes, whether recreational or professional, the goal in management is often to differentiate between injuries that need to be addressed with surgery versus those that may be managed nonoperatively. The athlete usually prefers to return to activity as soon as possible, and the treating hand surgeon needs to determine whether further injury is risked or if early return can be accomplished safely.

TRIQUETRAL FRACTURES

Triquetral fractures are the second most common carpal fracture following scaphoid fractures. They account for 4% to 29% of all carpal fractures.[3-7] Three primary patterns are noted: dorsal cortical or chip fractures, triquetral body fractures, and palmar cortical fractures.

Dorsal Cortical Fractures

Dorsal cortical, or chip fractures of the triquetrum are the most common, with reports indicating they may represent up to 93% of all triquetral fractures.[8] Proposed mechanisms of injury for these include an avulsion, impaction, or shear forces.[6,8,9] An avulsion of the radiotriquetral and triquetroscaphoid ligaments could occur with extreme palmar flexion with radial deviation.[7,10] Impaction occurs with a fall onto a dorsiflexed wrist in ulnar deviation, which is a common presentation. In this scenario, the ulnar styloid is driven into the dorsal cortex of the triquetrum causing the impaction.[8,11] An increased length in the ulnar styloid has been noted in patients with triquetral fracture.[9] Finally, a shearing force occurs from the proximal edge of the hamate during wrist dorsiflexion against the distal dorsal triquetrum.[6]

Body Fractures

Fractures of the body of the triquetrum are the second most common type of triquetral fractures. These are seen with high-energy injuries, and seen with greater arc perilunate type injury.[12] In fact, a triquetral body fracture should alert the treating physician to carefully evaluate for ligamentous injury of the carpus if no other fractures are noted. Perilunate fracture-dislocations are seen in 12% to 25% of triquetral injuries.[13] Fractures of the triquetral body may be categorized descriptively. Common patterns include sagittal fractures, fractures in the medial tuberosity, transverse fractures of the proximal pole, transverse fracture of the body, and comminuted fractures.[14]

Palmar Cortical Fractures

Avulsion fractures on the volar aspect of the triquetrum are secondary to the palmar ulnar triquetral ligament and the lunotriquetral interosseous ligament injuries. These carry a worse prognosis than dorsal cortical fractures.[15]

Clinical examination

Point tenderness at the site of injury will be present in cases of triquetral fractures. Careful examination should differentiate between tenderness at the triangular fibrocartilage complex, the lunotriquetral interval, and other ulnar wrist structures. In patients with dorsal avulsion fractures, pain with wrist flexion and extension will be present.[16]

Radiographic examination
Anteroposterior, lateral, and 45° pronated oblique radiographs of the wrist will identify most triquetral fractures, with the lateral 2 views being most helpful for dorsal cortical fractures. Palmar cortical fractures can be identified on radial deviation views.[14] Computed tomography (CT) scans are helpful for occult triquetral fractures.

Treatment
Dorsal cortical fractures are treated nonoperatively (**Fig. 1**). These are treated with immobilization for approximately 3 to 6 weeks, either in a short arm cast or other form of immobilization.[4,6,17,18] As the treatment is mainly for the underlying soft tissue injury, it is tailored specifically for each athlete, and he or she must understand that the fracture is of little consequence and will likely form a fibrous nonunion.[16] An MRI can identify extrinsic intercarpal ligament injuries or occult fractures. Initially, immobilization is achieved with a cast or splint and the patient is reexamined 1 week after the injury. If the soft tissue swelling is improved and the athlete can play his or her sport with a playing cast or splint, early return to play is allowed. However, vigilance and frequent reexamination should confirm that the soft tissue injury continues to heal.[16] Depending on the athlete's sport, return to play can be delayed until he or she can demonstrate safe return to play. Patients with dorsal cortical fractures have shown excellent return to motion and function.[6] If symptoms persist for greater than 6 to 8 weeks, further imaging to evaluate for concurrent intercarpal ligament injury or triangular fibrocartilage complex injury is necessary. Symptomatic nonunions may be treated with fragment excision.[18]

Treatment for triquetrum body fractures can be more involved (**Fig. 2**). In the setting of perilunate fracture-dislocations, treatment often involves either arthroscopic or open reduction of the fracture or carpal injury, fracture fixation and stabilization of the intercarpal ligament injuries, such as the scapholunate or lunotriquetral joints. Nonunion of the triquetral body is rare. The wrist must be immobilized for 8 to 12 weeks after a perilunate fracture-dislocation. Return to sport depends on if use of a playing

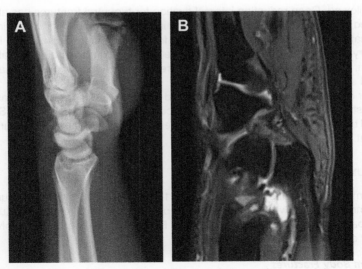

Fig. 1. A 26-year-old man being evaluated for a scapholunate ligament injury was incidentally found to have a previous, asymptomatic dorsal triquetral fracture (*A*). MRI shows an avulsion of the dorsal proximal aspect of the triquetrum (*B*).

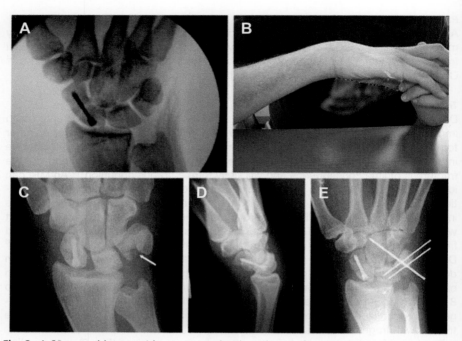

Fig. 2. A 22-year-old man with a transscaphoid perilunate fracture-dislocation (*A, B*) was treated with an ORIF of the scaphoid. Later, a displaced fracture of the triquetrum (arrow) (*C*) and a volar intercalated segmental instability deformity (*D*) was noted. Open reduction and pinning was then performed for this injury (*E*). (*From* Marchessault J, Conti M, Baratz M. Carpal Fractures in Athletes Excluding the Scaphoid. Hand Clin. 2009;25(3):371–88; with permission.)

cast is allowed. Open reduction internal fixation for triquetral fractures has also been described in displaced body fractures.[19,20] It is important to look for carpal instability when treating these fractures. The threshold for an MRI must be low as the ligamentous injury will determine return to sport. In the rare situation of a triquetral malunion or nonunion, pisiform excision can provide pain relief in the setting of posttraumatic pisotriquetral arthritis.[21,22]

Palmar cortical fractures must be evaluated with an MRI for the potential associate carpal instability, and treatment should be focused on any carpal instability. Similar to triquetral body fractures, return to sport is determined by the ligamentous injury and its treatment.

TRAPEZIUM FRACTURES

Trapezium fractures make up approximately 1% to 5% of carpal bone fractures.[23–26] They commonly occur with fractures of other bones, often with the distal radius or first metacarpal.[24,26,27] Isolated fractures are rare. Fractures of the trapezium involve either the body or the ridge.

Trapezium Body Fractures

Body fractures are more common, and these are described based on the fracture pattern (**Fig. 3**). Body fractures are most commonly a sagittal split fracture, or vertical

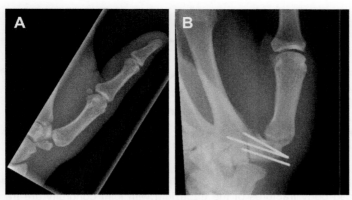

Fig. 3. An 18-year-old college football player sustained a trapezium body fracture (*A*) and underwent ORIF (*B*). The pins were removed at about 6 weeks and he gradually progressed to all activities by 10 weeks after ORIF. (*Courtesy of* Warren Hammert, MD, Rochester, NY.)

intraarticular pattern, and this frequently accompanies a Bennett fracture.[28] A dorsoradial tuberosity fracture is the next most common trapezium body fracture. Horizontal fractures and comminuted fractures are rare. Fractures of the body of the trapezium can occur during athletics from a fall onto an outstretched hand, resulting in an axial load from the first metacarpal.[18] This mechanism produces the sagittal split most commonly seen with a Bennett fracture. The lateral body fragment that is often attached to the first metacarpal will displace radially and proximally along with it due to the abductor pollicis longus.[13] A fall may also impact the radial styloid into the trapezium when the thumb is abducted and hyperextended, resulting in a dorsoradial tuberosity fracture.[16] Horizontal shear injury or a high-energy direct blow are required for horizontal fractures and comminuted fractures.

Trapezial Ridge Fractures

Palmar trapezial ridge fractures are classified either as occurring at the base of the ridge (type I) or an avulsion of the tip of the ridge (type II) (**Figs. 4** and **5**).[25] The ridge is a superficial structure and is palpable distal to the scaphoid tubercle. Thus, fractures are often the cause of direct trauma, which can occur when being struck by a ball or falling onto an outstretched hand. A fall onto an outstretched hand may also cause avulsion of the transverse carpal ligament.[14]

Clinical examination

In the acute setting, without the presence of other injuries, the trapezium is palpated distal to the volar tubercle of the scaphoid. The patient may also have pain with thumb motion, and weakness with pinch. Wrist flexion may cause pain as the flexor carpal radialis runs in a groove on the volar aspect next to the palmar ridge.[16]

Radiographic examination

Standard radiographic views usually identify trapezium body fractures. A pronated anteroposterior (AP) view, Bett's view, can be of further help as it shows the trapeziometacarpal articulation and help the surgeon identify any displacement.[13] For trapezial ridge fractures, a carpal tunnel view is used.[29] CT scans are very helpful for further detail on fractures noted in radiographs, or identifying rare fractures, such as horizontal, or coronal plane fractures.[30]

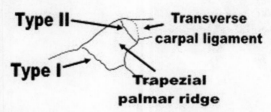

Fig. 4. Palmer trapezial ridge fractures. (*From* Vigler M, Aviles A, Lee S. Carpal fractures excluding the scaphoid. Hand Clin. 2006;22:501–16; with permission.)

Treatment

Nondisplaced body fractures of the trapezium with joint congruity are treated with thumb spica immobilization for 4 to 6 weeks. Close follow is required as these injuries are unstable and may displace. Displaced fractures are best managed with closed versus open reduction and internal fixation (ORIF) (see **Fig. 3**). If ORIF is required, a volar Wagner incision may be used, and the thenar muscle is elevated to expose the trapezium after capsulotomy. The radial artery should be identified and protected during the approach radially and the palmar cutaneous branch of the median nerve ulnarly.[31] Minifragment screws or Kirschner wires can be used for fixation.[27] The goal of reduction and fixation in the case of displaced fractures is to minimize deformity and posttraumatic arthritis. Depending on the injury, bone grafts (either allograft cancellous or autologous graft) can be considered to support the articular surface.[14]

Fractures of the volar ridge of the trapezium are classified as either base or avulsions of the tip as described earlier. Type I fractures occurring at the base may be treated nonoperatively with 4 to 6 weeks of casting. These should still be followed

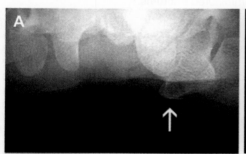

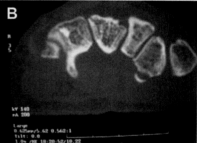

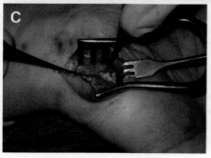

Fig. 5. A carpal tunnel view radiograph and CT scan showing a palmer trapezial ridge fracture (*A, B*), followed by an incision at the base of the thenar eminence for resection of the fracture (*C*). Arrow is pointing to a trapezial ridge fracture. (*From* Marchessault J, Conti M, Baratz M. Carpal Fractures in Athletes Excluding the Scaphoid. Hand Clin. 2009;25(3):371–88; with permission.)

as the pull of the transverse carpal ligament may prevent fracture healing.[32] Type II fractures occurring as an avulsion of the tip are treated with immobilization. If symptomatic nonunion occurs, the tip can be excised.

With all trapezium fractures, particularly in athletes trying to minimize time out of activity, one should remain vigilant of flexor carpi radialis irritation that may occur near the fracture site. This poses a theoretic risk for tendon rupture if ignored. Carpal tunnel syndrome may also develop following the fracture.[32] In cases of missed trapezium fractures, posttraumatic arthritis can be the first sign of the injury noted, but may also be asymptomatic and noted on radiographs incidentally.[27]

After 4 to 6 weeks of thumb immobilization with evidence of radiographic healing, the athlete begins practicing. Depending on the sport, splinting or taping may be used for comfort. Once safe return to play is demonstrated in practice, full activity is allowed 6 to 8 weeks after initiating treatment. Padded gloves may be useful as the palm can remain tender for several months.[14] Return to activity following fragment excision procedures can occur once the incision is healed and the patient has no other findings on examination (such as carpal tunnel syndrome or flexor carpi radialis irritation). For fixation of body fractures, return to activity occurs once immobilization for 4 to 6 weeks is complete and the patient demonstrates safe return to play.

HAMATE FRACTURES

Hamate fractures make up approximately 2% of all carpal fractures.[3,33,34] The unique anatomy of the hamate hook places the bone at risk, particularly if the palm is struck. The hook is the origin for the flexor digiti minimi muscles, opponens digiti minimi muscles, hypothenar muscles, pisohamate ligaments, and distal attachment of the transverse carpal ligament. It is the radial border of Guyon's canal and the ulnar border of the carpal tunnel.[16] Fractures of the hamate are classified as being hook of the hamate or body fractures.

Hook of the Hamate Fractures

Hook of the hamate fractures are likely underreported as they may not always be treated by a hand surgeon. These are more common in athletes compared with the general population.[18] They occur with direction compressive forces, shear forces, or a combination of both. In a batter or golf, sports involving two-handed swings, the nondomination hand is at more at risk. In one-handed swings, such as tennis or racquet sports, the dominant hand during forehand shots receives the force of impact. Shear forces from taut flexor tendons during power grip contribute to the fracture and displacement along with direct compression.[16]

Hamate Body Fractures

Hamate body fractures occur with high-energy axial load to the fourth and fifth digits, and can occur as a carpometacarpal fracture-dislocation.[17,35] In the athlete, these can occur with a direct fall causing an axial load at the fourth and fifth carpometacarpal joints. These joints are important for gripping and allow for about 30° of motion. Body fractures of the hamate are further divided into 4 categories: (1) proximal pole fractures, (2) fractures of the medial tuberosity, (3) sagittal oblique fractures, and (4) dorsal coronal fractures. Fractures of the medial tuberosity occur via a direct blow to the ulnar side of the wrist. The remainder are all a result of axial force transmission and high-energy trauma.[36,37]

Clinical examination

The most common sign of a hamate hook fracture is pain in the ulnar palm worsened with active gripping.[38] Tenderness to palpation is felt over the hamate hook, which is 2 cm distal and radial to the pisiform. The examiner may place his or her thumb interphalangeal joint on the patient's pisiform, direct his or her thumb toward the index metacarpophalangeal joint and roll the tip of his or her thumb directly onto the hook of the hamate. Patient's may also complain of ulnar nerve paresthesias.[38] Hamate hook fractures may also present late as chronic pain at the base of the hypothenar eminence. In this delayed presentation, median or ulnar nerve symptoms may accompany vague ulnar sided wrist pain.[38–40] Pain may occur with resistance of ring and small finger flexion, which is worse with ulnar deviation and lessened by radial deviation of the wrist. This happens since hamate hook fracture can irritate the flexor tendons of the ring and small finger. In a chronic setting, an untreated hamate hook fracture can lead to a rupture of the ring or small finger flexor tendons.

Radiographic examination

Hamate hook fractures are difficult to recognize on standard radiographic views. Clues on the posteroanterior radiograph include the absence of the hook, which appears as a cortical ring, or sclerosis in the region due to a nondisplaced nonunion.[41] A carpal tunnel view, a 45° supinated oblique view with the wrist dorsiflexed, and a lateral view projected through the first webspace are 3 difference specialized views to evaluate the hamate hook (**Fig. 6**).[42–45] The carpal tunnel is the most common used radiographic view, but with an acute injury this may be painful to obtain. A CT scan is a superior method over radiographs, and has been found to have 100% sensitivity and 94% specificity (**Fig. 7**).[46] This is in comparison with 72% sensitivity and 88% specificity for radiographs. Hamate body fractures are best identified on lateral and 45° pronated oblique radiographs, but are better defined with CT (**Fig. 8**).

Treatment

Treatment options for acute hamate hook fractures include immobilization, ORIF, and excision. Acute nondisplaced fractures can be treated nonoperatively with immobilization, particularly when diagnosed within the first week.[47] Less favorable results are noted if hamate hook fractures are treated nonoperatively after 1 week.[48] Support

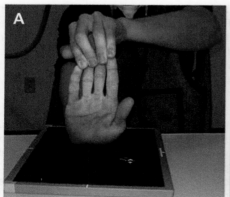
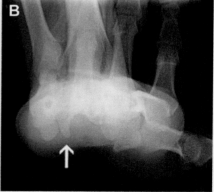

Fig. 6. Carpal tunnel view radiograph positioning (*A*), and image (*B*). Arrow is pointing to the hamate hook. (*From* Marchessault J, Conti M, Baratz M. Carpal Fractures in Athletes Excluding the Scaphoid. Hand Clin. 2009;25(3):371–88; with permission.)

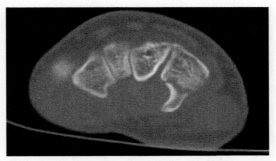

Fig. 7. An axial CT scan demonstrating a fracture through the base of the hook of the hamate. (*Courtesy of* Warren Hammert, MD, Rochester, NY.)

of open reduction internal fixation of hamate hook fractures is based on loss of the moment arm for flexor of the small fingers resulting in loss of strength.[49] Clinically, however, this has not been the case and there is little evidence to support an ORIF of the hook of the hamate.[50–52]

We recommend excision of acute hamate hook fractures as appropriate treatment in the athlete attempting earliest return to sport.[44] No adverse sequela with regards to wrist range of motion or grip strength are noted clinically.[44,53] Athletes can expect to return to full recovery and return to activity without further complications or deficits between 6 and 10 weeks after surgery.[44,53,54] A curvilinear excision centered over the hook of the hamate is used (**Fig. 9**). The ulnar nerve and artery are identified radial to the pisiform at the entrance of Guyon's canal and traced distally past the hook of the hamate to keep them protected. The distal portion of the transverse carpal ligament inserting on the hook of the hamate is release. The motor branch exits the ulnar nerve on the dorsal-ulnar aspect, and passes deep to the remaining ulnar nerve before diving beneath the flexor digiti minimi. It often lies at the fracture site at the base of the hamate, where fractures most commonly occur. It is critical to protect the ulnar nerve and its branches and the superficial vascular arch. Even if the fracture occurs at the tip or waist of the hook, we recommend complete excision with smoothing out of the remaining bone to prevent any remaining bone from irritating the flexor tendons.[16] The same surgical exposure and procedure is used for cases of symptomatic nonunions.

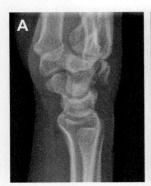
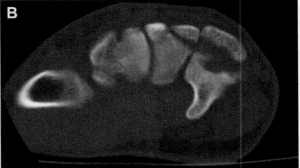

Fig. 8. A 25-year-old man with fractures at the base of the third metacarpal, dorsal hamate, and dorsal capitate, noted on radiographs (*A*), and more clearly visualized on CT scan (*B*). (*Courtesy of* Danielle Wilbur, MD, Rochester, NY.)

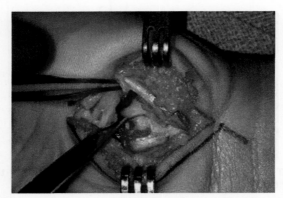

Fig. 9. Hook of the hamate excision with deep motor branch of the ulnar nerve passing around the base. (*From* Marchessault J, Conti M, Baratz M. Carpal Fractures in Athletes Excluding the Scaphoid. Hand Clin. 2009;25(3):371–88; with permission.)

Return to sport is relatively quick, with scar sensitivity being the limiting factor. Once the incision is healed in 10 to 14 days, and sutures are removed, a silicone patch, scar massage, and padded gloves can allow the athlete to return to play as soon as he or she is comfortable. Baseball players, golfers, and athletes playing racquet sports should gradually progress with dry swings, hitting off a tee and light contact, before moving to full swings. Although the scar sensitivity may last 4 to 6 months, and process of gradual progression means most athletes return to their sport in 4 to 6 weeks, or as they feel comfortable and capable.[16] Patients should be cautioned of the possible regrowth of the hook of hamate after fragment excision. The cause of this is unknown but has been postulated to be due to regrowth if the periosteum is sutured over the raw bony surface after fragment excision.

Displaced hamate body fractures are best treated with ORIF, particularly in the setting of carpometacarpal fracture-dislocation. A dorsal approach between the fourth and fifth extensor tendons provides a direction path to the joint. Care must be taken to identify and protect the dorsal sensory branch of the ulnar nerve. Kirschner wires or mini fragment screws can be used for anatomic reduction and fixation. Particular caution is advised when drilling dorsal to volar as the motor branch of the ulnar nerve is immediately volar to the hamate. Four to 6 weeks of immobilization is required with operative treatment of displaced hamate body fractures and nonoperative treatment of nondisplaced hamate body fractures. This is followed by a progression back to play similar to excision of the hamate hook. Return to play depends on whether use of playing cast is allowed. Functional outcomes are correlated with radiographic reduction, with about 75% of patients reporting good to excellent results.[55]

As mentioned earlier, chronic hamate hook fractures may cause irritation and rupture of the flexor tendons to the small and ring fingers. These require repair with palmaris tendon bridge or end-to-side repairs.[52] Reports of nerve injury following excision of the hamate hook indicate a 3% risk.[56]

CAPITATE FRACTURES

Capitate fractures make up 1% to 2% of all carpal fractures.[3,57] The capitate is centered within the carpus and typically well protected from injury. The capitate articulates with the scaphoid and lunate proximally and is well attached to the long finger metacarpal distally forming the central column of the hand and wrist. Capitate fractures can occur as part of a greater arc perilunate fracture-dislocation, although they may still occur in isolation.[58] The most common pattern for these remains a trans-caphoid, transcapitate perilunate fracture-dislocation.[59]

Isolate capitate fractures result from a direct blow or axial load down the third meta-carpal. The more common transcaphoid, transcapitate perilunate injury occurs with wrist hyperextension and the force initially being transmitted through the scaphoid. As the wrist continues to extend, the neck of the capitate may strike the dorsal ridge of the radius. The unattached proximal pole of the capitate may also rotate 180° with this proposed mechanism.[60,61]

Clinical Examination

Pain at the capitate with an appropriate index of suspicion is necessary for diagnosis. Cases of transcaphoid, transcapitate perilunate injuries will often have a clear trauma and event associated with them. A direct blow or axial load with an isolated capitate injury requires careful palpation and identifying localized tenderness at the capitate.

Radiographic Examination

Capitate fractures can often be seeing on standard AP, lateral and oblique radio-graphs. A nondisplaced fracture may be missed, but appropriate physical examination may lead one to order a CT scan in these cases. In cases of suspected ligament dam-age, an MRI can also be helpful. Advanced imaging is important to ensure that the capitate head is aligned as displacement or rotation can be seen that can lead to avas-cular necrosis of the capitate given its retrograde blood supply.[62,63]

Treatment

Nonoperative treatment is reserved for cases of nondisplaced capitate neck fractures occurring in isolation. Cast immobilization may take at least 6 to 8 weeks, and if radio-graphs are showing equivocal evidence of healing a CT scan is helpful. An MRI may also be used to evaluate the vascular supply of the proximal pole of the capitate, similar to a scaphoid fracture being treated nonoperatively. There is no agreement on what percentage of bony bridging on an isolated capitate neck fracture constitutes healing. However, the treating physician must combine his or her physical examination findings along with evidence of bony bridging to determine when to begin wrist motion and a gradual return to activity for athletes being treated nonoperatively.

Displaced fractures of the capitate in a transcaphoid, transcapitate perilunate in-juries should be treated with ORIF (**Fig. 10**). A dorsal incision between the third and fourth dorsal compartments, and in line with the radial border of the long finger, is used for access to the capitate.[18] A concomitant scaphoid fracture can also be addressed through this approach. Cannulated headless screws from proximal to distal provide appropriate stability. One may use 1 or 2 headless compression screws depending on the fracture. In the absence of a transcaphoid, transcapitate perilunate injury, range of motion of an isolated capitate fracture following fixation can begin as early as 2 weeks. More commonly, this injury will be in combination with either a scaphoid fracture or ligamentous injury and repair. As with other carpal fractures, re-turn to play depends on the ability to use a playing cast for their particular sport. Mid-carpal arthritis is a common consequence, and cases of transcaphoid, transcapitate perilunate injuries requiring ORIF are often season-ending injuries for athletes.[16] Once union is achieved with anatomic alignment, good outcomes along with return to all activities are noted.[16,64–66]

As noted earlier, an MRI is helpful to evaluate the vascular supply of the proximal pole of the capitate, which has a retrograde interosseous blood supply similar to the

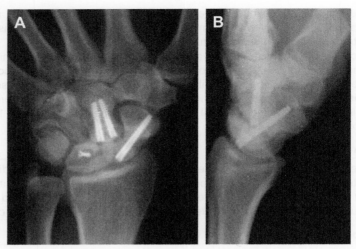

Fig. 10. A transcaphoid, transcapitate perilunate fracture-dislocation status after repair of the lunotriquetral ligament and ORIF of the capitate and scaphoid, noted both on AP (*A*) and lateral (*B*) radiographs. (*From* Lee S. Fractures of the Carpal Bones. In: Wolfe S, Hotchkiss R, Kozin S, Pederson W, Cohen M, editors. Green's Operative Hand Surgery. 7th ed. Philadelphia: Elsevier; 2017. p. 588–652; with permission.)

scaphoid. Although nonunions are not as common with the capitate as with the scaphoid, nonunions require addressing any collapse with a corticocancellous bone graft to restore carpal height. The potential of a nonunion and need for further surgery should be mentioned to athletes when they are first counseled about their injury.

PISIFORM FRACTURES

Fractures of the pisiform account for 1% to 2% of carpal fractures.[52,67] The pisiform is a prominent sesamoid bone within the flexor carpi ulnaris (FCU) tendon at the base of the hypothenar eminence. It also serves as an attachment point for the pisohamate, pisotriquetral, and transverse carpal ligaments, as well as the abductor digiti minimi muscle. About half of pisiform fractures are associated with other carpal injuries.[13] These fractures may be categorized as transverse, parasagittal, or comminuted.[14]

Pisiform fractures most commonly occur with a direct blow. Examples include being struck by a baseball, fall onto an outstretched hand, or in a marksmen as the force of a gun transmitted to the pisiform can also cause a fracture. Another mechanism is forceful FCU contraction while the pisiform is locked between the triquetrum and the floor in fall on an outstretched hand. This can create a transverse fracture, whereas a direct blow creates a comminuted fracture pattern. In a parasagittal pattern, the FCU tendon is not disrupted. As with all carpal fractures, the treating physician should have a high index of suspicion for fractures and injuries of other carpal.

Clinical Examination

Point tenderness over the pisiform or during a shuck maneuver of the pisiform is noted on clinical examination. Wrist flexion may also elicit pain as this is the attachment site for the FCU. One should carefully examine ulnar nerve function as the ulnar neurovascular bundle is in close proximity.

Radiographic Examination

The pisiform is difficult to visualize on standard radiographic views. The carpal tunnel view is helpful in visualizing the pisiform. In addition, an oblique radiograph with the wrist supinated 45° from the lateral position and in slight extension will also help visualize the pisiform. A CT scan is often used to further clarify the injury or if the plain radiographs are equivocal.

Treatment

Acute nondisplaced fracture of the pisiform can be treated nonoperatively with cast immobilization for 4 to 6 weeks (**Fig. 11**). Healing may occur via bony or fibrous union.[14] With any displacement, incongruity or for continued pain after nonoperative management, the treatment of choice is excision of the pisiform. Excision is usually performed through a volar zig-zag approached. The ulnar neurovascular bundle is identified and retracted and protected and the pisiform is shelled out of the FCU tendon. The FCU tendon is repaired side-to-side. This procedure has been shown to have no functional impairment.[68] Once the incision is healed and sutures removed, return to sport can begin occurring gradually. This may be as soon as 2 weeks after the surgery, and is limited primarily by scan sensitivity, similar to a hook of hamate

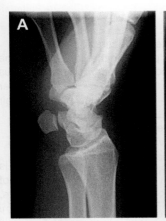
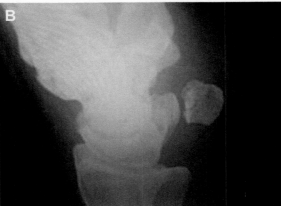
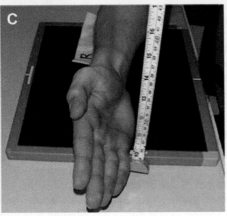

Fig. 11. An oblique 25° supinated view showing a normal pisotriquetral joint (*A*), a pisiform fracture (*B*), and proper position needed for the view (*C*). (*From* Marchessault J, Conti M, Baratz M. Carpal Fractures in Athletes Excluding the Scaphoid. Hand Clin. 2009;25(3):371–88; with permission.)

excision. Reports indicate good outcomes and return to activity following pisiformec-tomy, without any functional or range of motion deficits.[18,68,69]

Ulnar nerve injuries that occur with the initial injury are typically neuropraxias and resolve without intervention.[70] If a nerve defect persists for 12 weeks, nerve explora-tion and pisiform excision is recommended.[13] In the case of a nerve deficit after pisi-form excision, one may observe if the nerve was visualized and protected throughout the case. If the nerve was not visualized, exploration is appropriate. There is no evi-dence available to support the use of electrodiagnostic studies in the case of pisiform fractures.

TRAPEZOID FRACTURES

Trapezoid fractures make up less than 1% of all carpal fractures.[3,52] It is well sur-rounded and protected by the trapezium, scaphoid, capitate, and index metacarpal. Isolated fractures are extremely rare. The mechanism of injury is high-energy trauma, either an axial load or bending mechanism. This may be in combination with a fracture-dislocation of the index metacarpal.

The trapezoid is keystone shaped and has a dorsal surface twice as wide as the volar surface. The volar ligament are strong than the dorsal ligaments, and thus dorsal index metacarpal fracture-dislocations are more likely to occur with a high-energy axial load.[71]

Clinical Examination

On examination, point tenderness at the base of the index metacarpal, and pain with index metacarpal motion can help with the diagnosis. Palpation on the dorsum is most direct, although volar fracture-dislocations of the index metacarpal have been documented.[72]

Radiographic Examination

Fracture-dislocations of the index metacarpal and trapezoid are visualized on stan-dard AP, lateral, and oblique radiographs. The optimal view is often the AP as a dis-located trapezoid allows proximal migration and overlap of the index metacarpal. As with most carpal fracture, a CT scan if helpful to clarify the injury.

Treatment

In the case of an isolated nondisplaced trapezoid fracture, nonoperative management with immobilization is appropriate for 6 weeks after which a return to play program for the athlete's particular sport may be considered. In the case of displaced fractures or fracture-dislocations, closed versus ORIF is necessary. If during closed reduction there is residual joint incongruity, this should lead to ORIF, with care taken to identify and pro-tect the dorsal cutaneous nerves. Fracture-dislocations can result with avascular necro-sis of the trapezoid as 70% of the interosseous blood supply is through dorsal branches.[63,73] Severe comminution, symptomatic malunions, and nonunions can be treated with carpometacarpal arthrodesis. Blomquist and colleagues[74] reported excel-lent functional results with nonoperative management of nondisplaced trapezoid frac-tures and excellent union rates as well as functional outcomes with ORIF.

LUNATE FRACTURES

Acute traumatic lunate fractures make up about 1% of all carpal fractures[75] (**Fig. 12**). The lunate is well enclosed in the lunate fossa of the radius, and isolated acute frac-tures are rare. The challenge diagnosing an acute lunate fracture is whether it is truly

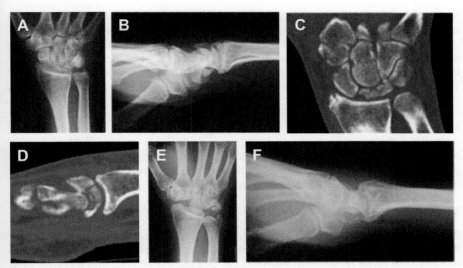

Fig. 12. A comminuted lunate fracture noted on posteroanterior and lateral radiographs (*A, B*), as well as coronal and sagital CT views (*C, D*). The patient underwent a proximal row carpectomy (*E, F*). (*From* Vigler M, Aviles A, Lee S. Carpal fractures excluding the scaphoid. Hand Clin. 2006;22:501–16; with permission.)

acute or a pathologic fracture in the setting of Kienböck disease. The proposed mechanism of injury for a lunate fracture is compression of the lunate between the distal radius and capitate. A direct blow to the lunate with a ball has also been described.[76] Lunate fractures may be categorized as volar pole fractures, dorsal pole fractures, osteochondral chip fractures, sagittal fractures, and transverse fractures.[75]

Clinical Examination

Tenderness to palpation dorsally at the lunate should raise the question of an injury. This is in close proximity to the scapholunate ligament, and an injury to this remains in the differential diagnosis as well.

Radiographic Examination

Fractures of the lunate are difficult to visualize on standard radiographs. If a clinical examination is concerning, a CT scan or MRI may be the next appropriate modality to use. However, x-rays should still be performed and scrutinized for dorsal intercalated segmental instability (DISI) or volar intercalated segmental instability (VISI) deformity. Small bone fragment off the lunate, may be pointing toward a major ligamentous injury that cannot be missed.

Treatment

Treatment of athletes with lunate fractures is similar to that of triquetral fractures noted earlier. Small chip fractures may be old injuries. Radiographs should be scrutinized for DISI or VISI deformity to rule out a ligamentous injury requiring specific treatment. Malalignment on radiographs however should result in further workup. In these cases, treatment of the ligamentous injury takes precedence.

Fractures that extend into the body of the lunate, and into the articular surface, should be evaluated with a CT scan. For displaced fractures, ORIF is necessary, and this is performed through a dorsal approach. Cancellous grafting may be needed for comminuted fractures and spanning external fixator or internal bridge plating may also be used to protect comminuted fractures from continuing to collapse.[16] Anticipated time to heal is 6 to 8 weeks and can be evaluated with a CT scan. Return to play depends on if a playing cast is allowed. Persistent pain and poor results may be due to avascular necrosis or midcarpal arthritis. They may also be as a result of VISI or DISI deformity. These all require further workup. There are no outcomes studies on isolated lunate fractures.

About 20% of lunates have only a volar nutrient artery.[73] Thus, displaced volar fragments may increase risk of avascular necrosis. There is no consensus on the causal relationship between acute lunate fractures and Kienböck disease.[16] There should remain a low threshold to pursue an MRI on an athlete with persistent pain after an acute lunate fracture. As with any intraarticular fractures, one has a risk of midcarpal arthritis with intraarticular lunate fractures.

SUMMARY

Although carpal fractures of bones other than the scaphoid occur at a much lower rate than scaphoid fractures, they remain an important diagnosis in athletes as well as non-athletes. The close relationship between the carpus, the intrinsic and extrinsic wrist ligaments, and wrist kinematics forces the physician to be thorough in the history, clinical examination, and to be attentive in interpreting imaging for carpal malalignment. Carpal malalignment should be addressed with reduction and fixation. Nondisplaced fractures are often treated nonoperatively and displaced intraarticular fractures are almost always treatment operatively. However, the physician should also keep in mind the athlete and his or her specific goals and needs. Treatment must be individualized. Options for early return to play should be discussed when possible.

DISCLOSURE

The authors have nothing to disclose.

REFERENCES

1. Botte M, Gelberman R. Fractures of the carpus, excluding the scaphoid. Hand Clin 1987;3(1):149–61.
2. Larsen C, Brondum V, Skov O. Epidemiology of scaphoid fractures in Odense, Denmark. Acta Orthop Scand 1992;63(2):216–8.
3. Garcia-Elias M. Carpal bone fractures (excluding scaphoid fractures). In: Watson H, Weinberg J, editors. The wrist. Philadelphia: Lippincott Williams & Wilkins; 2001. p. 174–81.
4. Bartone N, Greico R. Fractures of the triquetrum. J Bone Joint Surg Am 1956;38: 353–6.
5. Bryan R, Dobyns J. Fractures of the carpal bones other than the lunate and navicular. Clin Orthop Relat Res 1980;14:107–11.
6. Hocker K, Menschik A. Chip fractures of the triquetrum. J Hand Surg Br 1994;19: 584–8.
7. Bonnin J, Greening W. Fractures of the triquetrum. Br J Surg 1944;19:584–8.
8. Levy M, Fischel R, Stern G, et al. Chip fractures of the os triquetrum: the mechanism of injury. J Bone Joint Surg Br 1979;61-B(3):355–7.
9. Garcia-Elias M. Dorsal fractures of the triquetrum: avulsion or compression fractures? J Hand Surg Am 1987;12(2):266–8.
10. Greening W. Isolated fracture of the carpal cuneiform. Br Med J 1942;1:221–2.

11. Fairbank T. Chip fractures of the os triquetrum. Br Med J 1942;2:310–1.
12. Mayfield J, Johnson R, Kilcoyne R. Carpal dislocations: pathomechanics and progressive perilunar instability. J Hand Surg Am 1980;5:226–41.
13. Vigler M, Aviles A, Lee S. Carpal fractures excluding the scaphoid. Hand Clin 2006;22:501–16.
14. Lee S. Fractures of the carpal bones. In: Wolfe S, Hotchkiss R, Kozin S, et al, editors. Green's operative hand surgery. 7th edition. Philadelphia: Elsevier; 2017. p. 588–652.
15. Smith D, Murrary P. Avulsion fractures of the volar aspect of the triquetral bone of the wrist: a subtle sign of carpal ligament injury. AJR Am J Roentgenol 1996; 166(3):609–14.
16. Marchessault J, Conti M, Baratz M. Carpal fractures in athletes excluding the scaphoid. Hand Clin 2009;25(3):371–88.
17. Papp S. Carpal bone fractures. Orthop Clin North Am 2007;38:251–60.
18. Geissler W. Carpal fractures in athletes. Clin Sports Med 2001;20(1):167–88.
19. Culp R, Lernel M, Taras J. Complications of common carpal injuries. Hand Clin 1994;10(1):139–55.
20. Porter M, Seehra K. Fracture-dislocation of the triquetrum treated with a Herbert screw. J Bone Joint Surg Br 1991;73:347–8.
21. Suzuki T, Nakatsuchi Y, Tateiwa Y, et al. Osteochondral fracture of the triquetrum: a case report. J Hand Surg Am 2002;27(1):98–100.
22. Aiki H, Wada T, Yamashita T. Pisotriquetral arthrosis after triquetral malunion: a case report. J Hand Surg Am 2006;31(7):1157–9.
23. Garcia-Elias M, Henriquez-Lluch A, Rossignani P, et al. Bennett's fracture combined with fracture of the trapezium. A report of three cases. J Hand Surg Br 1993;18(4):523–6.
24. Cordrey L, Ferror-Torrells M. Management of fractures of the greater multangular. Report of five cases. J Bone Joint Surg Am 1960;42(A):1111–8.
25. Palmer A. Trapezial ridge fractures. J Hand Surg Am 1981;6(6):561–4.
26. Pointu J, Schwenck J, Destree G, et al. Fractures of the trapezium: mechanisms: anatomo-pathology and therapeutic indications. Rev Chir Orthop Reparatrice Appar Mot 1988;74(5):454–65.
27. McGuigan F, Culp R. Surgical treatment of intraarticular fractures of the trapezium. J Hand Surg Am 2002;27:697–703.
28. Walker J, Greene T, Lunseth P. Fractures of the body of the trapezium. J Orthop Trauma 1988;2(1):22–8.
29. McClain E, Boyes J. Missed fractures of the greater multangular. J Bone Joint Surg Am 1966;48:1525–8.
30. Binhammer P, Born T. Coronal fracture of the body of the trapezium. A case report. J Hand Surg Am 1998;23:156–7.
31. Checroun A, Mekhail A, Ebraheim N. Radial artery injury in association with fractures of the trapezium. J Hand Surg Br 1997;22:419–22.
32. Botte M, von Schroeder H, Gellman H, et al. Fracture of the trapezial ridge. Clin Orthop Relat Res 1992;276:202–5.
33. Milch H. Fracture of the hamate bone. J Bone Joint Surg 1934;16:459–62.
34. Adams B, Blair W, Reagan D, et al. Technical factors related to Herbert screw fixation. J Hand Surg Am 1988;13(6):893–9.
35. Thomas A, Birch R. An unusual hamate fracture. Hand 1983;15(3):281–6.
36. Hirano K, Inoue G. Classification and treatment of hamate fractures. Hand Surg 2005;10:151–7.

37. Chase J, Light T, Benson L. Coronal fracture of the hamate body. Am J Orthop 1997;26(8):568–71.
38. Bishop A, Beckenbaugh R. Fracture of the hamate hook. J Hand Surg Am 1988; 13:135–9.
39. Foucher G, Schuind F, Merle M, et al. Fractures of the hook of the hamate. J Hand Surg Br 1975;10(2):205–10.
40. Manske P. Fracture of the hook of the hamate presenting as carpal tunnel syndrome. Hand 1978;10:181–3.
41. Norman A, Nelson J. Fractures of the hook of hamate: radiographic signs. Radiology 1985;154:4953.
42. Hart V, Gaynor V. Roentgenographic study of the carpal canal. J Bone Joint Surg Am 1941;23:382–3.
43. Andress M, Peckar V. Fracture of the hook of the hamate. Br J Radiol 1970;43: 141–3.
44. Stark H, Jobe F, Boyes J, et al. Fracture of the hook of hamate in athletes. J Bone Joint Surg Am 1977;59(5):575–82.
45. Papilion J, DePuy T, Aulicino P, et al. Radiographic evaluation of the hook of the hamate: a new technique. J Hand Surg Am 1988;13(3):437–9.
46. Andresen R, Radmer S, Sparmann M, et al. Imaging of hamate bone fractures in conventional X-rays and high-resolution computed tomography. An in vitro study. Invest Radiol 1999;34(1):46–50.
47. Whalen J, Bishop A, Linscheid R. Nonoperative treatment of acute hamate hook fractures. J Hand Surg Am 1992;17:507–11.
48. Carroll R, Lakin J. Fracture of the hook of the hamate: acute treatment. J Trauma 1993;34(6):803–5.
49. Demirkan F, Calandruccio J, DiAngelo D. Biomechanical evaluation of flexor tendon function after hamate hook excision. J Hand Surg Am 2003;28:138–43.
50. Scheufler O, Andresen R, Erdmann D, et al. Hook of hamate fractures: critical evaluation of different therapeutic procedures. Plast Reconstr Surg 2005; 115(2):488–97.
51. Watson H, Rogers WD. Nonunion of the hook of the hamate: an argument for bone grafting the nonunion. J Hand Surg Am 1989;14(3):486–90.
52. Boulas H, Milek M. Hook of the hamate fractures. Orthop Rev 1990;19(6):518–22.
53. Devers B, Douglas K, Naik R, et al. Outcomes of hook of hamate fracture excision in high-level amateur athletes. J Hand Surg Am 2013;38(1):72–6.
54. Parker R, Berkowitz M, Brahms M, et al. Hook of the hamate fractures in athletes. Am J Sports Med 1986;14(6):517–23.
55. Wharton D, Casaletto J, Choa R, et al. Outcome following coronal fractures of the hamate. J Hand Surg Eur Vol 2010;35(2):146–9.
56. Smith P, Wright T, Wallace P, et al. Excision of the hook of the hamate: a retrospective survey and review of the literature. J Hand Surg Am 1988;13(4):612–5.
57. Adler J, Shaftan G. Fractures of the capitate. J Bone Joint Surg Am 1962;44: 1537–47.
58. Fenton R. The naviculo-capitate fracture syndrome. J Bone Joint Surg Am 1956; 38(3):681–4.
59. Rand J, Linscheid R, Dobyns J. Capitate fractures: a long-term follow up. Clin Orthop Relat Res 1992;165:209–16.
60. Stein F, Seigel M. Naviculocapitate fracture syndrome. A case report: new thought on mechanism of injury. J Bone Joint Surg Am 1969;51:391–5.

61. Vance R, Gelberman R, Evans E. Scaphocapitate fractures. Patters of disloca-
    tion, mechanisms of injury, and preliminary results of treatment. J Bone Joint
    Surg Am 1980;62:271–6.
62. Vander Grend R, Dell P, Leslie B, et al. Intraosseous blood supple of the capitate
    and its corrrelation with aseptic necrosis. J Hand Surg Am 1984;9(5):677–83.
63. Gelberman R, Panagis J, Taleisnik J, et al. The arterial anatomy of the human
    carpus. Part I: the extraosseous vascularity. J Hand Surg Am 1983;8(4):367–75.
64. Volk A, Schnall S, Merkle P, et al. Unusual capitate fracture: a case report. J Hand
    Surg Am 1995;20(4):581–2.
65. Freeman B, Hay E. Nonunion of the capitate: a case report. J Hand Surg Am
    1985;10(2):187–90.
66. Yoshihara M, Sakai A, Toba N, et al. Nonunion of the isolated capitate waist frac-
    ture. J Orthop Sci 2002;7(5):578–80.
67. McCarty V, Farber H. Isolated fracture of the pisiform bone. J Bone Joint Surg Am
    1946;28:390.
68. Carroll R, Coyle M. Dysfunction of the pisotriquetral joint: treatment by excision of
    the pisiform. J Hand Surg Am 1985;10(5):703–7.
69. Suh N, Ek E, Wolfe S. Carpal fractures. J Hand Surg Am 2014;39(4):785–91.
70. Matsunaga D, Uchiyama S, Nakagawa H, et al. Lower ulnar nerve palsy related to
    fracture of the pisiform bone in patients with multiple injuries. J Trauma 2002;
    53(2):364–8.
71. Garcia-Elias M, Dobyns J, Cooney W, et al. Traumatic dislocations of the carpus.
    J Hand Surg Am 1989;14(3):446–57.
72. Lewis H. Dislocation of the lesser multangular. J Bone Joint Surg Am 1962;44:
    1412–4.
73. Panagis J, Gelberman R, Taleisnik J, et al. The arterial anatomy of the human
    carpus. Part II: the intraosseous vascularity. J Hand Surg Am 1983;8(4):375–82.
74. Blomquist G, Hunt T III, Lopez-Benz R. Isolated fractures of the trapezoid as a
    sports injury. Skeletal Radiol 2013;42(5):735–9.
75. Teisen H, Hjarbaek J. Classification of fresh fractures of the lunate. J Hand Surg
    Br 1988;13:458–62.
76. Teisen H, Hjarbaek J, Jensen E. Follow-up investigation of fresh lunate bone frac-
    ture. Handchir Mikrochir Plast Chir 1990;22:20–2.

Ulnar-Sided Wrist Pain in the Athlete

Hannah A. Dineen, MD[a],*, Jeffrey A. Greenberg, MD, MS[b]

KEYWORDS

• Wrist • Ulnar • Pain • Athlete • Injury

KEY POINTS

- The athlete's wrist is subjected to high loads during activities that involve pronation/supination, radial/ulnar deviation, and flexion/extension.
- These activities stress stabilizing elements of the ulnar side of the wrist, including the triangular fibrocartilage complex, distal radioulnar joint, as well as the ulnocarpal region.
- Pathology along the ulnar side of the athlete's wrist can lead to pain, dysfunction, and difficulty participating in sport.

INTRODUCTION

Ulnar-sided wrist pain is a common problem in athletes that can be challenging owing to its frequent combination of overuse in conjunction with acute injury. Forceful forearm rotation, wrist flexion and extension, as well as radial and ulnar deviation can predispose the athlete to injury of ulnar stabilizing structures. Careful understanding of the sport-specific injuries as well as the underlying biomechanics are key to understanding and treating the athlete. In this article, we discuss the most frequent causes of ulnar-sided wrist pain in the athlete and focus on the anatomy and pathophysiology, presentation and diagnosis, as well as nonoperative and operative treatment options of:

1. Triangular fibrocartilage complex (TFCC)/distal radioulnar joint (DRUJ) injuries
2. Ulnocarpal impaction
3. Extensor carpi ulnaris (ECU) conditions
4. Flexor carpi ulnaris (FCU) calcific tendonitis

The management of hook of hamate fractures are not discussed in this article because it is detailed within Bilal Mahmood and Steve K. Lee's article, "Carpal Fractures Other than Scaphoid in the Athlete," in this issue.

[a] Indiana Hand to Shoulder Center, 8501 North Harcourt Road, Indianapolis, IN 46260, USA;
[b] All American Orthopedic and Sports Medicine Institute, 1045 Gemini Avenue, #100, Houston, TX 77058, USA
* Corresponding author.
E-mail address: handdr@mac.com

Clin Sports Med 39 (2020) 373–400
https://doi.org/10.1016/j.csm.2019.12.008
0278-5919/20/© 2019 Elsevier Inc. All rights reserved.

Triangular Fibrocartilage Complex and Distal Radioulnar Joint Injuries

Ulnar-sided wrist pain in athletes can be caused by injury to the TFCC. The TFCC is a group of interrelated anatomic structures that are integral to stability of the DRUJ. Traumatic injuries of the TFCC may occur from fall or hyper-rotational injuries to the forearm. Repetitive forceful movement of the athlete's wrist from supination to pronation can cause overload stress affecting components of the TFCC.

Anatomy and biomechanics

The TFCC is a group of structures that assist with load transmission from the hand and carpus, and is the primary stabilizer of the DRUJ. There are 6 main components of the TFCC that provide stability to the DRUJ (**Box 1, Fig. 1**). The volar and dorsal radioulnar ligaments are the major supportive structures of the joint. In particular, the deep ligamentum subcruentum fibers are the main stabilizing component of the DRUJ. These fibers insert at the fovea at a relatively obtuse angle of attachment onto the volar and dorsal margins of the sigmoid notch, facilitating rotational stability.[1] The superficial radioulnar ligaments insert at a more acute angle onto the styloid and provide secondary stability to the DRUJ, as well as support to the articular disc.[1]

Volarly, the TFCC is linked to the ulnar carpus through strong attachments to the lunotriquetral ligament and the ulnar extrinsic ligaments, as well as to the hamate and base of the fifth metacarpal.[2] Dorsally, there are weak attachments of the TFCC to the carpus, except where the TFCC blends with the ECU subsheath. The ulnar collateral ligament is a capsular structure that arises from the base of the ulnar styloid. The ulnocarpal meniscal homologue travels from the discoid section of the TFCC to the triquetrum, lunate, and fifth metacarpal. Both of these structures form the remainder of the TFCC in addition to the ECU subsheath and the articular disc.[3] The TFCC and distal ulna receive about 16% to 20% of wrist load in neutral variance, which increases with ulnar deviation of the hand and ulnar positive morphology. Heavy gripping activities, as well as the increased ulnar positive

---

Box 1
Components of the TFCC

- Central disc
  - Bound by the volar and dorsal superficial radioulnar ligaments and the distal sigmoid notch of the radius
  - Relative avascular central portion with significant peripheral vascularity

- Superficial radioulnar ligaments: volar and dorsal
  - Attach to the distal volar/dorsal edges of the sigmoid notch and the ulnar styloid
  - Narrow angle of attachment

- Deep radioulnar ligaments: volar and dorsal
  - Also attach to the distal volar/dorsal edges of the sigmoid notch, but at the fovea near the base of the ulnar styloid
  - Wide angle of attachment

- Ulnotriquetral and ulnolunate ligaments
  - Actually attach at the ulnar and volar aspect of the disc, not the ulna

- ECU subsheath
  - Course dorsally similar to the volar ulnocarpal ligaments

- Meniscal homologue
  - Ulnar side of the complex; a reflection of the joint capsule

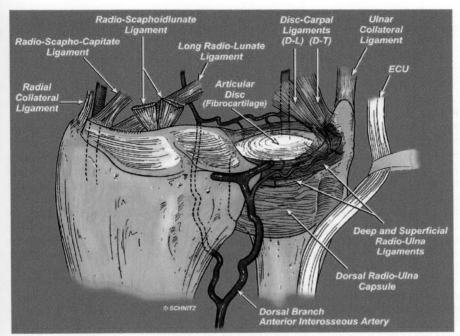

Fig. 1. Complex anatomy of the TFCC and surrounding structures. (*From* Kleinman WB. Stability of the distal radioulna joint: biomechanics, pathophysiology, physical diagnosis, and restoration of function: what we have learned in 25 years. J Hand Surg 2007; 32(7):1086-106; with permission.)

variance that occurs with wrist pronation, both serve to increase load transmission to the TFCC.[1,2]

The TFCC is supplied by terminal branches of the ulnar artery; in particular, the anterior and posterior interosseous arteries that insert around the periphery and provide a rich blood supply to the fovea.[3] The central articular disc, which can be likened to the central portion of the meniscus of the knee, is avascular and has limited healing potential.[4]

The DRUJ is inherently unstable through its bony configuration, where the sigmoid notch has a greater radius of curvature than the ulnar seat, providing approximately 20% of the stability.[1] The stability of the joint is achieved through extrinsic structures including the ECU tendon and its subsheath, the deep head of the pronator quadratus, and the distal interosseous ligament, which includes the distal oblique bundle that provides isometric stability during pronosupination.[5] Intrinsic stability of the DRUJ is provided largely by the radioulnar ligamentous components of the TFCC.[1]

Patient history

Athletes who participate in sports that use racquets, clubs, or bats are at risk for TFCC or DRUJ injures owing to the high torque loads transmitted, especially when moving from supination to pronation. Traumatic injuries from a fall with an extended and deviated wrist may cause an acute injury. The athlete may recall a specific event in which they experienced acute pain, or may have a more insidious onset. They may report a variety of symptoms:

- Mechanical symptoms of the ulnar wrist
- Pain located over the dorsal and ulnar wrist
- Pain with wrist loading
- Pain with forearm pronation or supination
- Pain with ulnar deviation
- Pain and feelings of instability

Physical examination

Knowledge of the anatomy of the TFCC is important to localize areas of pathology through the physical examination. Physical examination begins with examination of the wrist to assess for swelling or visual abnormality compared with the contralateral wrist. The patient is seated at the hand table with the elbow at 90° and fingers toward the ceiling. Range of motion, including flexion/extension, pronation/supination, and radial/ulnar deviation, is then assessed. The examination should be compared with the contralateral uninjured wrist. Tenderness to palpation over various components of the TFCC can help to focus on the pathologic area and should be performed in a stepwise fashion over each anatomic component. Dorsally, the TFCC is intimately associated with the ECU subsheath, which can make tenderness at this region difficult to isolate.

Tenderness at the ulnar fovea is a both highly sensitive and specific test for TFCC injuries or ulnotriquetral ligament injuries, with a sensitivity of 95% and specificity of 86% for detecting foveal disruptions or ulnotriquetral ligament tears.[6] The ulnar fovea is a soft spot that lies between the ulnar styloid process, the ECU and the FCU tendons, which is easily palpable with the forearm in neutral rotation.[6] This test is positive when pain is elicited and replicates the patient's pain when compared with the contralateral side. It is important to isolate the TFCC as the location of pain during the physical examination. The ECU synergy test, discussed within the ECU Tendonitis section, is helpful for distinguishing between intra-articular and extra-articular pathology.

Testing of the lunatotriquetral (LT) interval is important to determine LT instability as a cause of ulnar-sided pain. The LT shear test, as described by Kleinman, is performed with the wrist and fingers in the standard examining position.[7,8] To examine the patient's right hand, the examiner's left thumb is placed over the dorsal surface of the lunate with the remaining 4 fingers wrapping around the radial wrist to stabilize the hand–forearm unit. The right thumb is then placed over the pisiform, applying a dorsally directed force while the left thumb applies a volarly directed force across the lunate, to cause shearing at the LT interval and detect even mild pain.

The LT compression test, as described by Linscheid,[9] is performed with the hand and wrist in the standard position. The forearm is stabilized along the radial border, and the thumb of the examining hand pushes firmly on the triquetrum in an ulnar to radial direction. This causes compression across the LT joint and elicits pain in a positive test.[8,9]

As described by Kleinman,[1] the dorsal fibers of the deep ligamentum subcruentum are under maximum tension with the forearm in supination. Conversely, the palmar fibers of the deep ligamentum subcruentum are under maximum tension with the forearm in pronation. Testing of the dorsal fibers is performed by rotating the forearm to full supination, loading the distal ulna toward the patient and pulling the radiocarpal unit toward the examiner (**Fig. 2**). In an injury to these dorsal fibers, this maneuver causes pain or increased translation, depending on the degree of injury to the stabilizing complex. Palmar fiber testing is done similarly, with the forearm in full pronation. A dorsally directed force is then placed along the distal ulna while the radiocarpal unit is again

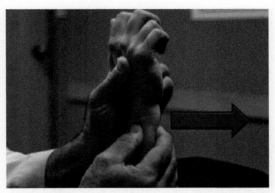

Fig. 2. Stress testing of the deep dorsal portion of the radioulnar ligament. The patient's wrist is positioned in supination and a volar-directed force is exerted (*arrow* depicts direction of applied load) on the ulna while stabilizing the radius and carpus.

pulled toward the examiner (**Fig. 3**). Pain or increased translation when compared with the contralateral arm results if there is an injury to the palmar fibers of the ligamentum subcruentum.[1]

The DRUJ compression test identifies inflammation or articular pathology within the DRUJ.[8] With the wrist and forearm in neutral rotation and fingertips toward the ceiling, the wrist is grasped proximal to the DRUJ at the junction of the distal and middle thirds of the forearm. The forearm is squeezed together to compress the radius and ulna, and the forearm is rotated.[8] Pain elicited when compared with the opposite side indicates a positive test.

Imaging

Plain radiographs are part of the initial workup and typically consist of zero-rotation posteroanterior and lateral radiographs (**Figs. 4** and **5**). In particular, ulnar variance, morphology, and degenerative changes of the DRUJ are assessed. It is important to also identify the presence of an ulnar styloid fracture or nonunion. MRI is commonly used for evaluation of the TFCC and associated soft tissues or for assistance in

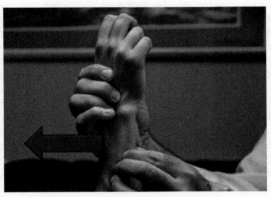

Fig. 3. Stress testing of the deep volar radioulnar ligament with the patient's wrist in pronation and a dorsally directed force (*arrow* depicts direction of applied load) on the ulna.

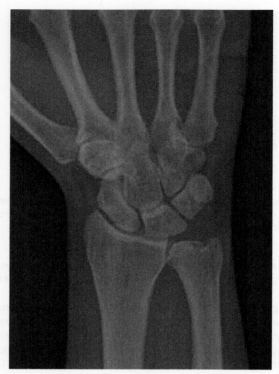

Fig. 4. Zero-rotation posteroanterior radiograph showing a profile of the DRUJ, normal forearm rotation, and standard radio/ulnar length relationship.

differentiating between extra-articular and intra-articular pathology. Conventional MRI has been shown to have sensitivity ranging from 44% to 100% and specificity of 60% to 100% in identifying TFCC injuries, depending on whether a 1.5 T or 3.0 T magnet is used.[10,11] MR arthrography has been shown to have increased accuracy in diagnosing both central and peripheral TFCC tears when compared with MRI, with sensitivity of up to 94% in central TFCC tears, 93% in peripheral tears, and specificity of 97% to 100% in a single study.[10] A systematic review of 21 studies demonstrated a pooled sensitivity of 75% and specificity of 81% for MRI in detecting full-thickness TFCC tears compared with 84% sensitivity and 95% specificity for MR arthography.[11] Arthroscopy, however, is considered to be the gold standard for diagnosing TFCC injuries. Confirmation of a tear can be performed with the assistance of arthroscopic tests. The trampoline test is done by using a probe to ballotte the articular disc and evaluate for loss of tension of the disc, which may occur with a peripheral tear. The hook test assesses the TFCC at its foveal insertion. This is done by placing a probe into the pre-styloid recess and applying a radial traction force. Displacement of the TFC off the ulnar head can be demonstrated when an unstable foveal tear is present. A recent cadaveric study demonstrated increased sensitivity, specificity, and reliability of the hook test in diagnosing TFCC tears when compared with the trampoline test.[12] Recently, the suction test has been described to identify peripheral TFCC tears as well as confirm integrity of a repair.[13] A shaver is placed arthroscopically and applies periodic suction, demonstrating a loss of tension along the TFCC in the presence of a tear, which is not seen after repair.

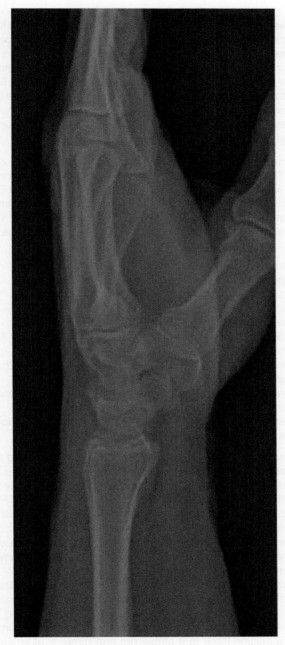

Fig. 5. Lateral wrist radiograph demonstrates the hand in a neutral position and overlap of the distal scaphoid over the pisiform.

Treatment

Nonoperative treatment In patients with an acute TFCC injury and a stable DRUJ, an initial period of nonoperative management should be initiated. This consists of the use of bracing to prevent forearm rotation. Taping of the DRUJ and the use of anti-inflammatories or intra-articular corticosteroid injections can be helpful for athletes that are trying to continue training. A retrospective study identified 57% of patients treated successfully with nonoperative treatment in 1 month in a volar wrist splint or cast.[14] Consideration of the athlete's activity level as well as time remaining in their season, as well as future career endeavors, must be taken into account when considering the duration of nonoperative treatment.

Operative treatment Operative treatment is considered for failure of nonoperative management or TFCC tears in the presence of DRUJ instability. Arthroscopic evaluation of the ulnar wrist is important for diagnosis and treatment of TFCC lesions. The Palmer classification is commonly used to describe TFCC injuries and is separated into both traumatic (class 1) and degenerative (class 2) injuries.[15] Class 2 injuries are often associated with ulnocarpal impaction and will be discussed further in that section.

Class 1: Traumatic[15]
    1A: Central perforation
    1B: Ulnar avulsion, with or without ulnar styloid fracture
    1C: Distal avulsion
    1D: Radial avulsion, with or without sigmoid notch fracture
Class 2: Degenerative[15]
    2A: TFCC wear without perforation or chondromalacia
    2B: TFCC wear with chondromalacia of the lunate or ulnar head, or both
    2C: TFCC perforation, with lunate/ulnar chondromalacia
    2D: TFCC perforation, with lunate/ulnar chondromalacia and lunotriquetral ligament perforation
    2E: TFCC perforation, with lunate/ulnar chondromalacia, lunotriquetral ligament perforation, and ulnocarpal arthritis

Class 1A lesions are the most common type of traumatic tears and are rarely associated with the instability that can be seen in class 1B and 1C injuries.[16] Although the Palmer classification is widely used, it does not offer a treatment-oriented approach. Atzei and Luchetti[17] described a classification system for peripheral TFCC injuries that incorporates stability of the DRUJ as well as offers a treatment algorithm (**Table 1**). This classification system divides the TFCC into the proximal component, which is composed of the proximal triangular ligament and ligament subcruentum, and the distal component, which is made up of the ulnar collateral ligament and distal hammock structure.[17]

For patients who have class 1A or traumatic central tears and fail nonoperative management, arthroscopic debridement is considered. Central tears of the TFCC lack the healing potential that is seen with peripheral tears owing to the relative avascularity of the central portion of the disc.[4] The goals of debridement are resection of the central portion back to a stable rim and removal of any loose flaps that may cause mechanical symptoms or irritation. Limited arthroscopic debridement for traumatic central tears has been shown to have good clinical results with success rates from 66% to 95%, without destabilization of the TFCC.[18–22] A biomechanical study demonstrated that partial excisions that compromised less than two-thirds of the disc region and left the peripheral 2 mm of the disc intact did

Table 1
Atzei and Luchetti classification of peripheral TFCC tears

Class	Injury Pattern	Treatment
0	Isolated ulnar styloid fracture without TFCC tear	Nonoperative (splinting) or fragment removal
1	Distal peripheral TFCC tear without DRUJ instability	TFCC suture or splinting acutely
2	Complete peripheral TFCC tear of both the proximal and distal components, with DRUJ instability	Fixation of TFCC to fovea
3	Proximal peripheral TFCC tear with DRUJ instability	Fixation of TFCC to fovea or styloid fixation if associated with avulsion fracture
4	Nonrepairable TFCC tear owing to large size or poor healing potential	Tendon graft reconstruction
5	TFCC tear and DRUJ arthritis	Arthroplasty

From Atzei A, Luchetti R. Foveal TFCC Tear Classification and Treatment. *Hand Clin*. 2011;27(3):263-272; with permission.

not result in any significant biomechanical changes.[23] In the setting of ulnar-positive variance, ulnar shortening osteotomy may also be considered. This will be discussed further in the Ulnocarpal Impaction section.

Peripheral tears, or type 1B lesions, are in the vascular region of the TFCC and are amenable to arthroscopic or open repair. A variety of arthroscopic techniques have been described and are often preferred in athletes to an open repair. Fixation options include repair of the torn fibers to capsule or to bone with suture anchors or transosseus fixation, the latter of which is performed if there is concomitant foveal injury resulting in DRUJ instability. Peripheral tears affecting the superficial fibers only have been described by Wysocki and colleagues[24] to have good results in treatment with outside-in repair of the TFCC to the ulnar capsule, with improvement in mean Disability of Arm Shoulder and Hand (DASH) scores from 38 to 9 at an average final follow-up of 31 months. Additionally, 64% of high-level athletes returned to sport at a similar level of competition. McAdams and colleagues[25] described arthroscopic repair of unstable TFCC tears in competitive athletes using an inside-out repair with good results and return to sport in all athletes at an average of 3.3 months. All-arthroscopic, all-inside fixation has also recently been described to decrease disadvantages such as extra incisions or prominent suture knots.[26,27] However, in our experience, peripheral stable tears are best treated with an arthroscopic repair using an outside-in suture tying technique. The postoperative protocol includes 6 weeks of immobilization followed by gradual return to activity. We have found that athletes are usually able to return to sport at 3 to 6 months postoperatively with the addition of circumferential compression support during activity.

For unstable peripheral tears associated with DRUJ instability or disruption of the deep radioulnar ligament, we feel that these injuries are best treated in an open fashion. This technique allows direct, secure fixation of the deep radioulnar ligaments to their anatomic site of bony origin. However, when comparing open versus arthroscopic repair of unstable peripheral TFCC repairs, neither approach has proven to be superior. A retrospective review comparing arthroscopic versus open foveal repairs showed no difference in pain, range of motion, grasping power, stability, or DASH scores.[28] Luchetti and colleagues[29] found no difference in postoperative outcomes when comparing functional outcomes of arthroscopic versus open repairs except for superior DASH scores in the arthroscopically treated group. Likewise, Anderson and colleagues[30] found no statistically significant differences between the 2 groups, but did observe a higher rate of postoperative superficial ulnar nerve pain in the open group as well as a slightly increased wrist range of motion.

Open Triangular Fibrocartilage Complex Repair

Preparation and patient positioning

The patient is placed supine and the operative extremity is prepped and draped. A sterile tourniquet is applied before placing the wrist in a commercial traction tower. Folded towels are used to pad the skin against the tower. Initial evaluation begins with establishment of a standard 3-4 portal; however, multiple portals are used depending on the site of pathology.

Surgical approach

Diagnostic arthroscopy is performed and confirmation of TFCC tear is visualized. The arm is then removed from the traction tower and placed onto the hand table in a pronated position. A longitudinal incision is made centered over the ECU tendon, with an ulnar angulation at the level of the DRUJ. Full-thickness skin flaps are then raised off the extensor retinaculum with care taken to identify and protect the dorsal sensory branch of the ulnar nerve. The retinaculum and dorsal ECU sheath are then opened sharply, the ECU is retracted ulnarly, the extensor digiti quinti proprius is retracted through the fifth dorsal compartment, and the location of the TFCC is localized with the placement of an 18-gauge needle distal to the pole of the distal ulna (**Fig. 6**). Proximally, the dorsal DRUJ capsule is elevated off the ulnar head using a radially based rectangular flap. Elevation of this exposes the proximal undersurface of the TFCC at its articulation with the pole of the ulna.

Procedure

The deep fibers of the ligamentum subcruentum are evaluated at their insertion onto the fovea (**Figs. 7** and **8**). A rongeur is used to debride any friable fibrous appearing tissue adjacent to the fovea, which is easily distinguishable from the healthy ligament, which is taut and has a stark white appearance. A scalpel is used to peel away any healthy remaining attachments of the deep fibers. A rongeur is again used to prepare the bony fovea for anchor placement.

We prefer to use a suture anchor placed directly into the anatomic foveal insertion because this technique restores the anatomy and facilitates repair. The suture anchor is typically double loaded to provide 4 suture limbs and is used to repair the TFCC with 2 horizontal mattress sutures (**Fig. 9**). Peripheral suture repairs can be added as necessary. More recently, fixation of unstable peripheral tears have been accomplished with knotless suture anchors. These devices provide strong, stable fixation and obviate the need for knots tied distal to the articular disc.

The dorsal capsule is then repaired, the ECU tendon is returned to its compartment, and the extensor retinaculum is repaired directly or with a step cut repair. The skin is then closed with 4-0 Prolene sutures.

Although stable, superficial radioulnar ligament tears are often treated with an arthroscopic outside-in technique, a similar open approach can be performed for these tears if preferred. Instead of a DRUJ capsulotomy as described, we perform an L-shaped capsulotomy over the ulnocarpal joint distal to the TFCC. The peripheral torn fibers from the styloid are then repaired to the ECU subsheath at the proximal ulnar margin of the TFCC.

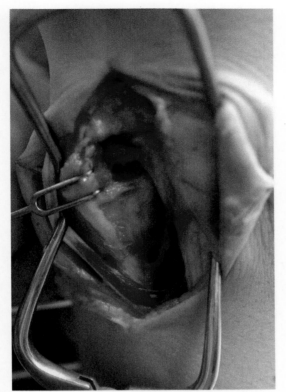

Fig. 6. The distal ulna approach through the fifth dorsal compartment. The extensor digiti quinti proprius has been retracted and a capsulotomy reveals the ulnar head with a large peripheral TFCC tear.

Postoperative care

A soft, well-padded bulky dressing is placed followed by a long arm splint with the elbow at 90° and the forearm in neutral rotation. This is considered the tightest position and shortest length of both the volar and dorsal radioulnar ligaments. Immobilization is continued until approximately 4 to 6 weeks, at which point range of motion is initiated. Strengthening is started at approximately 3 months postoperatively. We limit aggressive return forearm rotational activities until approximately 6 months after reconstruction of a destabilizing TFCC injury.

Complications

A lack of ligament healing and re-rupture are primary concerns. Stiffness may occur with prolonged immobilization and should be addressed with aggressive therapy after healing of the repair. Sensory paresthesias can occur if care is not taken to identify and protect the dorsal sensory branch of the ulnar nerve, which crosses the wrist obliquely just distal to the ulnar styloid.

Ulnocarpal Impaction

Ulnocarpal impaction is a degenerative condition that results from abutment of the distal ulna against the ulnar carpus and results in excessive load across the ulnocarpal joint. It occurs more commonly in patients with positive ulnar variance. Ulnar variance

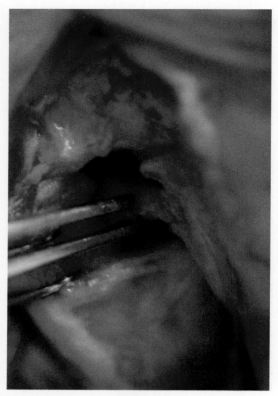

Fig. 7. The forceps grasps the periphery of the TFCC.

is dynamic, and ulnar length increases with grip and pronation.[31] Athletes who frequently perform repetitive pronation and power grip, as seen in baseball and racquet sports, may be affected by this condition.

Anatomy and biomechanics

In the ulnar neutral wrist, approximately 16% to 20% of the load across the wrist is received by the ulnocarpal joint. The TFCC helps with load bearing across the ulna, and increased thickness of the TFCC has been found to be associated with ulnar negative variance.[32] Increasing the length of the ulna by 2.5 mm has been shown to increase ulnocarpal loading to 42%. Conversely, decreasing the ulnar length by 2.5 mm has been shown to decrease ulnocarpal load to 4% of total load across the wrist.[2] Increased load across the ulnocarpal joint leads to progressive deterioration of the central TFCC, ulnar head, lunate, and lunotriquetral interface.

In young gymnasts, axial loads across the wrist can lead to progressive premature physeal closure of the distal radius.[33] This growth arrest may increase the risk for ulnar-positive variance and ulnocarpal abutment once skeletal maturity is reached.

Ulnar styloid impaction can be seen in patients with excessively long ulnar styloids; however, this condition is very distinct from ulnocarpal impaction (**Fig. 10**). Ulnar styloid impaction is different from ulnocarpal impaction in that the styloid impinges on the triquetrum during supination, causing wear of the meniscus homologue as well as chondromalacia at the tip of the styloid and triquetrum.[8]

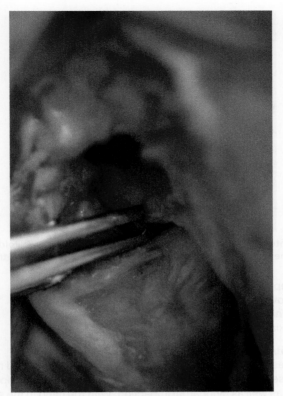

Fig. 8. The TFCC is not retracted and can easily be brought down to its anatomic location at the fovea.

Patient history

Ulnocarpal impaction tends to present in the absence of an acute injury, unlike acute TFCC injuries. Patients may present with more insidious onset of symptoms and vague ulnar-sided wrist pain.

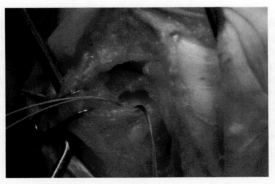

Fig. 9. Sutures have been placed in the fovea in preparation for anatomic repair of the TFCC to its foveal origin.

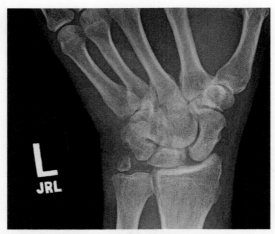

Fig. 10. Posteroanterior radiograph of the wrist showing an ulnar styloid nonunion with impaction onto the triquetrum and resultant cystic changes in the triquetrum.

- Pain with repetitive pronation
- Pain with power grip
- Pain with ulnar deviation
- Pain with axial loading across wrist

Physical examination
Patients often present with focal tenderness in the fovea or prestyloid recess. Tenderness may be present over the lunate. The ulnocarpal stress test is helpful to diagnosis TFCC pathology as well as ulnocarpal impaction. With the hand in the standard examining position with the forearm and wrist in neutral, the patient's wrist is brought into ulnar deviation and with an axial load. The wrist is then passively brought into pronation and supination. Pain or painful clicking or crepitation indicates a positive test.[34] With ulnar styloid impaction, the forearm is placed into neutral rotation, the wrist is then brought into full extension, and the forearm is maximally supinated to bring the dorsal triquetrum in closest proximity to the ulnar styloid. The triquetrum and styloid are separated by the ulnocarpal meniscal homologue. Reproduction of pain is considered a positive test for ulnar styloid impaction.[35]

Imaging
Zero-rotation posteroanterior and lateral radiographs are obtained and assessed for ulnar variance. A pronated or grip view can be helpful if dynamic ulnar variance is suspected. The lunate should be evaluated for presence of cystic changes or subchondral sclerosis that may occur with abutment. The length of the ulnar styloid can also be assessed for possible triquetral impingement. Although ulnocarpal impaction is largely a clinical diagnosis, MRI can be helpful to characterize changes to the lunate as well as evaluate for TFCC tears, which are most commonly central disc tears (**Fig. 11**). It can also help to differentiate from Kienbock's disease, which demonstrates edema within the lunate as opposed to impaction, where radiographic changes tend to be confined to the ulnar aspect of the lunate.

Treatment
Nonoperative treatment Delaying operative treatment for degenerative TFCC tears usually does not have any effect on long-term outcomes. Thus, symptom

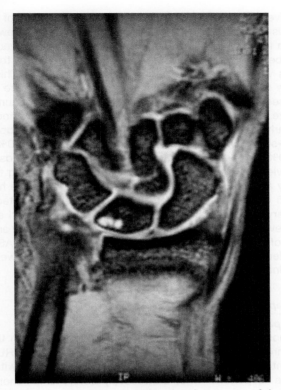

Fig. 11. Coronal T2 MRI scan showing cysts within the ulnar aspect of the lunate which can be consistent with ulnar impaction syndrome.

management to allow athletes to continue through their season is often attempted. Bracing or wrist taping is initiated as a first-line treatment. Semirigid bracing that blocks full ulnar deviation and full wrist extension can be used during play. Anti-inflammatories and injections can help with acute exacerbation of symptoms. The literature is scant regarding the outcomes of conservative treatment; however, a single study found that 60% of patients treated conservatively with a short arm cast for 4 weeks, followed by interval splinting and physical therapy, had improvements in their symptoms at 24 weeks.[36]

Operative treatment Treatment options for ulnocarpal impaction typically involve arthroscopic debridement of central TFCC tears and addressing ulnar positive variance in an attempt to decrease the load through the ulnocarpal joint. This goal can be accomplished via multiple treatment options, including an open or arthroscopic wafer procedure, ulnar shortening osteotomy, or distal ulnar metaphyseal closing wedge osteotomy. The wafer procedure entails partial excision of 2 to 3 mm of the distal ulna while preserving the styloid and TFCC.[37] The advantages of the wafer procedure include the avoidance of symptomatic hardware and nonunion, both of which are complications seen with the ulnar-shortening osteotomy. Ulnar shortening osteotomy is commonly performed and has the additional potential advantage of tightening the extrinsic ligaments in addition to decreasing ulnar length. It also preserves the ulnar articular cartilage. The ulnar shortening osteotomy involves resection of approximately 2 mm or more of the diaphyseal distal ulna. This is then fixed with a compression plate and lag screw. An alternative treatment option includes the distal ulnar metaphyseal closing wedge osteotomy, originally described by Slade.[38] This technique has been shown to be effective in treating athletes with ulnocarpal impaction without instability. This osteotomy is performed in the metaphysis just proximal to the articular surface and avoids the disadvantages seen in ulnar shortening osteotomy, such as nonunion and symptomatic hardware. The superiority of the specific treatment method has not been established clearly. In a systematic review comparing arthroscopic wafer, open wafer, and ulnar-shortening osteotomy, satisfaction rates were 100% for the arthroscopic wafer, 89% for open wafer, and 84% for ulnar-shortening osteotomy.[39] In a retrospective review by Constantine and colleagues[37] comparing the ulnar shortening osteotomy and open wafer procedure, all patients but one had satisfactory pain relief and 5 of 11 patients undergoing ulnar-shortening osteotomy required secondary surgery for painful hardware or delayed union. Khouri and Hammert[40] retrospectively reviewed the ulnar metaphyseal wedge osteotomy and found radiographic healing of all patients at 6 to 8 weeks and an average DASH score of 13. The authors prefer treatment with the ulnar metaphyseal closing wedge osteotomy or the oblique ulnar-shortening osteotomy.

Distal Ulnar Metaphyseal Closing Wedge Osteotomy

Preparation and patient positioning

The patient is positioned supine with the arm stretched out on the hand table. Frequently, arthroscopic evaluation is performed of the DRUJ and TFCC with debridement of the TFCC. It may be difficult in patients with severe ulnar positive variance to perform wrist arthroscopy before ulnar shortening osteotomy, and this procedure can be done after osteotomy to help gain access within the wrist.

Surgical approach

An approach to the DRUJ is made with a dorsal incision through the fifth dorsal compartment. The extensor digiti quinti proprius is retracted ulnarly, and an L-shaped capsulotomy is made through the dorsal DRUJ capsule proximal to the TFCC. If there are concomitant TFCC tears that are felt to be amenable to open repair, a distal ulnocarpal arthrotomy can also be made at this time to access the TFCC.

Procedure

After exposing the distal ulna and protecting the volar capsule as well as the volar neurovascular structures, a radially based closing wedge osteotomy is made. K-wires are used to help plan the location of the cuts. The distal cut is parallel to the distal ulnar pole articular cartilage, and the proximal diagonal cut is made anywhere from 2 to 5 mm to the distal cut (**Fig. 12**). A single headless compression screw is then passed through the dorsal radial corner, across the osteotomy, and into the diaphyseal ulnar cortex (**Fig. 13**). The capsule and extensor retinaculum are then closed, followed by skin closure.

Postoperative care

A soft, sterile bulky dressing is placed and the wrist is immobilized in a short arm splint. Immobilization is continue for 4 to 6 weeks or until bony union is achieved. Range of motion is initiated in a stepwise fashion once union is seen.

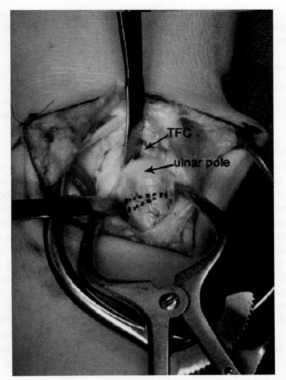

Fig. 12. Anatomic specimen showing osteotomy cuts for the distal ulnar metaphyseal closing wedge osteotomy.

Complications

Decrease in ulnar length alters the peak pressures seen by the DRUJ and can potentially lead to altered mechanics and resultant degenerative changes at the DRUJ. Care

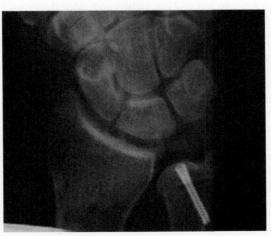

Fig. 13. Posteroanterior radiograph demonstrating headless compression screw fixation of closing wedge osteotomy of distal ulnar metaphysis.

must be taken to avoid overshortening. Additionally, specific care must be taken to identify and protect the dorsal sensory branch of the ulnar nerve. Complications such as nonunion are still possible.

Extensor Carpi Ulnaris Conditions

Disorders involving the ECU tendon can affect many athletes, especially those who participate in racquet or stick-handling sports. Injuries can range from tenosynovitis to subluxation or dislocation of the tendon associated with either acute or chronic overuse injuries.

Anatomy and biomechanics

The ECU tendon is contained within the sixth dorsal compartment within a groove along the dorsal ulna and is contained within its own fibro-osseous tunnel along the distal 1.5 to 2.0 cm of the ulna.[41] It is typically well-tethered in this location owing to its subsheath and contributions from the extensor retinaculum. The extensor retinaculum is composed of 2 layers, the supratendinous and infratendinous layers.[42] The ECU fibro-osseous tunnel includes its subsheath, formed from duplications of the infratendinous layer of the retinaculum and is covered by the supratendinous retinaculum superiorly. Ulnarly, it is bounded by the sixth septum and as well as by the linea jugata, which is the ulnar insertion of the retinaculum.[42] The ECU tendon inserts onto the base of the fifth metacarpal. Its direction of insertion depends on the position of the wrist: with the wrist in supination, the tendon exits the subsheath at approximately 30°, whereas in pronation, the ECU tendon exits the subsheath longitudinally.[43] Thus, with high supination, ulnar deviation and wrist flexion forces, the tension on the subsheath is greatest.[43] These loads placed on the ECU tendon can lead to tendonitis, subluxation or dislocation, and traumatic or attritional rupture.

Patient history

Athletes involved in racket or stick-handling sports are often affected; however, any athlete who performs repetitive pronation/supination as well as radial/ulnar deviation can have ECU pathology. Patients may report pain over the course of the ECU tendon, as well as pain with forceful gripping, wrist extension, or ulnar deviation. This pain may be associated with a single forceful supination and ulnar deviation event, or its onset may be more gradual. Patients with ECU tendonitis may report a chronic dorsal ulnar wrist pain and symptoms of tenosynovitis.

Physical examination

It is important when evaluating for ECU tendonitis to ensure that causes of intra-articular ulnar-sided wrist pain are ruled out before proceeding with treatment for extra-articular pathology.

With the forearm in the standard examining position, the ECU tendon should be palpated along its course for pain indicative of tendinopathy. With the wrist in extension, the forearm should be rotated into pronation and supination. Instability may present with painful subluxation of the tendon or frank dislocation out of the groove with wrist extension, ulnar deviation, and supination. Pain may be present with resisted wrist extension and ulnar deviation, and patients may demonstrate weakness of the ECU.

The ECU synergy test has been shown to be helpful in differentiating between intra-articular and extra-articular pathology. This test is performed with the forearm on the examining table with fingers to the ceiling and forearm in full supination. The examiner grasps the patient's thumb and middle finger with one hand and uses the other hand to palpate the ECU tendon, while the patient radially abducts the thumb against resistance (**Fig. 14**). A positive test results in reproduction of the patient's pain along the course of the tendon or bowstringing.[44] Another test recently described is the ice-cream scoop test, where the patient is asked to perform a scooping or hypersupination motion from the position of pronation, ulnar deviation, and extension. Subluxation of tendons is a positive test for ECU instability.[45,46]

Imaging
Zero-rotation posteroanterior and lateral radiographs are helpful for initial evaluation and for establishing ulnar variance. Recently, negative ulnar variance has been suggested to be associated with ECU pathology.[47] Ultimately, MRI is the most sensitive imaging modality to evaluate the ECU tendon and identify the presence of ECU tears, as well as

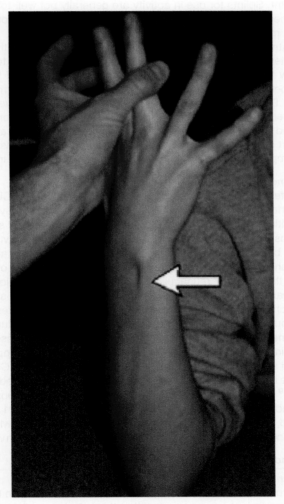

Fig. 14. ECU synergy test showing tendon bowstringing (*arrow* depicts prominent ECU tendon) under the skin.

tendonitis and tenosynovitis within the sixth dorsal compartment. Shallow ECU tendon grooves have been suggested to be associated with ECU pathology and can be evaluated on axial MRI; however, this connection has not been well-established.[47,48] Ultrasound examination has been found to be useful in identifying fluid around the tendon as well as its ability to perform a dynamic evaluation of tendon subluxation.[49] However, ECU abnormalities can be commonly seen on ultrasound in asymptomatic subjects. Therefore, caution must be used when interpreting ultrasound studies. A study of asymptomatic tennis players demonstrated static ECU tendon abnormalities in 75% of volunteers, with 92% of players exhibiting tendinosis and 42% of players demonstrating signs of instability, primarily in the form of subluxation.[50]

Nonoperative treatment

The mainstay of treatment for ECU tenosynovitis is nonoperative. Anti-inflammatories, ultrasound treatments, massage, and cold therapy may be helpful in addition to a resting wrist splint. Splints for use in activity are generally not well-tolerated and can alter shooting mechanics.[51] For refractory tendonitis, injection of corticosteroid into the ECU sheath may be helpful.

The initial treatment of ECU instability is typically nonoperative, with immobilization in pronation, extension, and slight radial deviation, for as long as 6 to 8 weeks in an attempt to allow the subsheath to scar down to the ulnar edge of the groove.[52,53] For athletes, operative treatment may be considered as first-line management for acute traumatic ECU instability; however, there are reports of athletes undergoing successful conservative treatment after an acute instability event. Montalvan and colleagues[54] treated 5 elite tennis players with complete, acute subluxation of the ECU tendon in a short arm cast in 15° of wrist extension for 2 to 3 months, with complete resolution of symptoms and return to play at 5 to 6 months after injury.

Operative treatment

For recalcitrant tenosynovitis despite nonoperative measures, an ECU tenosynovectomy can be performed. However, instability may coexist with tenosynovitis. If instability is the limiting symptom for sports participation, there are several surgical treatment options. Acute traumatic ECU dislocation may have an avulsed periosteal sleeve that can be addressed with transosseus fixation or suture anchors.[55] More commonly, the sheath may be torn and need to be directly repaired or reconstructed with the use of the extensor retinaculum. Multiple operative techniques have been described. Eckhardt and Palmer[56] described using a free graft of a strip of extensor retinaculum. Ruchelsman and Vitale[57] endorsed a radially based extensor retinacular sling passed around the tendon and secured to the native retinaculum near the fifth dorsal compartment. Other techniques include a slip of the FCU passed through an osseous tunnel in the distal ulna, or a strip of the retinaculum wrapped around the ECU tendon and secured into drill holes in the ulnar border of the ECU.[53,55]

Our preference is to perform an anatomic reconstruction as described by MacLennan and colleagues,[49] where the ECU groove is deepened and the ECU subsheath and retinaculum is then advanced and anchored into position. In their study of 21 patients treated with this method, 95% of patients returned to the activity during which their injury occurred and an increase in wrist range of motion as well as grip strength was observed.[49]

Anatomic Extensor Carpi Ulnaris Subsheath Reconstruction

Preoperative planning

MRI or dynamic ultrasound examination can be used to evaluate the ECU tendon as well as groove dysplasia; however, we feel that this is largely a clinical diagnosis and rarely use MRI to make the diagnosis.

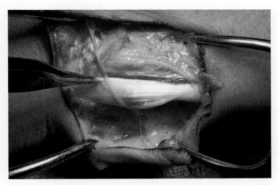

Fig. 15. The sixth dorsal compartment has been opened revealing a subluxated ECU tendon.

Preparation and patient positioning

The patient is placed supine with a nonsterile tourniquet on the upper extremity and the hand placed in pronation on the hand table.

Procedure

A dorsal approach to the wrist is performed with a longitudinal incision made centered over the ECU tendon. Full-thickness flaps are then raised above the extensor retinaculum. Care is taken to protect the dorsal sensory branch of the ulnar nerve. The retinaculum overlying the ECU is then incised along its ulnar margin and reflected radially. Alternatively, the retinaculum may be incised along its ulnar margin to use as a sling. The ECU subsheath is then elevated separately from the retinacular flap in a radial direction (**Figs. 15** and **16**). The ECU is inspected and debrided of any tenosynovium. The undersurface should be carefully inspected as tendinopathy is frequently noted on the deep surface despite a normal appearing superficial surface of the tendon (**Fig. 17**). A high-speed bur is then used to deepen the groove, about 2 to 3 mm, or as dictated by thickness of the tendon, and the subsheath is then repaired (**Fig. 18**). Suture anchors are then placed along the ulnar margin of the ECU groove, and the extensor retinaculum and the sheath are advanced to stabilize the tendon within its groove (**Fig. 19**). If a sling is created instead, deepening of the groove is not necessary, and the flap will be passed volar to the tendon and sutured back to itself to provide a stabilizing sling.

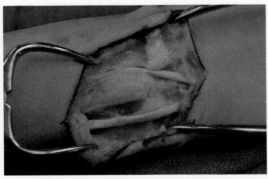

Fig. 16. In a different patient, the sixth compartment has been opened in preparation for an anatomic reconstruction and stabilization of the ECU.

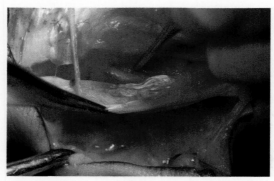

Fig. 17. The undersurface of the tendon reveals a significant area of tendinosis and delamination secondary to mechanical tendon irritation owing to subluxation over the bony prominence on the volar rim of the sixth compartment.

Postoperative care

A soft, well-padded bulky dressing is placed followed by a long arm splint for approximately 6 weeks. Wrist flexion and extension is started at 2 to 3 weeks, but pronation and supination are limited until 6 weeks. After recovery of range of motion, light activity is gradually initiated and progressed to strengthening, followed lastly by pronosupination strengthening. Return to sport is typically around 4 to 6 months postoperatively.

Complications

Instability is the major complication. Overtightening of the repair can strangulate the tendon. Aggressive retraction or lack of identification of the dorsal sensory branches of the ulnar nerve may result in paresthesias.

Flexor Carpi Ulnaris Conditions

Anatomy and biomechanics

The FCU tendon originates from the medial epicondyle and posteromedial ulna, and inserts onto the pisiform, hamate, and base of the fifth metacarpal. The FCU tendon helps to transfer ulnar wrist forces to the hand, as well as providing strong flexion

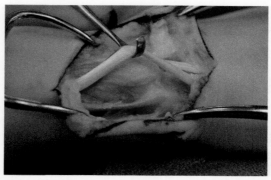

Fig. 18. The ECU tendon has been retracted and the groove deepened with a high-speed burr.

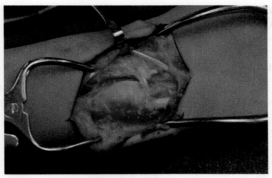

Fig. 19. The ECU has been relocated into the deepened groove and the retinaculum has been reefed to eliminate patulous tissue and provides an anatomic restraint to tendon instability.

and ulnar deviation of the wrist. Unlike the ECU tendon, it is not encased in a sheath and, thus, does not develop stenosing tenosynovitis. FCU tendonitis can present as calcific tendonitis or as a noncalcific tendinopathy.

Patient history
Patients may present with pain along the course of the FCU tendon that may be associated with a forceful ulnar deviating event, or may be more insidious and occur with

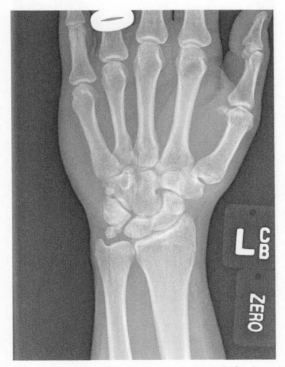

Fig. 20. Posteroanterior radiograph of wrist demonstrates calcific deposits along the ulnar aspect of the wrist.

repetitive flexion and ulnar deviation. Typically, the pain is activity related. In cases of calcific tendonitis, local inflammatory response may be so intense and acute that it may resemble gout or septic arthritis.

Physical examination

- Tenderness along the course of the FCU tendon. It is important to note that the pain along the FCU tendon is approximately 3 cm proximal to the pisiform, as to not confuse with pain at the pisotriquetral joint.[58]

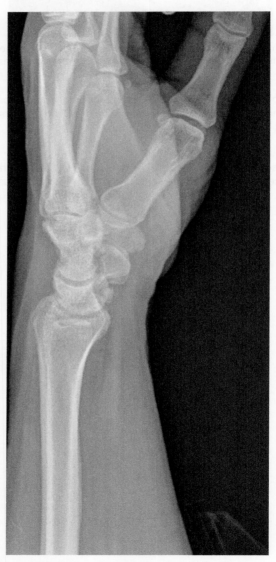

Fig. 21. Lateral radiograph of the wrist demonstrates calcific deposits just proximal to the pisiform along the course of the FCU tendon.

- Pain with resisted wrist flexion and ulnar deviation.
- Calcific tendonitis may present with swelling and erythema diffusely about the wrist.

Imaging
Radiographs of the wrist should include a pisotriquetral view to rule out the presence of pisotriquetral arthritis. Radiographs may demonstrate calcific deposits along the FCU tendon (**Figs. 20** and **21**).

Nonoperative treatment
Conservative management is the mainstay of treatment, and should consist of splint immobilization and anti-inflammatory medications, with physical therapy focusing on stretching and strengthening. Steroid injections may be indicated as well. Conservative treatment has been cited to result in symptom resolution in an average of 12 days with the use of a splint, and shortened to 1 week with the use of anti-inflammatories; however, no studies to the authors' knowledge have described rates of progression to operative treatment.[59]

Operative treatment
Operative debridement of the FCU tendon has been described for recalcitrant cases. As described by Budoff and associates,[58] this technique is performed with a longitudinal incision within the FCU tendon and removal of all degenerative tissue, followed by a side-side closure. Postoperatively, patients are splinted for a week and then allowed to start range of motion. At 1 year, all patients had complete or near complete relief of all symptoms.[58]

SUMMARY

Ulnar-sided wrist pain in athletes is common and can include a multitude of pathologies owing to the specific demands of the athlete. However, through careful diagnosis physical examination, and imaging modalities, the diagnosis can be made confidently and treatment can be initiated, taking into account the specific needs and goals of the athlete.

CONFLICT OF INTEREST

Each author certifies that he or she has no commercial associations that might pose a conflict of interest in connection with the submitted article. No funding or financial support was received for this project.

REFERENCES

1. Kleinman WB. Stability of the distal radioulnar joint: diagnosis, and restoration of function what we have learned in 25 years. J Hand Surg Am 2007;32(7): 1086–106.
2. Palmer AK, Werner FW. Biomechanics of the distal radioulnar joint. Clin Orthop Relat Res 1984;(187):26–35.
3. Sachar K. Ulnar-sided wrist pain: evaluation and treatment of triangular fibrocartilage complex tears, ulnocarpal impaction syndrome, and lunotriquetral ligament tears. J Hand Surg Am 2012;37(7):1489–500.
4. Bednar MS, Arnoczky SP, Weiland AJ. The microvasculature of the triangular fibrocartilage complex: its clinical significance. J Hand Surg Am 1991;16(6): 1101–5.

5. Moritomo H. The distal interosseous membrane: current concepts in wrist anatomy and biomechanics. J Hand Surg Am 2012;37(7):1501–7.

6. Tay SC, Tomita K, Berger RA. The "ulnar fovea sign" for defining ulnar wrist pain: an analysis of sensitivity and specificity. J Hand Surg Am 2007;32(4):438–44.

7. Kleinman WB. Diagnostic exams for ligamentous injuries. American Society for Surgery of the Hand, Correspondence Club Newsletter. Denver (CO): American Society for Surgery of the Hand; 1985. p. 51.

8. Kaplan FTD. Examination of the ulnar wrist. In: Greenberg JA, editor. Ulnar-sided wrist pain: a master skills publication. Chicago: American Society for Surgery of the Hand; 2013. p. 33–44.

9. Linscheid RL. Examination of the wrist. In: Nakamura RL, Miura T, editors. Wrist disord curr concepts challenges. Tokyo: Springer-Verlag; 1992. p. 13–25.

10. Lee YH, Choi YR, Kim S, et al. Intrinsic ligament and triangular fibrocartilage complex (TFCC) tears of the wrist: comparison of isovolumetric 3D-THRIVE sequence MR arthrography and conventional MR image at 3T. Magn Reson Imaging 2013;31(2):221–6.

11. Smith TO, Drew B, Toms AP, et al. Diagnostic accuracy of magnetic resonance imaging and magnetic resonance arthrography for triangular fibrocartilaginous complex injury: a systematic review and meta-analysis. J Bone Joint Surg Am 2012;94:824–32.

12. Trehan SK, Wall LB, Calfee RP, et al. Arthroscopic diagnosis of the triangular fibrocartilage complex foveal tear: cadaver assessment. J Hand Surg Am 2018; 43(7):680.e1–5.

13. Greene RM, Kakar S. The suction test: a novel technique to identify and verify successful repair of peripheral triangular fibrocartilage complex tears. J Wrist Surg 2017;6(4):334–5.

14. Park MJ, Jagadish A, Yao J. The rate of triangular fibrocartilage injuries requiring surgical intervention. Orthopedics 2010;33(11). https://doi.org/10.3928/01477447-20100924-03.

15. Palmer AK. Triangular fibrocartilage complex lesions: a classification. J Hand Surg Am 1989;14(4):594–606.

16. Ko JH, Wiedrich TA. Triangular fibrocartilage complex injuries in the elite athlete. Hand Clin 2012;28(3):307–21.

17. Atzei A, Luchetti R. Foveal TFCC tear classification and treatment. Hand Clin 2011;27(3):263–72.

18. Westkaemper JG, Mitsionis G, Giannakopoulos RN, et al. Wrist arthroscopy for the treatment of ligament and triangular fibrocartilage complex injuries. Arthroscopy 1998;14(5):479–83.

19. Whipple TL. The role of arthroscopy in the treatment of wrist injuries in the athlete. Clin Sports Med 1998;17(3):623–34.

20. Miwa H, Hashizume H, Fujiwara K, et al. Arthroscopic surgery for traumatic triangular fibrocartilage. J Orthop Sci 2004;9(4):354–9.

21. Minami A, Ishikawa J, Suenaga N. Clinical results of treatment of triangular fibrocartilage complex tears by arthroscopic debridement. J Hand Surg Am 1996; 21(3):406–11.

22. Arsalan-Werner A, Gruter L, Mehling IM, et al. Results after arthroscopic treatment of central traumatic lesions of the triangular fibrocartilage complex. Arch Orthop Trauma Surg 2018;5(138):731–7.

23. Adams BD. Partial excision of the triangular fibrocartilage complex articular disk: a biomechanical study. J Hand Surg Am 1993;18(2):334–40.

24. Wysocki RW, Richard MJ, Crowe MM, et al. Arthroscopic treatment of peripheral triangular fibrocartilage complex tears with the deep fibers intact. J Hand Surg Am 2012;37(3):509–16.

25. McAdams TR, Swan J, Yao J. Arthroscopic treatment of triangular fibrocartilage wrist injuries in the athlete. Am J Sports Med 2009;37(2):291–7.

26. Yao J, Lee AT. All-arthroscopic repair of palmer 1B triangular fibrocartilage complex tears using the FasT-Fix device. J Hand Surg Am 2011;36(5):836–42.

27. Geissler WB. Arthroscopic knotless peripheral ulnar-sided TFCC repair. Hand Clin 2011;27(3):273–9.

28. Abe Y, Fujii K, Fujisawa T. Midterm results after open versus arthroscopic transosseous repair for foveal tears of the triangular fibrocartilage complex. J Wrist Surg 2018;7(4):292–7.

29. Luchetti R, Atzei A, Cozzollino R, et al. Comparison between open and arthroscopic-assisted foveal triangular fibrocartilage complex repair for posttraumatic distal radio-ulnar joint instability. J Hand Surg Eur Vol 2014;39(8):845–55.

30. Anderson ML, Larson AN, Moran SL, et al. Clinical comparison of arthroscopic versus open repair of triangular fibrocartilage complex tears. J Hand Surg Am 2008;33(5):675–82.

31. Friedman SL, Palmer AK, Short WH, et al. The change in ulnar variance with grip. J Hand Surg Am 1993;18(4):713–6.

32. Palmer A, Glisson R, Werner FW. Relationship between ulnar variance, and triangular fibrocartilage complex thickness. J Hand Surg Am 1984;9:681–2.

33. Chawla A, Wiesler ER. Nonspecific wrist pain in gymnasts and cheerleaders. Clin Sports Med 2015;34(1):143–9.

34. Nakamura R, Horii E, Imaeda T, et al. The ulnocarpal stress test in the diagnosis of ulnar-sided wrist pain. J Hand Surg Br 1997;22(6):719–23.

35. Topper SM, Wood MB, Ruby LK. Ulnar styloid impaction syndrome. J Hand Surg Am 1997;22(4):699–704.

36. Roh YH, Kim S, Gong HS, et al. Prognostic value of clinical and radiological findings for conservative treatment of idiopathic ulnar impaction syndrome. Sci Rep 2018;8(1):9891.

37. Constantine KJ, Tomaino MM, Herndon JH, et al. Comparison of ulnar shortening osteotomy and the wafer resection procedure as treatment for ulnar impaction syndrome. J Hand Surg Am 2000;25(1):55–60.

38. Slade JF 3rd, Gillon TJ. Osteochondral shortening osteotomy for the treatment of ulnar impaction syndrome: a new technique. Tech Hand Up Extrem Surg 2007; 11(1):74–82.

39. Stockton DJ, Pelletier ME, Pike JM. Operative treatment of ulnar impaction syndrome: a systematic review. J Hand Surg Eur Vol 2015;40(5):470–6.

40. Khouri JS, Hammert WC. Distal metaphyseal ulnar shortening osteotomy: technique , pearls, and outcomes. J Wrist Surg 2014;1(212):175–80.

41. Spinner M, Kaplan EB. Extensor carpi ulnaris. Its relationship to the stability of the distal radio-ulnar joint. Clin Orthop Relat Res 1970;68:124–9.

42. Taleisnik J, Gelberman RH, Miller BW, et al. The extensor retinaculum of the wrist. J Hand Surg Am 1984;9(4):495–501.

43. Campbell D, Campbell R, O'Connor P, et al. Sports-related extensor carpi ulnaris pathology: a review of functional anatomy, sports injury and management. Br J Sports Med 2013;47(17):1105–11.

44. Ruland RT, Hogan CJ. The ECU synergy test: an aid to diagnose. J Hand Surg Am 2008;33(10):1777–82.

45. Pang EQ, Yao J. Ulnar-sided wrist pain in the athlete (TFCC/DRUJ/ECU). Curr Rev Musculoskelet Med 2017;10(1):53–61.
46. Ng CY, Hayton MJ. Ice cream scoop test: a novel clinical test to diagnose extensor carpi ulnaris instability. J Hand Surg Eur Vol 2013;38(5):569–70.
47. Chang CY, Huang AJ, Bredella MA, et al. Association between distal ulnar morphology and extensor carpi ulnaris tendon pathology. Skeletal Radiol 2014; 43(6):793–800.
48. Iorio ML, Bayomy AF, Huang JI. Morphology of the extensor carpi ulnaris groove and tendon. J Hand Surg Am 2014;39(12):2412–6.
49. MacLennan AJ, Nemechek NM, Waitayawinyu T, et al. Diagnosis and anatomic reconstruction of extensor carpi ulnaris subluxation. J Hand Surg Am 2008; 33(1):59–64.
50. Sole JS, Wisniewski SJ, Newcomer KL, et al. Sonographic evaluation of the extensor carpi ulnaris in asymptomatic tennis players. PM R 2015;7(3):255–63.
51. Smith DW. ECU tendonitis and subluxation in elite basketball. Hand Clin 2012; 28(3):359–60.
52. Iorio ML, Huang JI. Extensor carpi ulnaris subluxation. J Hand Surg Am 2014; 39(7):1400–2.
53. Burkhart SS, Wood MB, Linscheid RL. Posttraumatic recurrent subluxation of the extensor carpi ulnaris tendon. J Hand Surg Am 1982;7(1):1–3.
54. Montalvan B, Parier J, Brasseur JL, et al. Extensor carpi ulnaris injuries in tennis players: a study of 28 cases. Br J Sports Med 2006;40(5):424–9.
55. Inoue G, Tamura Y. Surgical treatment for recurrent dislocation of the extensor carpi ulnaris tendon. J Hand Surg Br 2001;26(6):556–9.
56. Eckhardt WA, Palmer AK. Recurrent dislocation of extensor carpi ulnaris tendon. J Hand Surg Am 1981;6(6):629–31.
57. Ruchelsman DE, Vitale MA. Extensor carpi ulnaris subsheath reconstruction. J Hand Surg Am 2016;41(11):e433–9.
58. Budoff JE, Kraushaar BS, Valley S, et al. Flexor carpi ulnaris tendinopathy. J Hand Surg Am 2005;30:125–9.
59. Dilley DF, Tonkin MA. Acute calcific tendonitis in the hand and wrist. J Hand Surg Br 1991;16(2):215–6.

Management of Metacarpal and Phalangeal Fractures in the Athlete

Elizabeth P. Wahl, MD*, Marc J. Richard, MD

KEYWORDS

- Hand injuries • Metacarpal fractures • Phalangeal fractures • Athlete

KEY POINTS

- Metacarpal and phalangeal fractures are common injuries in athletes and usually result from low-energy, direct hits to the fingers and thumb.
- Contact sports, in particular football, account for most metacarpal and phalangeal fractures.
- Consideration of the degree of injury, the specific sport, the timing of the injury, the level of play, and the athlete's goals must be made when developing a treatment plan.
- Return to play can be expedited with early fixation, playing casts, and an emphasis on early range of motion.

INTRODUCTION

Metacarpal and phalangeal fractures account for 18% and 23%, respectively, of below-elbow fractures in the general population in the United States and are the most common injuries of the upper extremity.[1–4] In the sporting world, injuries to the hand and wrist account for 2% to 9% of all injuries, with some studies reporting that metacarpal and phalangeal fractures account for 39.2% of all sports-related fractures.[5–7] These fractures are more likely to occur in male athletes between the ages of 10 years and 40 years.[2,3,7] Rates of injuries vary by sport, with higher rates in contact sports and approximately half occurring in football..[8,9]

Participation in sports during childhood and adolescence has nearly doubled in the United States in the past 4 decades, leading to a similar increase in sporting injuries.[8] Hand fractures are the most common fractures sustained by children, and hand and wrist injuries account for up to 17% of sporting injuries in children.[8,10]

Athletes represent a unique population due to the high level of physical demand for function and the potential significant monetary impact injury has on players, whether

Department of Orthopaedic Surgery, Duke University Medical Center, 4709 Creekstone Drive, Durham, NC 27703, USA
* Corresponding author.
E-mail address: elizabeth.wahl@duke.edu

Clin Sports Med 39 (2020) 401–422
https://doi.org/10.1016/j.csm.2019.12.002
0278-5919/20/© 2019 Elsevier Inc. All rights reserved.

scholarship opportunity for high school or collegiate athletes or loss of income for elite and professional athletes.[11] Not only are these opportunities at risk in the short term due to loss of playing time from injury recovery but also there is potential risk for long-term functional hand impairment after an athletic career.[12] Because of this, thoughtful consideration of the treatment plan and fixation method is warranted for these fractures. The treating surgeon must take into account the specific sport being played, whether the athlete will finish the season, and the return-to-play time in order to proceed with a plan that is in best interest of the athlete.

ANATOMY

The metacarpals form a concave, transverse arch that is fixed proximally via the strong articulations with the distal carpal row at the carpometacarpal (CMC) joints and is more mobile and adaptive distally at the metacarpophalangeal (MCP) joints.[13,14] There are 4 finger metacarpals and 1 thumb metacarpal. The finger metacarpals articulate with the neighboring metacarpal proximally; they are attached to each other via strong interosseous ligaments and distally via the deep transverse metacarpal ligament (**Fig. 1**).[9,13,14]

The index finger metacarpal is the largest in length and diameter whereas the ring finger metacarpal is the smallest in diameter and the small finger metacarpal is the shortest in length.[9] Furthermore, the index and long finger metacarpals essentially are fixed at the CMC joints whereas the ring and small finger CMC joints allow for 15° to 25° of ring and small finger CMC joints, respectively.[15] This discrepancy in CMC joint stability gives the hand the ability to have a strong grasp while at the same time accommodate different-shaped objects.

The increased mobility of the ring and small finger CMC joints places them at higher risk for fracture and/or dislocation yet also allows for a greater degree of acceptable angulation and displacement after fracture.[12,13,16] Additionally, the border (index and small finger) metacarpals are more likely to shorten compared with the long and ring finger because they have fewer soft tissue attachments.[9,12,13,17]

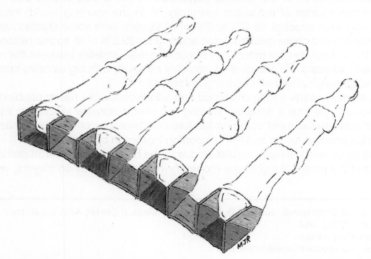

Fig. 1. The deep transverse metacarpal ligament (*green*) connects the nonthumb metacarpals (not shown) to each other at their distal end. The volar plates (*dark blue*) are interconnected via the deep transverse ligament.

The thumb metacarpal has a pronated position relative to the other metacarpals. It has a unique, saddle articulation with the trapezium featuring 2 biconcave surfaces, giving the thumb the unique motion of opposition as well as motion in the other 2 planes that helps provide 40% of hand function.[13,15,18,19]

The MCP joints consist of the metacarpal head and the base of the proximal phalanx. The metacarpal head has a cam-shaped appearance, with the head volar to the axis of the shaft. This results in the collateral ligaments changing length during range of motion. When the joint is flexed to approximately 90° degrees, the collateral ligaments are taut, firmly stabilizing the joint.[15] This multiaxial condyloid joint provides the fingers significant radioulnar movement when extended and stability when flexed to allow for power pinch and grip.[9,15] The volar plate is an important soft tissue structure at the MCP joint that prevents joint hyperextension. The volar plates of the nonthumb metacarpals are interconnected via the deep transverse ligament (see **Fig. 1**).[15,20]

Distal to the metacarpals are the proximal phalanges. The base of the proximal phalanx has insertion sites for the collateral ligaments of the MCP joint as well as a groove on the volar aspect for the flexor tendon sheath. The diaphysis is oval in shape and the head is bicondylar and broader volarly. The interossei insert onto the proximal phalanx whereas the central slip and terminal extensor tendon insert onto the middle phalanx and distal phalanx, respectively.[12,21] The pull from the interossei flexes the proximal fragment in proximal phalanx fractures, whereas the extensor mechanism extends the distal fragment and remaining finger, accounting for the apex volar angulation exhibited by most fractures of the proximal phalanx (**Fig. 2**).[22]

Unlike the MCP joint, the proximal interphalangeal (PIP) joint allows mainly for flexion and extension; however, the slight asymmetry of the proximal phalanx condyles allows for a few degrees of rotation of the fingers with flexion.[21,23] In addition to the stability from the bony articulation, the PIP joint has strong collateral ligaments that are taut throughout range of motion and a thick volar plate as well as the flexor and extensor tendons that contribute to stability.[21,22] The articular surface of the middle phalanx is biconcave with an intercondylar ridge, creating stability for the PIP joint.[13,23] Fractures of the middle phalanx have a less predictable angulation as the flexor digitorum superficialis (FDS) inserts onto the middle phalanx, countering the pull of the central slip.[9,12,21] If the fracture is proximal to the FDS insertion, the resulting deformity is apex dorsal as the FDS pulls the distal fragment into flexion and central slip extends the proximal fragment. If the fracture is distal to the FDS insertion, then the FDS flexes the proximal fragment and the extensor mechanism extends the distal fragment (**Fig. 3**).[9,12]

The distal phalanx base has tubercles that are the attachment sites for the collateral ligaments of the distal interphalangeal (DIP) joint. The distal phalanx is protected by the nail plate, which acts as a splint to prevent deformity with fracture.[9,12]

The classification of metacarpal and phalangeal fractures is best described by the name of the bone, the location of the fracture, the type of fracture, and whether the fracture is angulated, translated, rotated, or shortened (**Fig. 4**).

MECHANISM OF INJURY

In a review of the National High School Sports-Related Injury Surveillance Study of hand and wrist injuries over an 11-year period, the most frequent mechanism of injury was contact with another player (40.9%), followed by contact with sporting equipment, and, in football, 60% of metacarpal injuries occurred in player-to-player contact.[8] In the adult literature, injuries to the metacarpals and phalanges from athletic endeavors occurred from falls, direct hits, or a crush mechanism.[5,11,24]

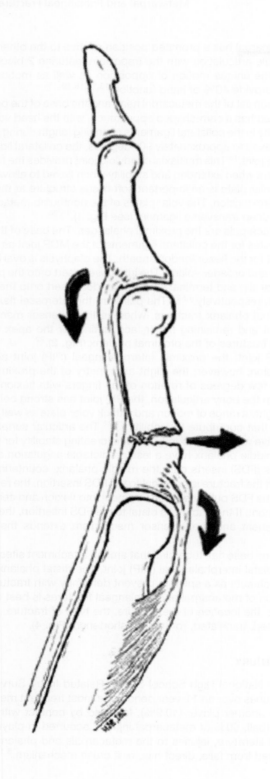

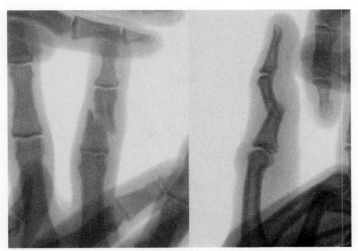

Fig. 3. Radiograph of a middle phalanx demonstrating apex volar deformity. The proximal fragment is flexed and the distal fragment is extended.

Consideration must be made to the specific sport being played because this may influence the location and type of fracture. For example, skiers are more likely to fracture the bones of the first ray whereas football players are more likely to fracture a bone of the fifth ray.[7] Weiss and Hastings[24] reported on 28 patients with unicondylar fractures of the proximal phalanx and found the most common mechanism of injury was during ball-handling sports. Less commonly reported are stress fractures of the upper extremity; however, there are case series reporting metacarpal stress fractures in racket sport athletes and epiphyseal stress fractures of the phalanges in rock climbers.[25–27]

EVALUATION AND MANAGEMENT

The initial management of hand and finger injuries may be performed first by an athletic trainer or sideline physician. The hand and fingers should be evaluated for any wounds suggestive of an open fracture, which require treatment more promptly than a closed injury.[9] Gross deformities, like apparent shortening or loss of normal knuckle contour, should clue the treating provider that a fracture or dislocation may have occurred. This may be confirmed by crepitus and/or instability felt by palpation if tolerated.[12] Not all fractures result in gross deformity; thus, careful examination of the hand and fingers for rotational deformity is necessary to avoid potential misalignment of the hand and fingers.[9,12]

If a dislocation is suspected or confirmed radiographically, joint reduction should be prioritized, followed by splint immobilization. The same is true for displaced extra-articular fractures. When immobilized, athletes are encouraged to mobilize the

Fig. 2. Deforming forces acting on proximal phalanx fractures. The curved arrows demonstrate the direction of pull on the distal fragment from the central slip dorsally and on the proximal fragment from the flexor digitorum superficialis tendon volarly, ultimately creating an apex volar deformity as demonstrated by the straight *arrow*. (*From* Cotterell IH, Richard MJ. Metacarpal and Phalangeal Fractures in Athletes. Clin Sports Med 2015 34(1):72; with permission.)

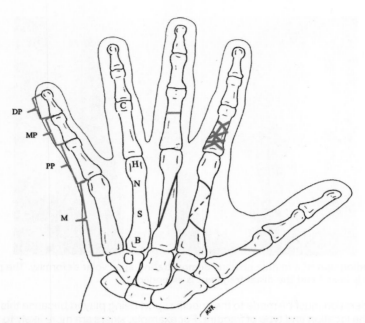

Fig. 4. Fractures of the metacarpals and phalanges are described by the name of the bone: metacarpal (M), proximal (PP), middle (MP), or distal phalanx (DP). The location of the fracture with in the bone: head (H), neck (N), shaft (S), base (B), and condyle (C). The fracture types are transverse (*green*), long oblique (*dark blue*), spiral (*purple*), comminuted (*orange*), and short oblique (*light blue*).

uninjured fingers as well as the shoulder, elbow, and wrist to prevent stiffness. Care should be taken if using ice for pain and swelling of the fingers to prevent vasospasm and potential vascular compromise.

Three views, posteroanterior, lateral, and oblique, of the injured finger and hand should be obtained for any suspected fracture. Oblique views of the hand allow for better visualization of the metacarpals and CMC joints due to the overlap of the metacarpals.[15,28] In addition to oblique views, there are specific views to better evaluate particular areas. A Brewerton view provides the best visualization of the MCP joints. The MCP joints are flexed 60° and the x-ray beam is directed 75° to the cassette. To adequately image the thumb, a Robert's view should be performed to get a true anteroposterior (AP) of the thumb. This is achieved with the arm in full pronation and the dorsum of the thumb on the x-ray cassette. A true lateral of the thumb is achieved with the hand pronated 30° and the beam angled 15° distally (**Fig. 5**).

Three-dimensional imaging, such as computed tomography (CT), usually is not necessary for simple or nondisplaced fractures; however, CT can be helpful for surgical planning for intra-articular or highly comminuted fractures. Magnetic resonance imaging and ultrasonography rarely are indicated for acute fractures of the metacarpals and phalanges.

FRACTURES
Metacarpal Fractures

Metacarpal fractures can be divided into base, shaft, neck, and head. Each metacarpal tolerates a different degree of angulation and displacement based on its

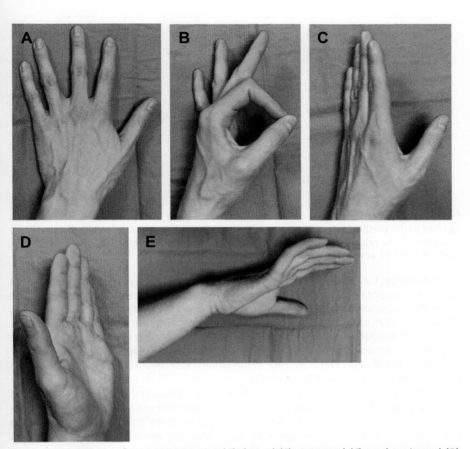

Fig. 5. Hand positions for posteroanterior (*A*), lateral (*B*), pronated (*C*), and supinated (*D*) oblique views of the hand. Robert's view of the thumb metacarpal with the hand fully pronated (*E*).

location due to the increasing mobility of the CMC joint from radial to ulnar.[9] Given this, the ring and small finger metacarpals can tolerate more angulation and displacement, whereas the index and long finger tolerate less.

In general, most metacarpal fractures are stable and can be treated successfully nonoperatively. This can be accomplished by buddy taping or splinting. Metacarpal neck fractures often can be successfully reduced via the Jahss maneuver (**Fig. 6**) and then immobilized.[29] Traditionally, metacarpal fractures were immobilized in the intrinsic plus position with the MCP joints in flexion and interphalangeal (IP) joint in extension to prevent contracture of the collateral ligaments.[1] A randomized controlled trial by Hofmeister and colleagues,[30] however, compared ulnar gutter casting of small finger metacarpal fractures with the MCP joint in neutral or flexion for 4 weeks in a young, active population and found no difference in range of motion, grip strength or aesthetics.[9,30] Additionally, another prospective study evaluated the difference between 3 different immobilization techniques—with the MCP joints in flexion with free IP joint motion, with the MCP joints in extension and full IP joint motion permitted, and with the MCP joints in flexion and the IP joints in extension without joint motion permitted—and found no difference at 9 weeks in range of motion, fracture reduction, and grip strength.[9,31]

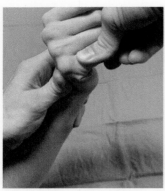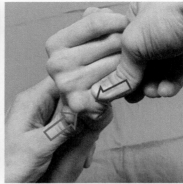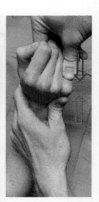

Fig. 6. Jahss maneuver. Flexion of the MCP joint to 90° (*left*). Then, a volarly directed force is applied to the metacarpal proximal to the fracture (*red arrows*) and a dorsally directed force is applied to the proximal phalanx (*blue arrows*) to reduce and stabilize the metacarpal neck fracture (*middle and right*).

Unstable fractures that demonstrate displacement or malalignment or are angulated more than accepted parameters[32] should undergo operative treatment. In a cadaveric study, Strauch and colleagues[33] reported that for every 2 mm of metacarpal shortening, an average of 7° of extensor lag was demonstrated.[5] Furthermore, metacarpal shortening leads to altered interosseous muscle anatomy resulting in changed force ratios and, thus, reduced grasp and grip strength.[34,35] In general, greater than 10° to 20° of angulation in the index finger and 40° in the small finger results in undesirable fingertip overlap and is an indication for operative treatment.[3,12,20,32]

A unique consideration for operative fixation of metacarpal fractures in athletes is return to play. Although a fracture may not meet operative criteria by radiographic parameters, surgical fixation may offer a more rapid recovery and minimize lost playing time. Similarly, operative management may lessen the immobilization requirements and allow for a sooner return to play. These decisions are specific to the sport, position, and time of season.

Metacarpal head
Metacarpal head fractures are best treated by headless compression screws via a dorsal, extensor-splitting approach.[15] Hand drilling can be useful to prevent further shearing or comminution of the fragments.[17] Head fractures require anatomic reduction and rigid fixation due to their intra-articular nature. Intra-articular head fractures that cannot be fixed in this manner pose a challenge in the athlete because the alternative treatment methods, arthrodesis and arthroplasty, can jeopardize an athlete's career.[17]

Metacarpal neck and shaft
There are multiple methods of operative fixation for metacarpal neck and shaft fractures. Percutaneous Kirschner (K)-wire fixation is a minimally invasive treatment option that provides fixation in multiple planes with cross-pinning in a retrograde fashion through the collateral recesses of the metacarpal head (**Fig. 7**).[12] Furthermore, the K-wire can be fixed to an intact, adjacent metacarpal for further stability.[12] This does not provide rigid fixation, however, and thus requires a period of protected, immobilization, delaying athletes' return to play.[15] There is a risk of pin tract infection from the exposed pins; however, this can be prevented by burying the pins under the skin whenever possible.[20]

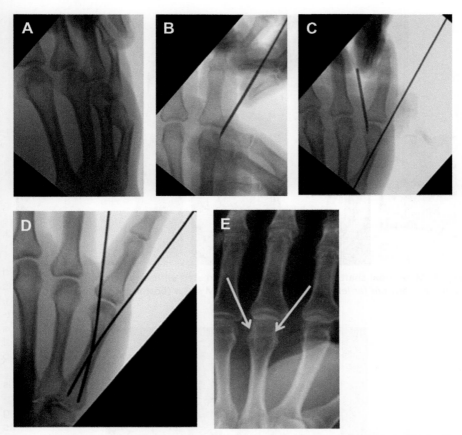

Fig. 7. Metacarpal neck fracture (*A*) treated with retrograde cross percutaneous K-wire fixation (*B–D*) through the recesses of the metacarpal head. The recesses of the metacarpal head are highlighted in *red* and the K-wire entry points are shown by the *yellow arrows* in (*E*).

Intramedullary (IM) fixation, whether via an IM screw or the IM bouquet pinning technique, is another option for metacarpal neck or shaft fractures. IM screw fixation is an attractive option for athletes for several reasons. The biomechanics of the construct allow for early motion and typically result in rapid callus formation from secondary bone healing. The technique can be performed percutaneously and minimize wound healing issues that affect the timing of return to play (**Fig. 8**). Bouquet pinning does not provide rigid fixation and is recommended for neck or shaft fractures of the ring and small finger metacarpals that can tolerate a greater degree of angulation.[15] The bouquet method has been shown to produce comparable results to transverse pinning of the small finger metacarpal.[20,36–38]

Lag screw fixation allows for interfragmentary compression if the screw is placed perpendicular to the fracture site. Lag screw fixation provides greater rigidity than cross–K-wire fixation,[15] which for an athlete means earlier range of motion and hence return to play. This technique, if used in isolation, is minimally invasive. Lag screws are useful particularly for long oblique fractures when the fracture line is at least twice the diameter of the bone (**Fig. 9**). Generally, 2.0-mm screws are used for this fracture pattern.[3]

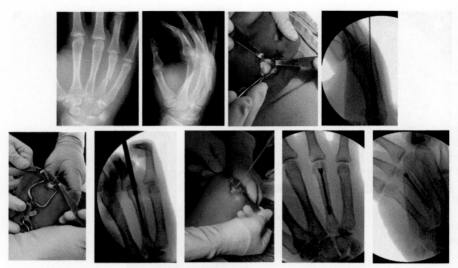

Fig. 8. Metacarpal shaft fracture (*top left two*) treated with a mini-open reduction (*top right two, bottom far left*) and placement of an IM screw (*bottom right four*).

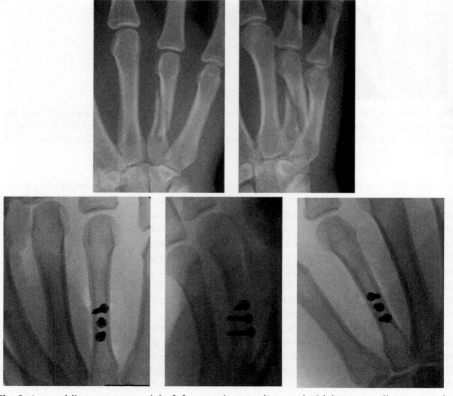

Fig. 9. Long oblique metacarpal shaft fracture (*top row*) treated with lag screws (*bottom row*).

Plate fixation often is required for comminuted fractures or for multiple metacarpal fractures.[3,9] Furthermore, plate fixation should be considered for athletes wishing to return to play during the season. The plate can be used alone or in conjunction with lag screws, depending on the fracture type (**Fig. 10**). Often, oblique fracture lines are too short for a lag screw and either require only plate fixation or lag screw for compression with supplementary plate fixation to protect the screw.[3,9]

Supplementary plate fixation should be considered for any athlete wishing to return to play within the same season. Plate fixation does require more extensive soft tissue dissection; thus, postoperative rehabilitation is paramount to prevent contractures and for the athlete to regain full active range of motion.[3,15] Early range of motion can be initiated to promote tendon gliding and prevent tendon adhesions, and return to play can be considered within 1 week to 3 weeks.[3,9,17]

Newer plate designs, including thinner locking plates, afford surgeon comparable reduction and fixation with less surgical trauma to the soft tissues.

Metacarpal base fractures

Intra-articular fractures of the CMC joints are more tolerated than fractures that extend to the MCP joint given the comparably limited range of motion at the CMC joint. Yet, intra-articular fractures of the ring and small finger CMC joint are less well tolerated than those of the index and long finger due to the increased mobility of the ring and

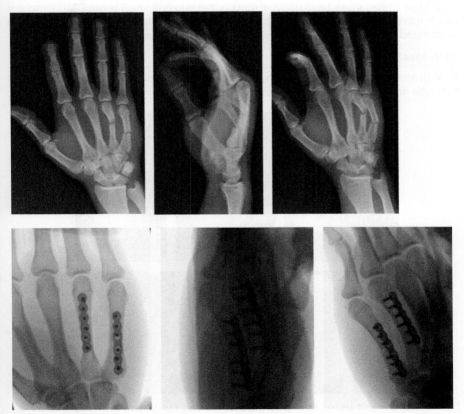

Fig. 10. Multiple metacarpal fractures (*top row*) treated with plate fixation (*bottom row*).

small finger CMC joints. CMC dislocations always should be ruled out and, if present, reduced. As previously stated, these are more common in the ring and small finger CMC joints, given their larger range of motion compared with the index and long finger CMC joints.[17] To appropriately image the CMC joints, the hand should be imaged with oblique laterals. The index and long finger CMC joints are seen best with a 45° pronated lateral.[39] Traditionally, the teaching was that the ring and small finger CMC joints are best seen with a 45° supinated lateral[39]; however, this has been questioned in the literature, as demonstrated by a recent cadaveric study by Johnson and colleagues.[28] Based off of their findings, the authors of this study recommends a 60° pronated view to evaluate the small finger CMC joint (**Fig. 11**).

Open reduction with plate-and-screw fixation is more likely to achieve anatomic reduction and thus has a smaller likelihood of developing posttraumatic arthritis for comminuted, intra-articular fractures or for fracture-dislocations. Percutaneous fixation also can be used, particularly in highly comminuted fractures, where axial traction with K-wires crossing the CMC joint and into adjacent metacarpals are used to maintain reduction of the joint.[17] In contrast to intra-articular fractures of the MCP joint, nonoperative management is a valid option for minimally displaced intra-articular fractures of the index or long finger CMC joints. Studies have demonstrated minimal functional impairment with nonoperative treatment. In this setting, the athlete uses pain as a guide for return to play and if pain limits the ability to play, CMC joint arthrodesis can be considered with minimal functional loss.[17] Although the CMC joints of the index and long finger metacarpals have minimal motion, the ring and small finger CMC joints are much more mobile. Intra-articular fractures at these joints are more susceptible to associated dislocation and the threshold for operative intervention is lower.

Phalangeal Fractures

As with metacarpal fractures, phalangeal fractures can be divided into base, shaft, and condylar fractures. If minimally displaced and without intra-articular involvement,

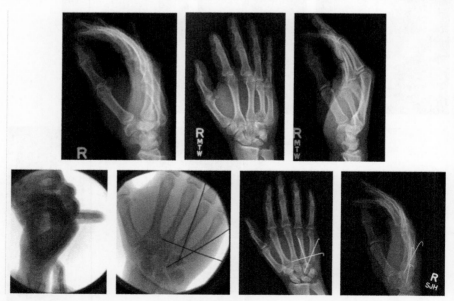

Fig. 11. Oblique and lateral radiographs demonstrating fourth and fifth CMC fracture dislocations (*top row*) treated with closed reduction and percutaneous pinning (*bottom row*).

these fractures can be treated with buddy taping and immobilization. The annular pulleys, fibro-osseous tendon sheaths, and osteocutaneous ligaments inherent to the fingers provide stability, minimizing immobilization time to less than 3 weeks after a fracture.[9,22] When a fracture is unstable or there are multiple phalangeal fractures, however, operative treatment may be indicated.[12]

Middle and proximal phalanges

Proximal and middle phalangeal shaft fractures with minimal displacement and no intra-articular involvement can be treated nonoperatively in a protective splint with the use of a playing cast for 4 weeks to 6 weeks.[22,40,41] If operative fixation is deemed necessary, however, treatment with K-wires, screws, plates, and external fixators may be considered.[3,22] As with metacarpal fractures, plate fixation allows earlier return to play than IM K-wire or external fixation methods.[3,22,42] Furthermore, placing the plate either radially or ulnarly instead of dorsally minimizes scarring of the extensor tendon (**Fig. 12**).

Distal phalanx

Fractures of the distal phalanx are the most common site of injury in an athlete's hand.[7] Tuft fractures are inherently stable due to the nail plate dorsally and the dense fibrous septa volarly in the pulp.[9,22] These can be treated with protective splitting, allowing prompt return of the athlete to competition. A mallet finger is the dorsal avulsion of the terminal extensor tendon insertion. This can be a boney avulsion and commonly is seen after an axial force to the fingertip causing forced flexion of the DIP joint from an extended position. As long as joint congruency is maintained, these injuries can be managed nonoperatively with full-time extension splinting. Temporary K-wire fixation across the DIP joint is considered for specific situations that require intermittent splint removal (**Fig. 13**). Joint incongruency is an indication for operative management and typically is achieved with K-wire fixation. Fixation can be achieved with either longitudinal or oblique K-wires. The advantage of an oblique K-wire is that it can be placed bicortically so that if the wire breaks, it can be easily removed from each end. The disadvantage of an oblique K-wire is that it tends to be more prominent in its subcutaneous position. The authors prefer a longitudinal K-wire cut below the level of the skin with careful attention to avoid the PIP joint. Return to play is sport-specific and position-specific. If a finger can be appropriately immobilized and protected for play, return is allowed as early as 2 weeks once the surgical wounds are appropriately healed.

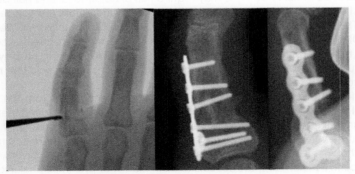

Fig. 12. Proximal phalanx fracture (*left*) treated with a radially based plate (*middle, right*).

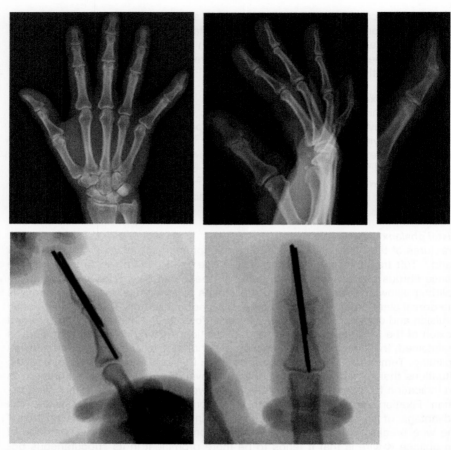

Fig. 13. Mallet finger (*top row*) treated with temporary K-wire fixation across the DIP joint (*bottom row*).

Minimally displaced diaphyseal shaft fractures of the distal phalanx may be treated nonoperatively with a thermoplastic or foam-laminated aluminum splint, leaving the PIP joint free.[22,43] For displaced diaphyseal shaft fractures, however, injury to the nail bed must be considered. This may require nail plate removal and nail bed repair in conjunction with longitudinal K-wire fixation of the shaft fracture after closed reduction.[22,43] The K-wire commonly is placed in a retrograde fashion to the middle phalanx with the DIP joint in extension. The distal end of the pin may be buried, allowing the athlete to return to play with a protective splint. If an athlete is using a playing cast or splint during sport, the athlete also should have a thermoplastic splint for nonsport activities to allow for early active range of motion.[43]

In a review of players who missed games due to a hand injury from the National Basketball Association (NBA) inactive list, Morse and colleagues[44] found that players with phalangeal fractures were out a mean 46 days and missed 13 games if they underwent surgery versus a mean 33 days and 11 games if they were treated nonoperatively. Although the time to return to play was higher in the operative players, this was not significant. Furthermore, the specific (distal, middle, or proximal) phalanx was not specified nor was a subgroup analysis performed.

Intra-articular fractures

Injuries of the PIP and DIP joints are commonly seen in ball-handling sports.[24] This usually is the result of an axial force, commonly referred to as jamming of the finger. These injuries can range from intra-articular fractures of the phalanges to fracture dislocations of the joint and can be divided into stable and unstable injuries.[22,23]

Unicondylar fractures of the head proximal phalanx can be unstable even if nondisplaced.[3,24] In athletes, operative treatment may be favorable given the intra-articular nature and the potential to progress to arthritis. Percutaneous methods are preferred to open methods, if possible, due to the significant soft tissue stripping necessary for exposure, with subsequent longer recovery time and potential for postoperative stiffness.[3,23] Furthermore, the vascular supply to the condyle travels with the collateral ligament, and excessive stripping risks osteonecrosis of the fracture fragment. Percutaneous screw fixation is a favorable option, with the possibility of returning to play within 1 week in a protective splint.[3,22]

Bicondylar fractures of the head of the proximal phalanx commonly are treated with lateral plate fixation (**Fig. 14**). Geissler, however, described a percutaneous, cannulated, headless, compression screw fixation method for unicondylar and bicondylar intra-articular fractures of the proximal phalanx that also can be used. This method provides maximal stability without the morbidity of open reduction and soft tissue stripping.[3,23,45]

Despite the inherent stability of the PIP joint, dorsal dislocations remain a common injury in athletes from a hyperextension or an axial force. Treatment is guided by the stability of the injury. In injuries with less than a 40% intra-articular fracture, closed reduction is the first line of treatment followed by a period of immobilization by buddy taping for 3 weeks to 6 weeks. Return to play usually can begin immediately if the fingers are adequately protected and there is no instability in full extension as noted on the lateral radiograph. If there is an articular fracture of the volar base of the middle phalanx that is greater than 40% of the surface, rendering the joint unstable, this may require dorsal extension block splinting or operative treatment.[22,43]

Operative options include open reduction and internal fixation, closed reduction and percutaneous pinning, dynamic external fixation, and volar plate arthroplasty.[43] When open reduction is necessary, preservation of the collateral ligament attachments is paramount to preserve the vascular supply to the condyles. A volar shotgun approach is used to expose the articular surface of the phalangeal base. The flexor tendon sheath is opened between the A2 and A4 pulleys, and the volar plate is released distally.[9] Internal fixation can be achieved with low-profile plates and screws (**Fig. 15**). Postoperatively, patients are placed into a dorsal-blocking splint at 30° for 1 week. At that time, patients initiate hand therapy for edema control and progressive active range of motion. Return to play is dependent on the sport and position. In many sports, the position of the finger in space can expose it to injury if there is limited range of motion. For sports, such as basketball, where there is a risk of reinjury from this loss of range of motion, return is delayed until full range of motion is achieved.

In highly comminuted, or pilon, fractures of the PIP joint, anatomic joint restoration may not be possible and distraction osteosynthesis with a dynamic external fixation device, such as a Suzuki frame, may be necessary to maintain reduction (**Fig. 16**). This can be a devastating injury because return to play is not recommended with the traction device, resulting in the athlete missing practice and games. If the traction device does not provide adequate reduction or stability, salvage procedures, such as hemi-hamate autograft, can be used.[9,22]

As with the PIP joint, dorsal dislocations of the DIP joint result from hyperextension and axial forces. DIP joint dislocations, however, are more likely to be accompanied by

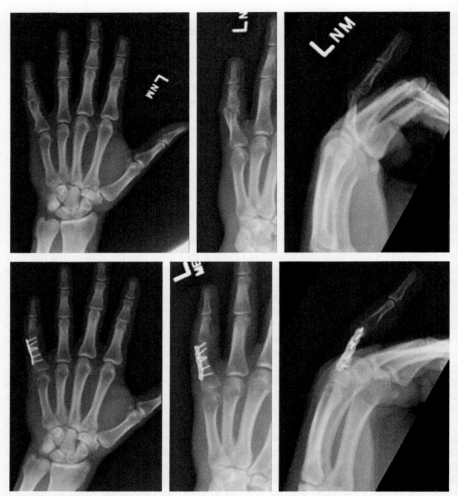

Fig. 14. Bicondylar fracture of the head of the small finger proximal phalanx (*top row*) treated with a lateral plate (*bottom row*).

fracture than are PIP joint dislocations.[22] A simple DIP joint dislocation that undergoes a successful closed reduction usually can be immobilized in a splint with the DIP joint in slight flexion for 2 weeks to 3 weeks. Depending on the sport, the athlete often can return to play immediately. If there are fractures that render the joint unstable, then operative treatment is warranted.

Thumb

The thumb phalanges and metacarpal can be treated similarly to the other digit injuries. The thumb phalanges and metacarpal can tolerate a comparably larger degree of angulation due to the large range of motion at the thumb CMC joint.[17] Intra-articular fractures of the CMC joint, however, referred to as Bennett fractures and Rolando fractures, may require operative treatment to preserve the range of motion at this joint.

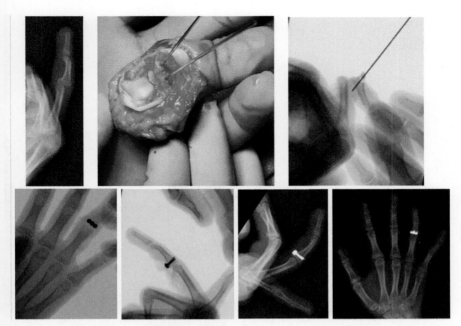

Fig. 15. An unstable base of middle phalanx fracture at the PIP joint (*top left*) treated with open reduction and internal fixation via a volar shot gun approach (*top middle and top right*) and a low-profile plate with screws (*bottom row*).

Bennett fractures are partial articular fractures and are more common than the comminuted, intra-articular Rolando fractures.[9] In a Bennett fracture, the smaller, volar-ulnar fragment is the stable piece, held in place by the anterior oblique ligament. The metacarpal shaft is displaced proximally, dorsally, and radially by the abductor pollicis longus (**Fig. 17**).[9,15,17] Rolando fractures tend to have a T-shaped or Y-shaped fracture pattern at the articular surface. Both of these fractures require operative fixation to prevent posttraumatic arthritis.

Bennett fractures can be treated with closed reduction and percutaneous fixation. The reduction maneuver is traction, abduction, pronation, and extension (TAPE) of the metacarpal shaft. This is then held with a K-wire from the metacarpal to the volar-ulnar fragment and another K-wire from the metacarpal to the trapezium or index finger metacarpal.[9,15] Alternatively, internal screw fixation with 1.5-mm to 2.0-mm screws via a Wagner approach can be used. Open reduction and internal fixation allow for shorter immobilization compared with K-wire fixation.[17] Rolando fractures most often are treated with open reduction and internal fixation using a plate-and-screw construct. Sometimes bone grafting is necessary to maintain the reduction.[15,17] In the highly comminuted Rolando fracture, external fixation may be required, which in turn may have a detrimental effect to an athlete's season and possibly career.[17]

Rolando and Bennett fractures both require thumb spica splint immobilization. The return to play is often longer for the thumb than the other digits, sometimes up to 6 weeks to 8 weeks, because these injuries, in particular Rolando fractures, are at greater risk for loss of reduction or persistent instability due to the high stresses concentrated at this joint in athletes.

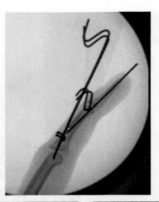

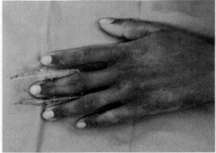
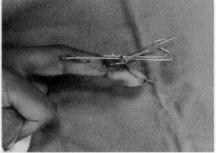

Fig. 16. Dynamic external fixation device (Suzuki frame) used for a dorsally unstable volar base fracture of the middle phalanx at the PIP joint (*top row*). The bottom row are clinical photographs of the dynamic external fixation device on the long finger for an unstable volar base fracture of the middle phalanx at the PIP joint.

REHABILITATION AND RETURN TO PLAY

When treating an athlete, the physician must consider the appropriate initial management and method of fixation as well as the circumstances surrounding the timing of return to play. Expectations of the athlete and coaching staff may differ depending on the level of play as well as the type of sport played. Athletes who play contact sports or upper-extremity ball sports depend on intact hand biomechanics.

For the metacarpal and phalangeal shaft fractures treated nonoperatively, initial immobilization with a cast glove or similar hand-based immobilization that protects the fractures yet still allows wrist motion can be applied.[46,47] Athletes can return to protected play at 2 weeks or when fracture callus is visible and full play at approximately 4 weeks.[46] In a study evaluating return to play in NBA players, NBA players with metacarpal and phalangeal fractures treated nonoperatively returned to play at means 26 days and 33 days after injury for metacarpal and phalangeal fractures, respectively.[44] A survey of United States hand surgeons treating professional athletes demonstrated that approximately half waited 3 weeks to 4 weeks to start protective play and 4 weeks to 8 weeks to allow unprotected play.[48] If treated surgically, plate fixation allows for earlier range of motion and thus return to play. Most athletes can return to play with a cast or semirigid splint (protected) within 2 weeks yet should wait 6 weeks to 10 weeks to progress to full unprotected play.[43]

Because a vast majority of metacarpal neck fractures can be treated nonoperatively, after reduction of the fracture, an ulnar gutter splint followed by a functional

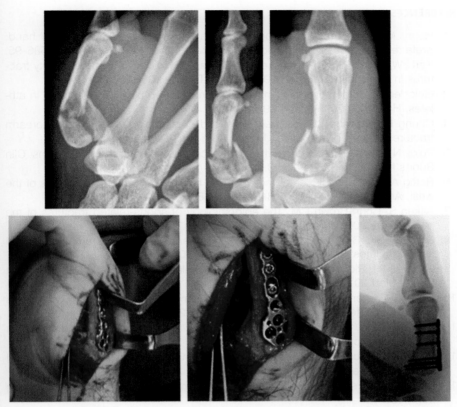

Fig. 17. Rolando fracture of the first metacarpal with a Y-shaped pattern (*top row*). This was treated with open reduction and internal fixation with a plate (*bottom row*).

brace that leaves the IP joints free often is the modality of choice.[17] The functional brace allows for early range of motion and athletes are often back to full unprotected play at 5 weeks to 6 weeks.[43,47] In contrast, phalangeal base fractures, both intra-articular and extra-articular, often require operative treatment. Similar to metacarpal shaft fractures, rigid immobilization should continue for 2 weeks[43] with protected play, and then the athlete should wait up to three months if there is a dislocation injury for full unprotected play because the risk of recurrent injury or dislocation with axial forces remains high in athletes.[17,47]

SUMMARY

Metacarpal and phalangeal fractures are common in athletes. Often these injuries can be treated nonoperatively; however, consideration of operative treatment is warranted for early return to play. The overarching theme throughout the literature is the emphasis on tailoring the treatment plan to the specific injury as well as to an athlete's sport and level of play. Close collaboration with the athlete, surgeon, trainer, and coaching staff is necessary to set expectations as well as determine the best treatment plan.

DISCLOSURE

M.J. Richard is a consultant for Acumed, DePuy Synthes, and Extremity Medical.

REFERENCES

1. Henry MH. Fractures of the proximal phalanx and metacarpals in the hand: preferred methods of stabilization. J Am Acad Orthop Surg 2008;16(10):586–95.
2. Karl JW, Olson PR, Rosenwasser MP. The epidemiology of upper extremity fractures in the United States, 2009. J Orthop Trauma 2015;29(8):e242–4.
3. Geissler WB. Operative fixation of metacarpal and phalangeal fractures in athletes. Hand Clin 2009;25(3):409–21.
4. Chung KC, Spilson SV. The frequency and epidemiology of hand and forearm fractures in the United States. J Hand Surg Am 2001;26(5):908–15.
5. Pulos N, Kakar S. Hand and wrist injuries: common problems and solutions. Clin Sports Med 2018;37(2):217–43.
6. Rettig AC. Athletic injuries of the wrist and hand. Part I: traumatic injuries of the wrist. Am J Sports Med 2003;31(6):1038–48.
7. Aitken S, Court-Brown CM. The epidemiology of sports-related fractures of the hand. Injury 2008;39(12):1377–83.
8. Johnson BK, Brou L, Fields SK, et al. Hand and wrist injuries among US high school athletes: 2005/06-2015/16. Pediatrics 2017;140(6):1–9.
9. Cotterell IH, Richard MJ. Metacarpal and phalangeal fractures in athletes. Clin Sports Med 2015;34(1):69–98.
10. Chew EM, Chong AK. Hand fractures in children: epidemiology and misdiagnosis in a tertiary referral hospital. J Hand Surg Am 2012;37(8):1684–8.
11. Avery DM 3rd, Rodner CM, Edgar CM. Sports-related wrist and hand injuries: a review. J Orthop Surg Res 2016;11(1):99.
12. Kozin SH, Thoder JJ, Lieberman G. Operative treatment of metacarpal and phalangeal shaft fractures. J Am Acad Orthop Surg 2000;8(2):111–21.
13. Panchal-Kildare S, Malone K. Skeletal anatomy of the hand. Hand Clin 2013; 29(4):459–71.
14. Watt AJ, Chung KC. Surgical exposures of the hand. Hand Clin 2014;30(4): 445–57, vi.
15. Chin SH, Vedder NB. MOC-PSSM CME article: metacarpal fractures. Plast Reconstr Surg 2008;121(1 Suppl):1–13.
16. Nakamura K, Patterson RM, Viegas SF. The ligament and skeletal anatomy of the second through fifth carpometacarpal joints and adjacent structures. J Hand Surg Am 2001;26(6):1016–29.
17. Fufa DT, Goldfarb CA. Fractures of the thumb and finger metacarpals in athletes. Hand Clin 2012;28(3):379–88, x.
18. Cooney WP 3rd, Lucca MJ, Chao EY, et al. The kinesiology of the thumb trapeziometacarpal joint. J Bone Joint Surg Am 1981;63(9):1371–81.
19. Moran SL, Berger RA. Biomechanics and hand trauma: what you need. Hand Clin 2003;19(1):17–31.
20. Kollitz KM, Hammert WC, Vedder NB, et al. Metacarpal fractures: treatment and complications. Hand (N Y) 2014;9(1):16–23.
21. Leversedge FJ, Goldfarb CA, Boyer MI. A pocketbook manual of hand and upper extremity anatomy : primus manus. Philadelphia: Wolters Kluwer/Lippincott Williams & Wilkins; 2010.
22. Chen F, Kalainov DM. Phalanx fractures and dislocations in athletes. Curr Rev Musculoskelet Med 2017;10(1):10–6.
23. Blazar PE, Steinberg DR. Fractures of the proximal interphalangeal joint. J Am Acad Orthop Surg 2000;8(6):383–90.

24. Weiss AP, Hastings H 2nd. Distal unicondylar fractures of the proximal phalanx. J Hand Surg Am 1993;18(4):594–9.
25. Balius R, Pedret C, Estruch A, et al. Stress fractures of the metacarpal bones in adolescent tennis players: a case series. Am J Sports Med 2010;38(6):1215–20.
26. Fukuda K, Fujioka H, Fujita I, et al. Stress fracture of the second metacarpal bone in a badminton player. Kobe J Med Sci 2008;54(3):E159–62.
27. Merritt AL, Huang JI. Hand injuries in rock climbing. J Hand Surg Am 2011; 36(11):1859–61.
28. Johnson J, Fowler J, Costello J, et al. Optimal oblique radiographs to identify fifth carpometacarpal dorsal subluxations: a cadaveric study. J Hand Surg Am 2018; 43(12):1139.e1-5.
29. Day CS. Fractures of the metacarpals and phalanges. In: Wolfe SW, Hotchkiss RN, Pederson WC, et al, editors. Green's operative hand surgery. 7th edition. Philadephia: Elsevier; 2017. p. 231–77.
30. Hofmeister EP, Kim J, Shin AY. Comparison of 2 methods of immobilization of fifth metacarpal neck fractures: a prospective randomized study. J Hand Surg Am 2008;33(8):1362–8.
31. Tavassoli J, Ruland RT, Hogan CJ, et al. Three cast techniques for the treatment of extra-articular metacarpal fractures. Comparison of short-term outcomes and final fracture alignments. J Bone Joint Surg Am 2005;87(10):2196–201.
32. Stern PJ. Fractures of the metacarpals and phalanges. In: Green DP, Hotchkiss RN, Pederson WC, et al, editors. Operative hand surgery. New York: Churchill Lingstone; 2005. p. 277–342.
33. Strauch RJ, Rosenwasser MP, Lunt JG. Metacarpal shaft fractures: the effect of shortening on the extensor tendon mechanism. J Hand Surg Am 1998;23(3): 519–23.
34. Marjoua Y, Eberlin KR, Mudgal CS. Multiple displaced metacarpal fractures. J Hand Surg Am 2015;40(9):1869–70.
35. Freeland AE, Orbay JL. Extraarticular hand fractures in adults: a review of new developments. Clin Orthop Relat Res 2006;445:133–45.
36. Winter M, Balaguer T, Bessiere C, et al. Surgical treatment of the boxer's fracture: transverse pinning versus intramedullary pinning. J Hand Surg Eur Vol 2007; 32(6):709–13.
37. Wong TC, Ip FK, Yeung SH. Comparison between percutaneous transverse fixation and intramedullary K-wires in treating closed fractures of the metacarpal neck of the little finger. J Hand Surg Br 2006;31(1):61–5.
38. Schadel-Hopfner M, Wild M, Windolf J, et al. Antegrade intramedullary splinting or percutaneous retrograde crossed pinning for displaced neck fractures of the fifth metacarpal? Arch Orthop Trauma Surg 2007;127(6):435–40.
39. Buren C, Gehrmann S, Kaufmann R, et al. Management algorithm for index through small finger carpometacarpal fracture dislocations. Eur J Trauma Emerg Surg 2016;42(1):37–42.
40. Ginanneschi F, Milani P, Mondelli M, et al. Ulnar sensory nerve impairment at the wrist in carpal tunnel syndrome. Muscle Nerve 2008;37(2):183–9.
41. Gaston RG, Chadderdon C. Phalangeal fractures: displaced/nondisplaced. Hand Clin 2012;28(3):395–401, x.
42. Kodama N, Takemura Y, Ueba H, et al. Operative treatment of metacarpal and phalangeal fractures in athletes: early return to play. J Orthop Sci 2014;19(5): 729–36.
43. Morgan WJ, Slowman LS. Acute hand and wrist injuries in athletes: evaluation and management. J Am Acad Orthop Surg 2001;9(6):389–400.

44. Morse KW, Hearns KA, Carlson MG. Return to play after forearm and hand injuries in the national basketball association. Orthop J Sports Med 2017;5(2). 2325967117690002.
45. Geissler WB. Cannulated percutaneous fixation of intra-articular hand fractures. Hand Clin 2006;22(3):297–305, vi.
46. Toronto R, Donovan PJ, Macintyre J. An alternative method of treatment for metacarpal fractures in athletes. Clin J Sport Med 1996;6(1):4–8.
47. Halim A, Weiss AP. Return to play after hand and wrist fractures. Clin Sports Med 2016;35(4):597–608.
48. Dy CJ, Khmelnitskaya E, Hearns KA, et al. Opinions regarding the management of hand and wrist injuries in elite athletes. Orthopedics 2013;36(6):815–9.

Management of Finger Joint Dislocation and Fracture-Dislocations in Athletes

Erin A. Miller, MD, MS, Jeffrey B. Friedrich, MD, MC*

KEYWORDS

- PIP fracture-dislocation • Finger dislocation • IP dislocation • DIP dislocation
- Athlete • Return to play

KEY POINTS

- Finger joint dislocations encompass a range of injury severities from benign to permanently disabling if improperly treated; therefore, appropriate diagnosis in athletes is key to ensure maximal function is retained.
- Simple dislocations should be reduced with the appropriate maneuver and most athletes can return to play with protective buddy taping in days.
- Volar proximal interphalangeal (PIP) joint dislocations are important to diagnose and treat with immediate extension splinting to prevent subsequent boutonnière deformity secondary to central slip injury.
- PIP joint fracture-dislocations all require treatment by a hand surgeon to determine whether extension block splinting or open reduction with internal fixation is indicated.
- Untreated PIP joint fracture-dislocations require reconstruction of the joint and may include hemihamate grafting to replace the articular surface and restore joint congruity and stability.

INTRODUCTION

Finger injuries are a known risk in athletes, especially in ball-related sports and high-impact sports such as gymnastics.[1] Specifically, a 2008 review of professional football injuries found that 24% of hand injuries were to the fingers, and 49% of those were joint subluxations or dislocations.[2] Both amateur and professional competitors are at risk for these injuries, especially in early season when conditioning may not be optimal.[1] Often, finger injuries are perceived as minor and athletes encouraged to play through the injury,[3] which is where the role of coaches and team physicians is especially critical in early recognition of more complicated dislocations and fracture-dislocations, to ensure that proper treatment is initiated early. Timely

Division of Plastic Surgery, Department of Surgery, University of Washington, Harborview Medical Center, 325 9th Avenue, Box 359796, Seattle, WA 98104, USA
* Corresponding author.
E-mail address: jfriedri@uw.edu

Clin Sports Med 39 (2020) 423–442
https://doi.org/10.1016/j.csm.2019.10.006
0278-5919/20/© 2019 Elsevier Inc. All rights reserved.
sportsmed.theclinics.com

treatment of complex fracture-dislocations ensures optimal outcome, both in range of motion and overall hand function. This article reviews these injuries with a focus on fracture-dislocations; other fractures and finger injuries are covered elsewhere in this issue.

INTERPHALANGEAL JOINT ANATOMY

A brief review of interphalangeal (IP) joint anatomy is needed to set the stage for examining the mechanism and treatment of finger joint injuries. The proximal IP (PIP) and distal IP (DIP) joints are both bicondylar hinge joints with motion in 1 plane. The middle phalanx (P2) base has a midline ridge that articulates with the trough between the proximal phalanx (P1) condyles to limit rotation.[4] because IP joints are constrained to flexion and extension, they are more susceptible to injury than joints with greater degrees of freedom.

The DIP joint has an arc of motion from 0° to 80°, whereas the PIP joint has a slightly greater range, from 0° to 110°. The PIP joint plays the largest role in functional grasp, contributing 85% of the motion required.[4] In addition to the constraint of bony interface, stabilization is provided by stout ligamentous structures. Radial and ulnar stability is provided by the proper collateral ligaments and dorsal capsule in flexion, and the volar plate and accessory collateral ligaments in extension.[5] The volar plate provides resistance to any hyperextension force and subsequent dislocation. Dorsally, the joint is less protected, because the central slip is the primary support of the PIP joint and is significantly less robust than the volar plate. The DIP joint dorsally is supported by the terminal tendon[6] (**Fig. 1**).

This anatomy leads to specific vulnerabilities in the IP joints; during end-on loading in hyperextension, the weaker dorsal support leads most commonly to dorsal dislocation. The longer lengths of P1 and P2 compared with P3 creates a longer lever arm, which likely explains the increased incidence of PIP joint dislocations compared

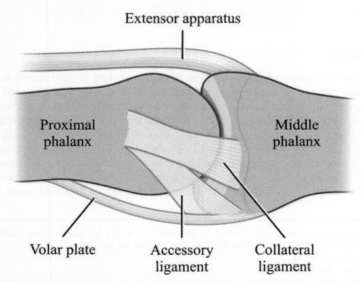

Fig. 1. Soft tissue support of the PIP joint. (*From* Bindra, R. R. & Foster, B. J. Management of proximal interphalangeal joint dislocations in athletes. Hand Clinics 25, 423–435 (2009); Figure 1 p424. With Permission.)

with the DIP joint.[1,6] In fracture-dislocations, the insertion of the proper collateral ligaments onto the volar lip of P2 dictates the relative stability of the joint: fractures volar to the insertion leave the collateral ligaments intact and are more likely to be stable because the ligaments remain on the base, as opposed to fractures that are more dorsal (involving a greater percentage of the joint surface), which disassociate the ligaments from the phalanx (discussed in more detail later).

With all finger injuries, early motion is key to final function. Both PIP and DIP joint injuries develop rapid stiffness when immobilized, which may lead to irreversible contracture of the previously discussed ligamentous supports of the joint.[7] Although hand surgeons often delay motion or select treatment courses because of concerns of patient noncompliance, athletes are typically motivated to achieve the best possible result and are dedicated to their therapy. Thus, in athletes, the authors advocate selection of the treatment option that allows earliest return to motion given their overall adherence to a structured, supervised hand therapy program.

FINGER-JAM ASSESSMENT

The common clinical complaint for dislocations and fracture-dislocations may be nonspecific: the athlete reports jamming the finger. Many athletes instinctually pull on a dislocated finger after injury and reduce the joint in the field,[1] presenting for follow-up days later with edema and stiffness. Unless evaluated shortly after injury, swelling may preclude easy visualization of an ongoing dislocation.

History should proceed per routine evaluation of the patient with a hand injury. Additional evaluation of the athlete should include sport, position, training/competition schedule, and previous injuries to the finger. The physician must also elicit the patient's expectations in timing of return to play and final range of motion. The injured finger should be assessed and compared with the contralateral normal side. A digital block may be used to facilitate full examination.

Key examination points include:

- Gross deformity of the finger
- Resting posture (flexion vs extension)
- Stability of PIP and DIP joints to radial and ulnar stress
- Hyperextensibility
- Range of motion at both IP joints

Significant bruising under the nail may indicate a concurrent soft tissue mallet. Posture of the finger gives clues to the type of dislocation: a PIP joint fixed in extension is typically seen with a dorsal dislocation, whereas a flexed PIP joint with limited motion indicates a fracture-dislocation. In reduced dislocations, radial and ulnar stress enables assessment of the integrity of the ligaments. This portion of the examination should be performed with the PIP extended to assess the accessory collateral ligaments and volar plate as well as in 30° of flexion to assess the proper collateral ligaments and dorsal capsule.[8] Gentle pressure applied dorsally on the PIP while supporting the DIP volarly can elicit hyperextensibility, indicating volar plate injury from a recent dislocation. Range of motion should be smooth; any catch or clunk alerts the examiner to the diagnosis of a fracture-dislocation. Joint subluxation may only be seen as a slight limitation in range of motion or subtle scissoring.[4] If fluoroscopy is available, it is a useful adjunct to evaluate whether the joint is stable throughout the full range of motion.

Differential diagnoses of these injuries can include:[9]

- Collateral ligament sprain
- Volar plate avulsion
- Central slip disruption
- Simple dislocation
- Fracture-dislocation

Before any reduction, imaging should be obtained to guide the appropriate maneuver. Especially in delayed presentation of an injury, imaging may help confirm reduction because swelling may obscure any ongoing deformity. Dedicated views of the finger are essential, and hand films do not suffice. The lateral view must show alignment of the condyles to support joint assessment. Reduction is confirmed with presence of a true concentric joint. The dorsal V sign (**Fig. 2**) indicates ongoing subluxation of the phalangeal base.[4] Fractures should be assessed for the percentage of articular surface involved. Advanced imaging such as a computed tomography scan may be used to delineate complex injuries such as middle phalanx base fracture-dislocations.

SIMPLE DISLOCATIONS

In the fingers, any immobilization beyond 3 weeks is undesirable because stiffness will occur. Dislocations without any associated fractures should be mobilized early unless

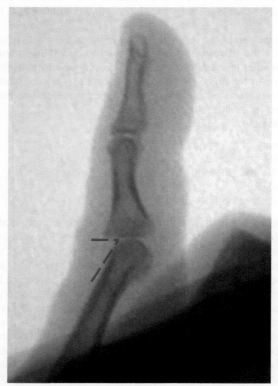

Fig. 2. Dorsal V sign indicated by red dashed line; note loss of congruency between proximal and middle phalanges.

grossly unstable: in a retrospective study of PIP joint dislocations comparing splinting for 4 weeks with early motion, 92% of the early motion group regained full range compared with 36% of immobilized patients.[10] Motion should be initiated 2 to 3 days after injury (allowing 24–48 hours of soft tissue rest) with buddy taping to an adjacent finger.[11] Buddy taping should avoid including the border digits (index and small fingers) unless they are the injured digits. Athletic tape may be used, or specialized Velcro loops may be fabricated by a therapist or purchased online (**Fig. 3**). Additional sport-specific orthoses may be available.

Edema control in the immediate postinjury period can significantly improve range of motion. Coban (3M Science, Maplewood, MN) wrapping is an effective treatment and may be adjusted by the patient serially. Although custom sleeves and gloves are available and may be used in select cases, most patients benefit from the simplicity of digit wrapping. A dislocation may develop a mild flexion contracture; however, these are rarely functionally significant, with the exception of specific pitching grips.[12]

IP joint dislocations vary slightly in the disorder and treatment based on the direction of dislocation; each permutation is considered subsequently (**Fig. 4, Table 1**).

Dorsal Distal Interphalangeal Joint

Dorsal dislocations of the DIP joint are the most common and result from a hyperextension impact on the finger.[1] They are seen more frequently in sports with forceful ball handling, such as basketball and volleyball. On presentation, the finger is extended with an inability to flex. Reduction of these dislocations is performed by longitudinal traction and direct pressure on the dorsal P3 base.[9] The collateral ligaments are likely to be torn and splinting in slight flexion for 2 to 3 weeks promotes stable healing.[13] A dorsal or a volar splint may be applied with the PIP left free (see **Fig. 3**). These dislocations are more likely to be open than PIP or volar DIP given the paucity of tissue between the joint and skin, and thus may require operative debridement.[13–15]

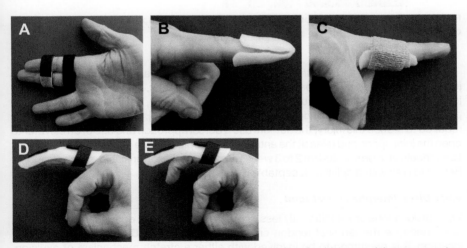

Fig. 3. Occupational therapy devices. (*A*) Reusable Velcro buddy tape. (*B*) DIP extension splint for mallet finger; the valves allow for swelling and Coban, tape, or Velcro straps are used to secure splint with appropriate tension. (*C*) PIP extension splint for volar dislocation (presumed central slip rupture); the open dorsal half allows for swelling. (*D*) Dorsal blocking splint for PIP fracture-dislocations; (*E*) allows range of motion within splint.

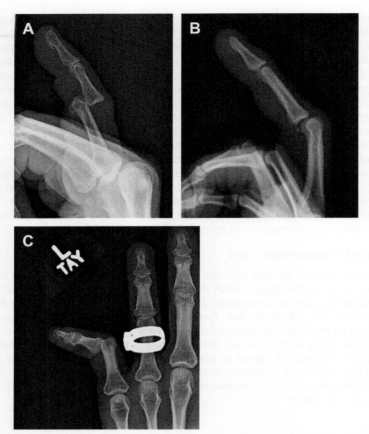

Fig. 4. Directional PIP dislocations. (*A*) Dorsal is the most common direction. (*B*) Volar dislocation. (*C*) Lateral dislocation.

If irreducible, a dorsal DIP joint dislocation may have an entrapped volar plate within the joint space. This finding may be subtle on lateral radiographs, with several millimeters of joint space widening, and should thus be evaluated carefully, especially in patients with persistent limitation in motion despite lack of deformity (**Fig. 5**).[1] An operative approach is required to reduce this injury; the authors use a dorsal approach and use of an elevator to open the joint space and release the entrapped volar plate. Once reduced, these dislocations should also be splinted for 2 to 3 weeks in extension before initiating range of motion. Return to play with a splint is acceptable if the sport allows.

Volar Distal Interphalangeal Joint

Volar dislocations are significantly less common and are most commonly seen in softball.[1] Because the terminal tendon crosses the joint at the DIP immediately before insertion, it is presumed to be involved with either a stretch mechanism or avulsion, with or without a small bony fragment. Extension splinting for 6 weeks is required to prevent chronic mallet deformity, and any flexion of the DIP during this period necessitates restarting the period of immobilization.[16,17] Splinting should be in slight hyperextension with the PIP free.

Table 1
Reduction maneuvers for interphalangeal joint dislocations

Dislocation	Reduction Maneuver	Additional Tips	After Reduction
Dorsal DIP	Volarly applied pressure on P3 base + axial traction	If irreducible, consider entrapped volar plate	Recommend splinting 2–3 wk in extension
Volar DIP	DIP flexion + axial traction	Least likely to need reduction	Needs assessment for bony mallet (fracture-dislocation)
Dorsal PIP	PIP extension + axial traction	Use thumb to hook base of P2 longitudinally	Needs assessment for PIP fracture-dislocation
Volar PIP	PIP flexion + axial traction	Flex metacarpophalangeal and wrist, may require slight rotation	Presume central slip injury and splint PIP in extension
Lateral PIP	Radial or ulnar force in direction of dislocation + axial traction	Easiest dislocation to reduce	Assess collateral ligament stability after reduction

Although splinting is adequate in treatment of mallet fingers during daily activities, it is unlikely to be robust enough for sports. If absolutely necessary for an athlete to return to play, a splint may be transitioned to a finger-based cast during games for additional protection and swapped for a splint during all other times to allow motion of the PIP joint. Five-year outcomes of soft tissue mallets treated with splinting alone showed an average 8° extension lag and 55° of active motion, with 25% showing arthritis.[18]

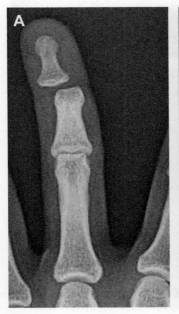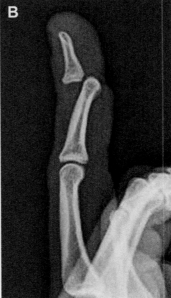

Fig. 5. Simple DIP dislocation. (*A*) Posteroanterior view of the DIP. (*B*) Lateral view of the DIP.

Longer duration of full-time splint wear is also associated with decreased extension lag; however, additional nocturnal splinting has not been found beneficial.[19] For non-compliant patients, oblique pinning across the DIP into extension is an alternative; however, unprotected return to play with a Kirschner wire in place may lead to a bent or broken pin.

Dorsal Proximal Interphalangeal Joint

Dorsal dislocations represent a spectrum of injury. Type I is a hyperextension injury with avulsion of the volar plate but intact accessory and proper collateral ligaments preventing full dislocation (**Fig. 6**). Type II injuries involve a split in the accessory and proper collateral ligaments leading to a true dorsal dislocation.[4] When hyperextension is accompanied by a significant axial loading force, a type III injury occurs as a dorsal dislocation with a volar fracture of P2.[6] The joint remains stable in flexion in all but the worst type 3 injuries, because of the support of the proper collateral ligaments.

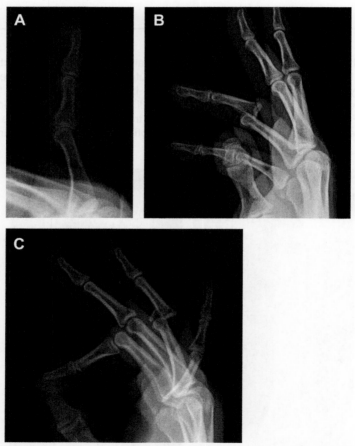

Fig. 6. Spectrum of PIP injuries. (*A*) Hyperextension injury without dislocation shows middle phalangeal extension beyond neutral, indicating volar plate injury. (*B*) Frank PIP dislocation. (*C*) PIP fracture-dislocation.

To reduce the injured joint, physicians should wrap their fingers around the patient's finger distal to the PIP and apply an extension force across the joint while using the thumb to hook around the base of P2 and pull the phalanx distally. A straight traction maneuver may lead to entrapment of the condyles in the collateral ligaments, pulling the volar plate into the joint and creating an irreducible dislocation.[9,11] Motion and return to play can be immediate if there is no concurrent fracture; the finger should be protected with buddy taping for the next week or until motion is normal.

Open PIP joint dislocations should be treated with more caution and be presumed unstable, because a soft tissue injury indicates significantly greater force. Irreducible dorsal PIP joint dislocations are similarly secondary to volar plate entrapment. They should be first approached dorsally through a small longitudinal incision with distraction of the joint to allow entrapped structures to fall volarly. Stability is typically present on reduction, and early active motion with protected return to play may happen once incisions heal. A retrospective review of 75 hyperextension injuries treated conservatively with buddy tape showed average range of motion of 85°.[20] A randomized trial of patients with dorsal PIP joint dislocations compared cast immobilization with dorsal splint allowing early motion; final range of motion in the cast group was limited in 60% of patients, whereas in the early motion group only 15% showed limitation.[21] A larger trial of buddy taping versus aluminum splinting in 15° of flexion showed less pain and faster return of motion in the buddy tape group with no difference in final outcome.[22]

Volar Proximal Interphalangeal Joint

A volar PIP dislocation is frequently the result of a combined flexion and radial or ulnar stress; there is usually a rotatory component with complete tear of one of the collateral ligaments. During the dislocation, the volar movement of the P2 creates a central slip avulsion.[11] Although the joint is stable on reduction, this injury requires treatment of the central slip injury with extension splinting of the PIP for 4 weeks. The DIP should be left free to allow mobilization of the lateral bands and terminal tendon (see **Fig. 3**).[4,23]

The reduction maneuver attempts to recreate the force applied to the cause the injury. Offloading the flexor tendons with flexion of the wrist and metacarpophalangeal, the PIP is further flexed while distal traction and rotation counter to the direction of the deformity is applied. These dislocations are more likely to be irreducible.[5,11]

There is a lack of outcomes data on closed central slip injuries; the largest study, by Souter[24] in 1967, reviewed 29 closed central slip injuries, of which 24 were treated with 4 weeks of PIP joint extension splinting, with a satisfactory result in 71%. Missed or untreated injuries that develop boutonnière deformity may require operative intervention.

Lateral Proximal Interphalangeal Joint

A tangential force causes lateral PIP dislocations, and although most are easily reduced, an underlying complete collateral ligament tear persists. Careful assessment of radial and ulnar stability should be undertaken under local anesthetic. Pain (grade I) and mild laxity (grade II) are treated with a week of extension splinting followed by 3 weeks of motion with buddy taping; grade III injuries do not have an end point, and can be especially debilitating in border digits.[4,14] Grade III injuries in athletes should be treated operatively: although range of motion at 1 year was similar in grade III collateral ligament injuries treated with splinting as opposed to those with surgery, recovery of motion is quicker with operative treatment, with Lee and colleagues[25] noting 40° versus 80° arc of motion at 1 month respectively.

Operative treatment is performed through a lateral approach and a suture anchor placed to repair the ligament to its proximal origin, where the avulsion most commonly occurs.[26] The finger is immobilized for 3 days and then motion protection by buddy taping is initiated. Return to play should be delayed 4 to 6 weeks until adequate motion has been restored to prevent the finger from exposure to repeat injury.

Thumb Interphalangeal Joint

The thumb IP joint has a larger arc of motion than both DIP and PIP joints, with the ability for significant hyperextension. With greater flexibility, it is less prone to dislocation than its counterpart in the fingers. Dorsal instability is the most common direction of dislocation. Reduction may be performed with simple longitudinal traction in most cases. Irreducible thumb IP joint dislocations may be secondary to flexor tendon interposition or condyle entrapment in the flexor tendon.[1,6,9]

Double Joint Dislocations

Simultaneous dislocations of both DIP and PIP can occur, with limited case reports within the literature.[27–30] Nearly all such injuries are associated with ball sports. Dawson[1] hypothesizes that these double dislocations are fairly common, and athletes self-reduce 1 of the joints before presentation to a physician for reduction of the other. The distribution of force over 2 joints may indicate a less severe soft tissue injury, because these joints are typically stable on reduction, and the athletes may start early range of motion and protected return to play.

FRACTURE-DISLOCATIONS OF DISTAL INTERPHALANGEAL JOINT

The short lever arm of the distal phalanx as well as the need for nearly 50% of the joint surface to be fractured to enable a dislocation renders this injury pattern uncommon.[31] Time between injury and initiation of immobilization has been shown as a risk factor for developing subluxation or dislocation.[32] When subluxation occurs, it is frequently secondary to a mallet injury, in which a large fragment of bone avulsed with the terminal tendon allowing volar subluxation/dislocation of the main body of the distal phalanx (**Fig. 7**).

These injuries are easily reduced in the acute setting and may be maintained in a hyperextension splint for 6 weeks (see **Fig. 3**); if unable to maintain the reduction, a Kirschner wire should be placed across the joint. This treatment yields equivalent outcomes to hook plate fixation, and thus is our treatment of choice; final DIP joint range of motion ranges from 50° to 80° in several studies, with extensor lag from 0° to 10°.[33,34] As discussed earlier, return to play depends on the ability to wear a splint or finger cast to prevent any flexion of the DIP joint.

FRACTURE-DISLOCATIONS OF PROXIMAL INTERPHALANGEAL JOINT

Management of fracture-dislocations of the PIP joint are differentiated from other phalangeal fractures, including unicondylar and other intra-articular fractures, in the unique mechanism and resultant instability they impart. A dorsal fracture-dislocation at the PIP occurs as a result of axial loading in conjunction with either flexion or hyperextension, which creates a coronal fracture of the volar lip of the middle phalanx.[35] The significance of this fracture location is belied by the anatomy: the volar plate as well as accessory collateral ligaments insert onto the volar lip, whereas the proper collateral ligaments insert onto the volar base of the phalanx. Volar fracture-dislocations are significantly less common, and similarly result from an axial load directed palmarly

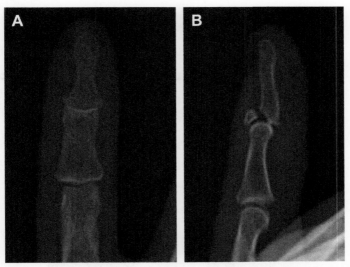

Fig. 7. Dorsal DIP fracture-subluxation creating mallet finger. (*A*) Posteroanterior view. (*B*) Lateral view.

while the finger is in extension. They represent an avulsion of the central slip with a fragment of bone, and are more likely to be stable.

The pilon fracture may be in the category of fracture-dislocation depending on the individual injury. A result of a straight axial load, the middle phalanx is compressed onto the proximal phalangeal head. The pilon fracture involves both the dorsal and volar lips with impaction of the central fragments, leading to subsequent widening of the articular surface.[35] These injuries are most frequent in athletes whose hands are exposed to significant end-on forces in not only ball-handling sports but other high-energy sports in which the hands may be outstretched, such as gymnastics.

Imaging assessment plays a key role in management. Lateral radiographs should be assessed closely for concentric joint reduction. The dorsal V sign (see **Fig. 2**) indicates an incomplete reduction because the joint is not concentric.[15] Live fluoroscopy allows visualization of the joint through range of motion and is recommended when available.

The fracture fragment should be assessed for size and noted as a percentage of the articular surface. Fracture fragments involving 10% to 15% of the joint surface represent a bony avulsion from the volar plate injury and are stable throughout the arc of motion. Unstable fractures typically involve more than 40% of the joint surface and do not maintain reduction, because the volar and lateral PIP joint stabilizers remain attached to the fracture fragment and only the central slip provides support to the remaining phalanx. Fragments between 15% and 40% are variable: they are usually well aligned in flexion but unstable when moved into extension (**Fig. 8**).[1,4,6,8,12,35] Volar fracture-dislocations tend to be unstable if more than 50% of the joint surface is involved.

A frequent problem with these injuries is delay in treatment. Many athletes and trainers assume that the initial benign appearance of the finger does not necessitate evaluation. When they are ignored or treated as a simple sprain or dislocation, articular degeneration, pain, and fixed deformity may develop. Operative treatment becomes necessary, and outcomes are significantly worse with lifelong limitation in range of motion.[1,8]

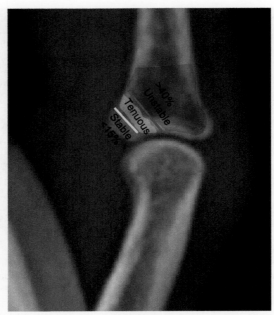

Fig. 8. Percentage joint involvement and relative stability of PIP fracture. Less than 15% of joint surface fractured is stable (*green*), 15% to 40% is tenuous (*yellow*), and greater than 40% is unstable (*red*).

Treatment of Stable Proximal Interphalangeal Joint Fracture-Dislocations

Stable fractures show a congruent joint throughout the range of motion. Although there are varying reports in the literature about the involved percentage of the articular surface that leads to an unstable joint, from 10% to 30%,[1,9,15,31,35] these numbers are only useful in general terms because the assessment of stability depends on each individual patient's examination and imaging. If there is any evidence of hinging of the joint or subluxation with full extension on the lateral radiograph, regardless of joint percentage involved, the injury should be treated as tenuous.

Those fractures that are truly stable may be treated with buddy taping, immediate active range of motion, and early return to play once pain permits (see **Fig. 3**). Tape may be weaned and passive range of motion started at 3 to 4 weeks; aggressive passive stretching should be avoided in the immediate postinjury period. The goal of early motion is to prevent flexion contracture, which develops within weeks of continual splinting.

Treatment of Tenuous Proximal Interphalangeal Joint Fracture-Dislocations

Fractures with a larger volar lip fragment are often stable in flexion, only showing subluxation when ranged into varying degrees of extension. These patients usually have a fracture fragment that is too small for fixation. If the fracture is stable with 30° or less of flexion, they are candidates for nonoperative treatment with dorsal blocking (see **Fig. 3**). The dorsal blocking splint should be fabricated by a hand therapist and the degree of flexion decreased weekly (either by 25% or 10°) until full extension is achieved; transition to buddy taping is then initiated.[4,9] These injuries must be followed with weekly imaging to ensure no further displacement or subtle joint incongruity occurs.

In general, studies report good range of motion, with an average total range of 87° at the PIP in 1 series.[36] Immediate return to play is an option with secure protection; blocking splint may be transitioned to a cast for activity to provide extra stability.[37] Although some investigators advocate a dorsal blocking pin and report excellent motion (average of 93° after treatment),[38] this does not allow weekly increase in range of motion, and consequently delays return to full range of motion.

Treatment of Unstable Proximal Interphalangeal Joint Fracture-Dislocations

In fractures that are grossly unstable or require more than 30° of flexion for stability, operative treatment may be required for optimal function. The goal of any procedure of the PIP joint is adequate stability to initiate early range of motion and prevent joint contracture. With these injuries, there is little difference in the operative treatment between athletes and lay persons, because the importance of a congruent joint to maintain range of motion supplants any desire for early return to play.[39]

When large volar fragments exist, open reduction with internal fixation (ORIF) is the ideal choice to allow early active motion, 3 to 5 days postoperatively (**Fig. 9**). The joint

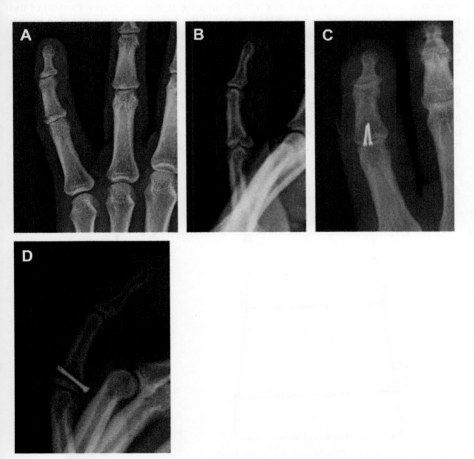

Fig. 9. Demonstration of ORIF of a PIP fracture-dislocation with miniscrews. (*A*) Preoperative posteroanterior view. (*B*) Preoperative lateral view. (*C*) Postoperative posteroanterior view. (*D*) Postoperative lateral view.

is exposed via a volar approach for adequate exposure. Use of 1.2-mm screws allows stable fixation and does not require a second procedure for removal,[8,39,40] although some investigators advocate a minihook plate or trimmed T plate.[35] With any fixation, the joint should be checked through full range of motion to ensure smooth gliding and absence of fracture gapping. To avoid a boutonnière deformity, which is often seen in athletes postoperatively, the joint may be pinned for 3 weeks in slight hyperextension.

Multiple series present varying postoperative motion arcs after ORIF from 70° to 100° with increasing range noted in patients with fewer fracture fragments.[7,41–43] Hamilton and colleagues[41] reported a series of 9 patients treated with miniscrew fixation and achieved an average arc of 70° (range, 55°–90°) more than 1 year after surgery and symmetric grip strength when compared contralaterally; only 2 patients modified activity because of the injury. Giugale and colleagues[44] found similar motion using miniscrews in 5 patients, with an average arc of 84° and range of 60° to 100°. Volar plating can have good results but greater variability in outcomes are seen. A series of 13 patients found an average motion arc of 75° with a range from 10° to 100°; 30% of patients had severe loss of motion and 3 of these underwent removal of hardware in an attempt to increase motion.[45] Percutaneous Kirschner wire fixation of the fragments has generated more reliable results if the fragments are amenable to this form of stabilization; in a series of 9 patients, an average arc of 106° (range from 80°–110°) was found.[46] This increased motion was attributable to avoidance of additional soft tissue injury from an open exposure.

Fractures with severe comminution are not candidates for ORIF because the fragments are too small to hold fixation. Dynamic external fixation may be considered if longitudinal traction restores a congruent joint surface (**Fig. 10**). Described by Badia and colleagues[47] in 2005, Kirschner wires and rubber bands are used to hold the joint out to length and allow range of motion throughout the healing period. Because the hardware traverses the skin, pin site infections are common complications. In a series

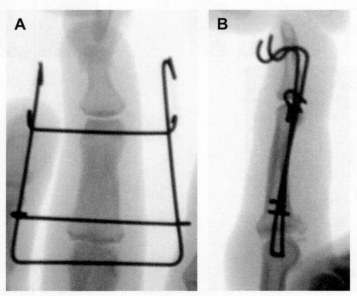

Fig. 10. Dynamic external fixator created with Kirschner wires for a comminuted PIP fracture-dislocation. (*A*) Posteroanterior view. (*B*) Lateral view.

of 34 patients, a final range of motion arc of 88° was achieved at the PIP.[48] The other options in severe comminution of the volar fragment are volar plate and hemihamate arthroplasties (discussed later).

Pilon fractures may be treated with either ORIF or dynamic external fixation, and often require bone graft to support the impacted central joint fragments.[35] Lag screws are usually able to adequately narrow the articular widening and provide a good result.[4]

The literature reports good outcomes in comminuted or delayed presentation of PIP joint fracture-dislocations using volar plate arthroplasty. Lin and colleagues[49] presented a series of 5 patients with average motion of 75° (range of 60°–85°). The largest series, of 17 patients, reports an average motion of 73° but finds worse motion when the series is subdivided into acute and chronic injuries: 85° versus 61°, respectively. Average extension lag (flexion contracture) was 22°, again worse in chronic injuries (29°).[50] Volar plate arthroplasty is no longer a staple in our treatment algorithm for unstable PIP fracture-dislocations, because the resultant flexion contracture from significant advancement of the volar plate is limiting to highly functioning patients.

Patients with delayed presentation, chronic injuries, or severely comminuted PIP fracture-dislocations should be considered for hemihamate arthroplasty. Introduced by Hastings in 1999, the procedure may be used in involvement of 40% to 80% of the volar joint surface of the middle phalanx. The hamate has a similar ridge that mirrors the normal articular anatomy of the P2 base, allowing resection of injured or diseased bone and replacement en bloc. Although technically challenging, it provides restoration of motion with excellent motion outcomes across multiple series: Williams and colleagues[51] reported on 11 patients with average PIP motion of 85° (range from 65°–100°) and average flexion contracture of 9°, Calfee and colleagues[52] reported on 22 patients with an average motion arc of 70°. However, hemihamate arthroplasty does have complication; in the Williams and colleagues[51] series, 2 patients (19%) had recurrent dorsal subluxation, but no intervention was required. The other series reported 2 complications: an 80° flexion contracture attributed to lack of participation in therapy, and a 10° coronal deviation that the patient was dissatisfied with despite a motion arc of 90°.[52]

The key to the hemihamate procedure is restoration of a concave joint surface (Fig. 11). A flattened appearance of the middle phalanx base on lateral imaging is a risk factor for dislocation. This deformity results from harvesting a graft that is too short, but it may be corrected by bone grafting distally between the graft and phalangeal shaft to rotate the hamate segment to recreate concavity. Rigid fixation with screws is necessary to allow early range of motion, starting 3 to 5 days postoperatively.

Palmar fracture-dislocations are often stable, unless more than half the joint surface is involved. In those cases, open reduction with lag screw placement through a dorsal approach or buttress plate fixation is sufficient to allow stability for early motion and return to play once imaging shows healing (average time of 5–8 weeks).[8]

CONSEQUENCES OF DELAYED DIAGNOSIS

Failure to receive proper treatment of complex fracture-dislocations inevitably leads to poor outcomes. Flexion contractures are prevalent even if the joint is reducible at the time of treatment. With chronically dislocated IP joints, joint destruction and chronic pain may result. Frequently, the only option left in these cases is fusion to relieve pain. Although this is not ideal for athletes because it obviates all motion, consideration of the patient's specific functional demands and placement in a position

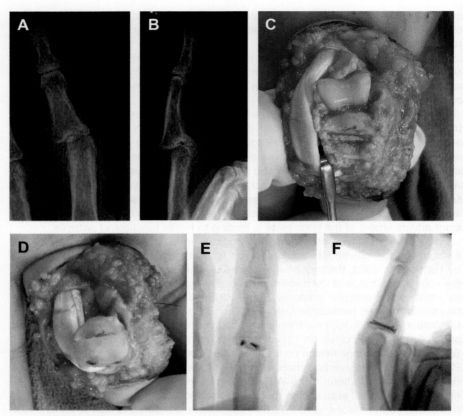

Fig. 11. Hemihamate reconstruction for a chronic PIP fracture-dislocation. (*A*) Preoperative posteroanterior view. (*B*) Preoperative lateral view. (*C*) Intraoperative view of the middle phalanx following excision of diseased articular surface. (*D*) Intraoperative view of the middle phalanx after placement of the hamate autograft. (*E*) Postoperative posteroanterior view. (*F*) Postoperative lateral view.

satisfying these needs provides a better outcome; the standard fusion recommendations may be impractical.[15] Athletes are typically not candidates for arthroplasty, given the risk for dislocation of the implanted joint with high-impact activities.

Improperly treated volar dislocation leads to boutonnière deformity. When seen in a delayed manner, surgical repair of the central slip or rebalancing of the lateral bands is more likely required to restore finger motion, necessitating 6 to 8 weeks off play for the recovery period.[3,53]

It is essential that coaches, trainers, and athletes alike recognize the potential complications of what may seem like a minor injury to avoid downstream consequences resulting in loss of motion and extended recovery. Evaluation should be sought with any jam or dislocation injury.

RETURN TO PLAY

Although the operative treatment of IP joint injuries is similar in athletes and the lay persons, the rehabilitation after injury is specifically tailored to athletes. Regular hand therapy with a certified hand therapist (CHT) should be initiated as soon as possible (in 1–3 days) with both operatively and nonoperatively managed injuries. Additional sport-specific conditioning should be initiated once adequate healing has been achieved, roughly at 1 week for simple dislocations and between 4 to 8 weeks for fracture-dislocations, depending on radiographic evidence of healing.[12,39] Rehabilitation with a CHT and a trainer should be synergistic and proceed concurrently.

Range of motion needs to improve before allowing return to play; a stiff finger protrudes and is easily reinjured. Initial return should be in a protected manner using buddy taping or splinting of the injured finger. Simple dislocations that are reduced are eligible for immediate return.[16] In more complicated injuries, early return may be facilitated by splinting or protective casting as discussed earlier.[40] Additional factors, such as position and hand dominance, may dictate timing. An outfielder with a nondominant stable PIP fracture-dislocation is protected by a glove and could return 1 week after injury, as opposed to the same injury in the dominant hand of a pitcher, in whom return at 3 to 4 weeks with buddy taping is more realistic.[39] Serial imaging should be obtained during the first 3 weeks of return to play for any injuries involving fractures.

Regardless of injury, return to play is an evolving discussion with the athlete, trainer, coach, and treating hand surgeon. Establishing realistic expectations at the initial consultation and continual communication with all involved parties is essential to overall patient satisfaction.

SUMMARY

Finger injuries can often be disregarded in the heat of the game; references to so-called coach's finger abound in sports and the literature. However, subtle findings that indicate a more serious injury can often be missed if proper treatment is not sought promptly after play is finished. Given the implications for final range of motion on hand function, the authors advocate early assessment of all finger dislocations to ensure that ligamentous injuries, tendinous injuries, and fractures are not missed and to ensure the best results for the players.

DISCLOSURE

The authors have no relevant interests to disclose.

REFERENCES

1. Dawson WJ. The spectrum of sports-related interphalangeal joint injuries. Hand Clin 1994;10(2):315–26.
2. Mall NA, Carlisle JC, Matava MJ, et al. Upper extremity injuries in the National Football League: part I: hand and digital injuries. Am J Sports Med 2008; 36(10):1938–44.
3. McDevitt ER. On-site treatment of PIP joint dislocations. Phys Sportsmed 1998; 26(8):85–6.
4. Bindra RR, Foster BJ. Management of proximal interphalangeal joint dislocations in athletes. Hand Clin 2009;25(3):423–35.
5. Carruthers KH, Skie M, Jain M. Jam injuries of the finger: diagnosis and management of injuries to the interphalangeal joints across multiple sports and levels of experience. Sports Health 2016;8(5):469–78.

6. Palmer RE. Joint injuries of the hand in athletes. Clin Sports Med 1998;17(3): 513–31.
7. Watanabe K, Kino Y, Yajima H. Factors affecting the functional results of open reduction and internal fixation for fracture-dislocations of the proximal interphalangeal joint. Hand Surg 2015;20(1):107–14.
8. Williams CS. Proximal interphalangeal joint fracture dislocations: stable and unstable. Hand Clin 2012;28(3):409–16, xi.
9. Merrell G, Slade JF. Dislocations and ligament injuries in the digits. In: Wolfe SW, editor. Greens operative hand surgery, vol. 1, 6th edition. New York: Elsevier; 2011. p. 291–320.
10. Arora R, Lutz M, Fritz D, et al. Dorsolateral dislocation of the proximal interphalangeal joint: closed reduction and early active motion or static splinting; a retrospective study. Arch Orthop Trauma Surg 2004;124(7):486–8.
11. Saitta BH, Wolf JM. Treating proximal interphalangeal joint dislocations. Hand Clin 2018;34(2):139–48.
12. Birman MV, Rossenwasser MP. Proximal interphalangeal joint fracture dislocations in professional baseball players. Hand Clin 2012;28(3):417–20.
13. Chung S, Sood A, Lee E. Principles of management in isolated dorsal distal interphalangeal joint dislocations. Eplasty 2014;14:ic33.
14. Chen F, Kalainov DM. Phalanx fractures and dislocations in athletes. Curr Rev Musculoskelet Med 2017;10(1):10–6.
15. Prucz RB, Friedrich JB. Finger joint injuries. Clin Sports Med 2015;34(1):99–116.
16. Halim A, Weiss AP. Return to play after hand and wrist fractures. Clin Sports Med 2016;35(4):597–608.
17. Peterson JJ, Bancroft LW. Injuries of the fingers and thumb in the athlete. Clin Sports Med 2006;25(3):527–42, vii–viii.
18. Okafor B, Mbubaegbu C, Munshi I, et al. Mallet deformity of the finger. Five-year follow-up of conservative treatment. J Bone Joint Surg Br 1997;79(4):544–7.
19. Gruber JS, Bot AGJ, Ring D. A prospective randomized controlled trial comparing night splinting with no splinting after treatment of mallet finger. Hand (N Y) 2014;9(2):145–50.
20. Adi M, Diaz JJH, Botero SS, et al. Results of conservative treatment of volar plate sprains of the proximal interphalangeal joint with and without avulsion fracture. Hand Surg Rehabil 2017;36(1):44–7.
21. Lutz M, Reinhart C, Kathrein A, et al. [Dorsal dislocation of the proximal interphalangeal joints of the finger. Results after static and functional treatment]. Handchir Mikrochir Plast Chir 2001;33(3):207–10.
22. Paschos NK, Abuhemoud K, Gantsos A, et al. Management of proximal interphalangeal joint hyperextension injuries: a randomized controlled trial. J Hand Surg 2014;39(3):449–54.
23. Grandizio LC, Klena JC. Sagittal band, boutonniere, and pulley injuries in the athlete. Curr Rev Musculoskelet Med 2017;10(1):17–22.
24. Souter WA. The boutonniere deformity: a review of 101 patients with division of the central slip of the extensor expansion of the fingers. J Bone Joint Surg Am 1967;49(4):710–21.
25. Lee SJ, Lee JH, Hwang IC, et al. Clinical outcomes of operative repair of complete rupture of the proximal interphalangeal joint collateral ligament: comparison with non-operative treatment. Acta Orthop Traumatol Turc 2017;51(1):44–8.
26. Kato H, Minami A, Takahara M, et al. Surgical repair of acute collateral ligament injuries in digits with the Mitek bone suture anchor. J Hand Surg Br 1999; 24(1):70–5.

27. Panchal AP, Bamberger HB. Dorsal dislocation of the distal interphalangeal joint and volar dislocation of the metacarpophalangeal joint in the same finger: a case report. Hand (N Y) 2010;5(2):200–2.
28. Abdelaal A, Edwards T, Anand S. Simultaneous dislocation of both the proximal and distal interphalangeal joints of a little finger. BMJ Case Rep 2016;2016 [pii: bcr2015213914].
29. Uysal MA, Akçay S, Öztürk K. Simultaneous double interphalangeal joints dislocation in a finger in a teenager. J Clin Orthop Trauma 2014;5(2):107–9.
30. Loupasis G, Christoforakis J, Aligizakis A. Simultaneous double interphalangeal dislocation in a finger. J Orthop Trauma 1998;12(1):70–2.
31. Calfee RP, Sommerkamp TG. Fracture-dislocation about the finger joints. J Hand Surg 2009;34(6):1140–7.
32. Kim JK, Kim DJ. The risk factors associated with subluxation of the distal interphalangeal joint in mallet fracture. J Hand Surg Eur Vol 2014;40(1):63–7.
33. Toker S, Türkmen F, Pekince O, et al. Extension block pinning versus hook plate fixation for treatment of mallet fractures. J Hand Surg 2015;40(8):1591–6.
34. Acar MA, Güzel Y, Güleç A, et al. Clinical comparison of hook plate fixation versus extension block pinning for bony mallet finger: a retrospective comparison study. J Hand Surg Eur Vol 2015;40(8):832–9.
35. Caggiano NM, Harper CM, Rozental TD. Management of proximal interphalangeal joint fracture dislocations. Hand Clin 2018;34(2):149–65.
36. Hamer DW, Quinton DN. Dorsal fracture subluxation of the proximal interphalangeal joints treated by extension block splintage. J Hand Surg 1992;17(5):586–90.
37. Williams CS. Football commentary: PIP fracture. Hand Clin 2012;28(3):423–4.
38. Vitale MA, White NJ, Strauch RJ. A percutaneous technique to treat unstable dorsal fracture-dislocations of the proximal interphalangeal joint. J Hand Surg 2011;36(9):1453–9.
39. Clinkscales C. Sports-specific commentary on PIP joint fracture dislocations in professional basketball players. Hand Clin 2012;28(3):421–2.
40. Gaston RG, Chadderdon C. Phalangeal fractures: displaced/nondisplaced. Hand Clin 2012;28(3):395–401, x.
41. Hamilton SC, Stern PJ, Fassler PR, et al. Mini-screw fixation for the treatment of proximal interphalangeal joint dorsal fracture-dislocations. J Hand Surg Am 2006;31(8):1349–54.
42. Tekkis PP, Kessaris N, Gavalas M, et al. The role of mini-fragment screw fixation in volar dislocations of the proximal interphalangeal joint. Arch Orthop Trauma Surg 2001;121(1–2):121–2.
43. Komura S, Yokoi T, Nonomura H. Mini hook plate fixation for palmar fracture-dislocation of the proximal interphalangeal joint. Arch Orthop Trauma Surg 2011;131(4):563–6.
44. Giugale JM, Wang J, Kaufmann RA, et al. Mid-term outcomes after open reduction internal fixation of proximal interphalangeal joint dorsal fracture-dislocations through a volar, shotgun approach and a review of the literature. Open Orthop J 2017;11:1073–80.
45. Cheah AEJ, Tan DMK, Chong AKS, et al. Volar plating for unstable proximal interphalangeal joint dorsal fracture-dislocations. J Hand Surg Am 2012;37(1):28–33.
46. de Haseth KB, Neuhaus V, Mudgal CS. Dorsal fracture-dislocations of the proximal interphalangeal joint: evaluation of closed reduction and percutaneous Kirschner wire pinning. Hand (N Y) 2015;10(1):88–93.
47. Badia A, Riano F, Ravikoff J, et al. Dynamic intradigital external fixation for proximal interphalangeal joint fracture dislocations. J Hand Surg 2005;30(1):154–60.

48. Ruland RT, Hogan CJ, Cannon DL, et al. Use of dynamic distraction external fixation for unstable fracture-dislocations of the proximal interphalangeal joint. J Hand Surg 2008;33(1):19–25.
49. Lin S-Y, Chuo C-Y, Lin G-T, et al. Volar plate interposition arthroplasty for posttraumatic arthritis of the finger joints. J Hand Surg Am 2008;33(1):35–9.
50. Dionysian E, Eaton RG. The long-term outcome of volar plate arthroplasty of the proximal interphalangeal joint. J Hand Surg 2000;25(3):429–37.
51. Williams RMM, Kiefhaber TR, Sommerkamp TG, et al. Treatment of unstable dorsal proximal interphalangeal fracture/dislocations using a hemi-hamate autograft. J Hand Surg 2003;28(5):856–65.
52. Calfee RP, Kiefhaber TR, Sommerkamp TG, et al. Hemi-hamate arthroplasty provides functional reconstruction of acute and chronic proximal interphalangeal fracture-dislocations. J Hand Surg 2009;34(7):1232–41.
53. Ruby LK. Common hand injuries in the athlete. Clin Sports Med 1983;2(3): 609–29.

Thumb Metacarpophalangeal Ulnar and Radial Collateral Ligament Injuries

Dane Daley, MD[a], Michael Geary, MD[b],
Raymond Glenn Gaston, MD[c],*

KEYWORDS

- Ulnar collateral ligament (UCL) • Radial collateral ligament (RCL)
- Thumb metacarpophalangeal joint injuries (MCP)
- Collateral ligament injury in athlete • Skier's thumb • Gamekeeper's thumb

KEY POINTS

- Ulnar collateral ligament (UCL) and radial collateral ligament (RCL) have an accessory and proper component.
- Grade I or II and certain grade III UCL injuries can be managed with nonoperative immobilization with good long-term results.
- Grade III UCL injuries with a Stener lesion and avulsion fractures involving greater than 30% of the articular surface are best treated with surgery.
- Treatment considerations need to take into account the level of athletic participation, hand dominance, demands on the thumb during the athlete's respective sport, the practicality of playing with thumb immobilization, the duration of season remaining, and patient's/athlete's specific goals.
- There are various methods of repair and reconstruction of both UCL and RCL injuries with comparable outcomes.

INTRODUCTION

Thumb metacarpophalangeal (MCP) joint collateral ligament injuries are among the most common injuries to the hand. Previous reports show an incidence of collateral ligament injuries as high as 86% of the injuries to the thumb.[1,2] These injuries are

ª Department of Orthopedics and Physical Medicine, Medical University of South Carolina, 96 Jonathan Lucas Street, Suite 708, Charleston, SC 29425, USA; ᵇ Atrium Musculoskeletal Institute, Charlotte Medical Center, 1000 Blythe Boulevard, Charlotte, NC 28203, USA; ᶜ Atrium Musculoskeletal Institute, OrthoCarolina, 1915 Randolph RD, Charlotte, NC 28207, USA
* Corresponding author.
E-mail address: Glenn.gaston@orthocarolina.com

Clin Sports Med 39 (2020) 443–455
https://doi.org/10.1016/j.csm.2019.12.003
0278-5919/20/© 2019 Elsevier Inc. All rights reserved.

sportsmed.theclinics.com

especially common in athletes.[3] Ulnar collateral ligament (UCL) injuries occur 10 times more frequently than radial collateral ligament (RCL) injuries.[4] UCL injuries occur via thumb MCP hyperabduction or hyperextension[5–11]; in contrast, RCL injuries result from a forced or sudden thumb MCP adduction moment.[12] Of note, complete injury of either the UCL or RCL can lead to MCP instability; disability; future degenerative changes; and, in athletes, missed time from play.

An acute UCL injury, often termed a skier's thumb because of its high prevalence in the sport,[13] occurs secondary to a fall onto an outstretched hand with the abducted thumb around the ski pole imparting a significant valgus stress to the thumb MCP joint. An 11-year study out of a Wyoming ski resort found that 7% of all injuries sustained were related to UCL injuries about the thumb. Other studies report UCL injuries to be the second most common ski injuries behind medial collateral ligament injuries of the knee.[14–16] A chronic UCL injury is termed gamekeeper's thumb, which was found to be a common attritional rupture of the UCL in Scottish gamekeepers.[17]

Thumb collateral ligament injuries are a frequent injury found in the National Football League (NFL). In a review of 10 years of injuries in the NFL, nearly one-third of all hand injuries involved the thumb, with 25% of those affecting the MCP joint.[18] In collegiate football, the subsequent impact of these injuries to the athletes resulted in approximately 3 weeks' loss of playing time.[3]

ANATOMY

The thumb MCP joint is a diarthroidal joint with motion primarily in the sagittal plane allowing flexion and extension but also some degree of abduction, adduction, and circumduction.[19] Stability of the thumb MCP joint is provided through both static and dynamic restraints. Static stabilizers include the bony anatomy of the MCP joint, the RCL and UCL, volar plate, and dorsal capsule. Dynamic stabilization is provided by the extrinsic and intrinsic muscles of the thumb crossing the MCP joint.[11] Of the intrinsic muscles, the adductor pollicis is the most pertinent to the thumb's MCP joint stability as it resists valgus forces.[20]

The UCL and RCL each consist of a proper and accessory collateral ligament, traveling in a proximal-dorsal to distal-volar direction. Cadaveric studies have shown that the UCL, on average, originates 4.2 mm from the dorsal surface and 5.3 mm proximal to the articular surface of the metacarpal head, and inserts 2.8 mm from the volar surface and 3.4 mm distal to the base of the proximal phalanx.[21] The proper collateral ligament runs approximately 30° in a dorsal to volar trajectory to insert at the base of the proximal phalanx. The accessory collateral ligament is volar to the proper collateral ligament, and inserts on the volar aspect of the proximal phalanx and volar plate at an approximately 90° trajectory from its origin.[22] With the MCP in approximately 30° flexion, the proper collateral ligaments and dorsal capsule provide stability to radial and ulnar deviation of the thumb MCP joint; therefore, this is the optimal position for testing the integrity of the proper UCL and RCL. With the MCP in full extension, stability is provided primarily by the accessory collateral ligament and volar plate.[23] The UCL is important in MCP joint stability and is critical for gripping, key pinch, and activities of daily living. It also provides resistance to volar subluxation.[24,25] In addition, the RCL and UCL accompany the dorsal capsule in providing dorsal support to the MCP joint.[12]

Variation exists in the population regarding the morphology of the thumb MCP joint, with round and flat types having been described.[26] The different morphology types have been linked to MCP joint range of motion as well as to the mode of failure of the UCL. Rounder MCP joint morphology shows increased range of motion with concomitant greater elasticity and creep before load to failure. In contrast, a flatter morphology has less range of motion and less creep before load to failure.[27]

Forced palmar abduction (radial deviation) at the thumb MCP joint may injure or rupture the UCL, with avulsion off the proximal phalanx occurring in approximately 90% of cases.[11] In addition to the collateral ligament injury, the dorsal capsule and/ or volar plate can also be injured, leading to volar and radial subluxation of the proximal phalanx. This subluxation is secondary to the pull of abductor pollicis brevis (APB) and flexor pollicis brevis.[8,11,28] The UCL most commonly tears at the distal insertion either as an avulsion or purely ligamentous injury, although proximal avulsions and midsubstance tears are described,[28–30] most likely because the UCL is narrower distally than proximally. The abduction force can be significant enough to displace the torn UCL ligament superficial to the adductor aponeurosis, creating the eponymous Stener lesion[28] (**Fig. 1**). A Stener lesion has been noted to occur in 60% to 90% of cases and portends a poorer prognosis without operative treatment.[7,28]

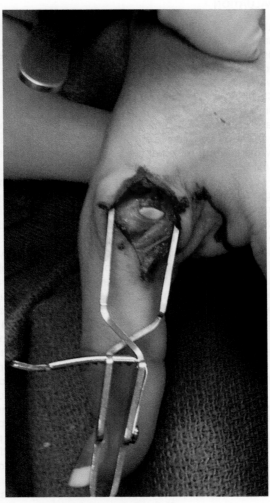

Fig. 1. UCL injury showing intraoperative Stener lesion.

On the radial side of the thumb MCP joint, the average footprint of the RCL origin is found 3.3 mm proximal to the articular surface and 3.5 mm from the dorsal surface of the metacarpal. The RCL insertion is 2.5 mm distal to articular surface and 2.8 mm from the volar cortex of the proximal phalanx.[21] The width of the RCL origin is often greater than its insertion, which is thought to contribute to the higher incidence of avulsions off the metacarpal. In 1 study, 55% of RCL injuries were proximal, 29% distal, and 16% midsubstance, which is notably different from UCL injury patterns.[31] Stener-equivalent lesions are much less frequently seen following RCL injuries because of the broader and more dorsal position of the APB aponeurosis, although they have been described on rare occasions.[31,32] Joint subluxation is more commonly seen with RCL injuries, in which the proximal phalanx subluxates in a volar and ulnar direction because of the powerful deforming pull of the adductor pollicis insertion on the proximal phalanx and ulnar sesamoid.[33]

PREOPERATIVE EVALUATION

A thorough evaluation should begin with careful history taking, in which the patient describes the mechanism of injury emphasizing the direction of force applied to the thumb. In addition to skiing, other common mechanisms to consider in athletes include forceful radial or ulnar deviation of the thumb from collision with other players, or from contact with balls or other equipment. In baseball, for example, a common mechanism of UCL injury includes sliding into a base head first with an outstretched and abducted thumb.[34]

Acute injuries are commonly accompanied by ecchymosis, swelling, and point tenderness along the radial or ulnar side of the MCP joint. It is also important to attempt to identify the point of maximal tenderness, remembering that UCL injuries typically occur distally at its insertion site and RCL injuries commonly occur proximally at the metacarpal origin. In more chronic conditions, players may complain of weakness with gripping equipment or difficulty with throwing or grasping. The examiner should palpate for the presence of a Stener lesion, which would indicate a complete tear of the UCL with retraction superficial to the adductor aponeurosis. However, absence of a palpable Stener lesion does not definitively rule out its presence.[2,7]

AP and lateral radiographs should be obtained evaluating for bony avulsions, fractures, presence of osteoarthritis, or subluxation of the MCP joint. Stability of the MCP joint should then be assessed by testing the integrity of the collateral ligaments and comparing them with the uninjured thumb. Stress examination should be performed in full extension to evaluate the accessory collateral ligament and volar plate, and at 30° of flexion to test the proper collateral ligament. The metacarpal head should be stabilized with the opposite hand, and the examiner must be careful to avoid MCP joint rotation, which may falsely mimic lateral instability, especially in patients with round metacarpal head morphology.[35] In the setting of suspected RCL injury, the thumb may lie in an ulnarly deviated position from the pull of the adductor pollicis and should be corrected to a neutral position before testing. If the patient is showing significant guarding that interferes with the ligamentous examination, local anesthetic may be a useful adjunct.[36] Degrees of laxity as well as the presence or absence of a firm end point should be noted. In suspected RCL injuries, anterior and posterior drawer testing should be performed as well.[11] A study of 100 asymptomatic thumbs found that it was common to have greater than 10° of variability between sides when testing lateral stability.[37]

Grading of both UCL and RCL injuries follows the same 3 stage classification. Grade 1 denotes pain along the collateral ligament without laxity to stress. Grade 2 injuries represent partial tears with asymmetric laxity and a firm end point. In addition, grade 3 injuries are complete tears with increased laxity and no discernible end point.[23] Values to consider when evaluating laxity in complete tears is greater than 30° of coronal plane deviation and greater than 15° relative to the uninjured side.[37] As discussed later, differentiating between partial and complete tears is critical to guiding treatment.

Debate exists regarding the role of stress radiographs in evaluating collateral ligament injuries, with opponents concerned that it may displace or complete a partial injury. A cadaveric study showed that stress radiographs can differentiate between partial and complete UCL tears, in which more than 2 mm of radial translation of the proximal phalanx is only possible with a complete tear.[38] Another important consideration is that fractures at the base of the proximal phalanx may occur separate from, or in combination with, tears of the collateral ligaments.[39] In this setting, clinical examination to assess coronal stability should be used in combination with radiographic findings for accurate diagnosis. Fracture of the proximal phalanx is not a contraindication to stress testing of the MCP joint.[34] MCP joint subluxation on a lateral radiograph is more commonly seen with RCL injuries, in which palmar subluxation greater than 3 mm is often a sign of a complete RCL tear with a dorsal capsular disruption.[33]

MRI may be useful in the setting of an equivocal clinical diagnosis to evaluate for collateral ligament injury or to identify the presence of a Stener lesion; however, MRI is not required to make the diagnosis in the setting of a clear history and physical examination (**Fig. 2**). The sensitivity and specificity of MRI for UCL injuries has been found to be as high as 100%, and it is the most reliable imaging modality to establish the diagnosis.[40,41] Ultrasonography has been used and studied as a diagnostic modality for diagnosing collateral ligament injuries. It is less expensive and often quicker

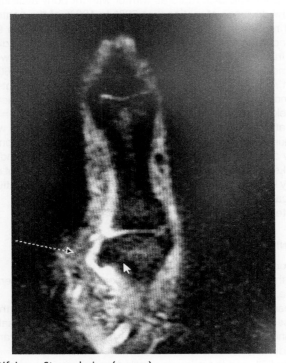

Fig. 2. MRI identifying a Stener lesion (*arrows*).

than MRI, with a sensitivity between 76% and 88% and a specificity between 81% and 83%.[40,41]

TREATMENT CONSIDERATIONS

Treatment considerations need to take into account the level of athletic participation, hand dominance, demands on the thumb during the athlete's respective sport, the physical ability to play with a splint/cast, the amount of time left in the season, and the patient's/athlete's specific goals.

- Nonoperative treatment:
  - Grade I or II injuries: initial thumb spica immobilization for a minimum of 4 weeks is the gold standard.[33,42,43]
- Operative treatment:
  - Grade III UCL tear with Stener lesion.
  - Grade III RCL: rationale for surgical treatment is based on the unopposed ulnar deviation at proximal phalanx from the adductor pollicis and extensor pollicis longus (EPL), which may lead to RCL healing in an elongated and displaced position. Repair may allow it to heal in a more anatomic position.[12,44]
  - Articular fracture involving greater than 30% of the articular surface or articular incongruity.[45]
- Controversy surrounds the treatment of:
  - Grade III UCL injuries without Stener lesion or joint subluxation: there is potential for healing without surgery if the ligament disruption is nondisplaced. Landsman and colleagues[46] showed successful nonoperative immobilization for 34 out of 40 acute complete UCL ruptures with or without bony avulsion. Furthermore, final follow-up range of motion was 60% to 100% of the contralateral thumb, 28 of 34 reported no pain, the average pinch strength was 92% compared with the contralateral thumb, and all bony avulsions united radiographically.
  - Avulsion fractures at UCL origin: good results have been shown with nonoperative management if there is no instability with stress despite 25% to 60% radiographic nonunion rates.[47,48] Kuz and colleagues[47] identified 30 patients with both displaced and nondisplaced avulsion fractures treated in thumb spica immobilization for 4 weeks. Subjectively, 29 patients reported mild pain (N = 10) or no pain (N = 19) at final follow-up and 23 patients reported their thumb was as strong as before injury. Objectively, 20 were available for clinical examination, with 3 showing instability and 15 with radiographic union, and none were found to have loss of grasp or key pinch strength. In contrast, minimally displaced but malrotated fractures may lead to persistent pain and thus do better with operative fixation.[49]
- Contraindications to surgery:
  - Chronic tears with associated MCP osteoarthritis.

SURGICAL TECHNIQUE

Acute UCL procedure[34]
1. Supine with an arm board and a well-padded tourniquet with general or regional anesthesia.
2. A curvilinear skin incision is made over the dorsal ulnar aspect of thumb MCP joint.
3. Blunt dissection is performed to identify and protect the dorsal radial sensory nerve branch followed by gentle dorsal retraction of this branch throughout the procedure.
4. Identify the EPL and the adductor pollicis aponeurosis.

5. Incise the aponeurosis longitudinally approximately 2 to 3 mm volar to its insertion to provide a cuff for later repair.
   a. At this point, a Stener lesion will be apparent with the UCL being superficial and proximal to the aponeurosis.
6. Isolate the torn UCL and mobilize:
   a. Subacute or chronic cases: the UCL may adhere to surrounding tissue and require further dissection.
7. Identify and roughen the insertion site with a curette.
8. Repair the UCL with suture only, suture anchor, or suture tape augmentation:
   a. Place sutures or anchor at the anatomic insertion point paralleling the joint surface.
   b. Avulsion fragments can be excised if small enough. If greater than 20% articular surface, retain and stabilize fragment with Kirschner wires or screw.
9. Repair dorsal capsular rent with 3-0 absorbable suture ideally with the MCP joint in flexion.
10. Repair adductor pollicis aponeurosis.
11. Assess stability of MCP joint in both full extension and 30° flexion.
12. Close wound and place patient in thumb spica splint.

POSTOPERATIVE PROTOCOL

Acute UCL tears:
- Thumb spica splint/cast for up to 4 weeks, interphalangeal joint free.
- At 4 to 6 weeks, removable thumb spica splint, and protected range-of-motion exercises.
- At 6 to 12 weeks, begin adductor and interossei strengthening, avoiding valgus stress on thumb MCP.
- At 10 to 12 weeks, return to full activity without brace.

Chronic UCL tears:
- Casting for 6 weeks.
- At 6 to 8 weeks, removable thumb spica splint, protected range-of-motion exercises.
- At 8 to 12 weeks, begin adductor and interossei strengthening, avoiding valgus stress on thumb MCP.
- At 12 to 16 weeks, return to full activity without brace.

Chronic Ulnar Collateral Ligament Considerations

In chronic cases in which the ligament is deemed irreparable, and there is no evidence of arthritis, the ligament remnants are excised to expose the UCL origin and insertion. In this case, an autograft tendon (palmaris longus if present) is used in a triangular configuration with the apex proximal with a distal bone tunnel or it is placed anatomically into the origin and insertion of the proper collateral ligament with interference screws. The MCP joint dorsal capsular rent is repaired with 3-0 absorbable suture, the adductor pollicis aponeurosis reapproximated, then the wound is closed and a thumb spica splint is applied.[34]

SURGICAL TECHNICAL CONSIDERATIONS

- Direct primary repair: when feasible, if native tissue is robust and easily identified.
  - Christensen and colleagues[50] performed a retrospective review of patients who underwent primary repair for a chronic UCL injury (>6 weeks). They

identified 24 patients who met their inclusion criteria and 12 were available for long-term follow-up. They reported excellent patient-reported outcomes in terms of satisfaction, overall pain relief, function, and stability. In the chronic setting, primary repair may be considered as an alternative to reconstruction.

- Transosseous suture: historical description in which the repair is tied over a button on the radial side of the thumb.[29]
- Suture anchors or interference screws: efficient, shorter surgical times, minimal soft tissue complications.
  - A 2014 retrospective review of collegiate football athletes with UCL injuries treated with suture anchor had quicker return to play, reliable return to same level of activity, and excellent long-term outcomes.[3] Skilled players were permitted to return to play in a fabricated orthosis or with taping after an initial 5-week period of immobilization. Non–skill-position athletes were allowed to practice and play in thumb spica cast after the 1-week wound check. All athletes returned to same level of play, without any postoperative complications, and with an average Quick-DASH score of 1 out of 100 (95% confidence interval, 0.4 to 2.3).[3]
- Suture tape augmentation (Arthrex Internal Brace): emerging technique for UCL repair/augmentation. A recent cadaveric study found the maximum load and load to clinical failure in the UCL repair group with suture tape augmentation to be 5 times and 4 times higher compared with the UCL repair–only specimens, respectively. Caution is needed to avoid overtightening the repair with this technique.
  - De Giacomo and colleagues[51] showed successful return to practice drills with removable thumb spica splint at 1 week and full unrestricted professional basketball play at 5 weeks postsurgery with this technique.[51,52] This technique requires larger drill holes within the metacarpal and proximal phalanx and, as such, concerns exist regarding possible fracture (**Fig. 3**).
- Reconstruction with autograft/allograft: generally indicated for chronic UCL/RCL injuries in which the ligament is unrepairable (**Fig. 4**).
- Acute and chronic RCL surgical considerations
  - Grade III RCL injuries are prone to healing in an elongated position secondary to the strong pull of the adductor and EPL and/or not healing at all. This position can lead to instability and degenerative changes at the MCP joint. However, they can heal with thumb spica immobilization because there is rarely intervening aponeurosis, provided the joint is congruently reduced. However, most surgeons advocate surgical repair or reconstruction for acute grade III and chronic RCL injuries, respectively.[12,44] RCL chronic injuries may be repaired with direct repair, RCL tissue advancement, soft tissue imbrication, RCL advancement with APB, or tendon graft reconstruction.[12] Limited literature exists analyzing the outcomes following acute and chronic RCL repair and reconstruction, respectively. Studies regarding the outcomes of both RCL and UCL repair and reconstruction have noted satisfactory outcomes.[12]

OUTCOMES IN ATHLETES/RETURN TO SPORT

Outcomes in athletes have varied depending on the sport-specific position, return-to-play timeline, the grade of collateral ligament injury, and the subsequent treatment performed. Familiarization with sport-specific regulations helps determine proper management and immobilization guidelines.[34]

Grade I and II UCL injuries treated nonoperatively are permitted to return to play if the sport and player position allow participation with immobilization. Following the

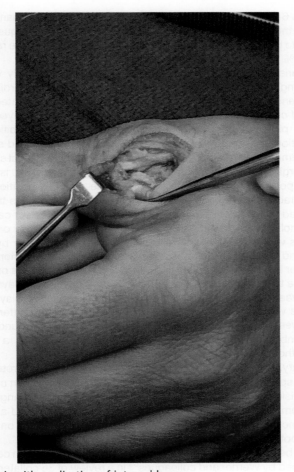

Fig. 3. UCL repair with application of internal brace.

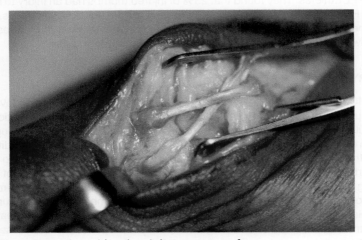

Fig. 4. RCL reconstruction with palmaris longus autograft.

initial 4-week to 6-week period of cast immobilization, a removable hand-based splint or dorsal radial thumb splint is recommended for play for the subsequent 4 weeks. In general, return to play without protection is considered once pain-free range of motion and at least 80% of grip strength are restored.[34]

Grade III injuries are typically treated with surgical repair, ideally within the first 3 weeks following injury; however, joint decision making is held regarding postponing surgery to the end of season. Werner and colleagues[53] in 2017 stated that surgical management of collateral ligament injuries in NFL athletes was delayed until the end of season with players immobilized in a customized position-specific splint in the interim. In addition, irrespective of length of time between injury and surgical repair, all collateral ligaments tolerated primary repair and all obtained clinical stability. Return to play after surgical intervention, as in nonoperative management, is based on the specific sport, position, time of the season, and the athlete's position-specific demands.[34] For grade III injuries in which the ligament is retracted less than 2 mm, the authors have had success with nonoperative management in select cases.

Werner and colleagues[3] in 2014 performed a retrospective study on 18 collegiate football athletes with UCL injuries treated with suture anchor repair by a single surgeon. They found 9 injuries in skill-position players and 9 injuries in non–skill-position players. A Stener lesion was identified in 4 athletes in each group. The only differences were earlier time to surgery in skill-position players (12 days vs 43 days) and later return to play (7 weeks vs 4 weeks) compared with non–skill-position players. Non–skill-position players were allowed to practice in a thumb spica cast after sutures were removed at 1 week. Skill-position players were allowed to play around 4 to 6 weeks after initial thumb spica immobilization for 4 weeks. At that point, a thermoplastic thumb spica orthosis was made for play.[3]

On the contrary, surgical repair of thumb UCL ruptures with early protected return to play in a thumb spica cast in collegiate football lineman has also been complicated by adjacent joint dislocations. One series identified proximal interphalangeal joint dislocations in 3 linemen who returned to play in thumb spica casts and a simple elbow dislocation in another. Early return to play may place added stress on the ipsilateral extremity with potential for further injury.[54]

It should also be mentioned that UCL and RCL injuries may occur in combination, as recently described by Werner and colleagues[53] in a review of 36 collateral ligament injuries in NFL athletes. They found that 25% of injured thumbs had an injury to both the UCL and RCL, and went on to operative treatment of both collateral ligaments. As previously mentioned, all athletes requiring surgery did so at the end of their respective seasons without detriment to the ability to perform a primary repair.[53]

SUMMARY

Thumb MCP joint collateral ligament injuries are common in athletes at all levels. The UCL is much more commonly injured and generally occurs at the distal insertion either as an avulsion injury or purely ligamentous injury. Determining the grade of injury and presence or absence of a Stener lesion is critical to guiding treatment. In addition, the level of athletic participation, hand dominance, demands on the thumb during the athlete's particular sport, the feasibility of playing immobilized, the length of season remaining, and the athlete's specific goals need to be considered. Surgical management is considered for grade III UCL/RCL injuries with ligament retraction, injuries with an associated Stener lesion, and avulsion fractures with involvement of greater than 30% of articular surface. Collateral ligaments may be repaired via transosseous sutures, suture anchors, suture tape augmentation, primary repair, or reconstruction.

Operative and nonoperative management in athletes has varied depending on the sport-specific position, the grade of collateral ligament injury, and the timing of injury. Outcomes have also varied regarding the return-to-play timeline, type and length of immobilization, and the treatment performed. It is our opinion that the treatment algorithm of collateral ligament injuries should continue to be handled on a patient-by-patient basis while considering all aspects associated with these injuries in athletes.

DISCLOSURE

The authors certify that they have no commercial associations (eg, consultancies, stock ownership, equity interest, patent/licensing arrangements) that might pose a conflict of interest in connection with this article.

REFERENCES

1. Rhee PC, Jones DB, Kakar S. Management of thumb metacarpophalangeal ulnar collateral ligament injuries. J Bone Joint Surg Am 2012;94(21):2005–12.
2. Baskies MA, Lee SK. Evaluation and treatment of injuries of the ulnar collateral ligament of the thumb metacarpophalangeal joint. Bull NYU Hosp Jt Dis 2009; 67(1):68–74.
3. Werner BC, Hadeed MM, Lyons ML, et al. Return to football and long-term clinical outcomes after thumb ulnar collateral ligament suture anchor repair in collegiate athletes. J Hand Surg Am 2014;39(10):1992–8.
4. Keramidas E, Miller G. Adult hand injuries on artificial ski slopes. Ann Plast Surg 2005;55(4):357–8.
5. Bostock SH, Morris MA. Rupture of the ulnar collateral ligament of the metacarpophalangeal joint of the thumb. Injury 1993;24(10):697.
6. Chuter GS, Muwanga CL, Irwin LR. Ulnar collateral ligament injuries of the thumb: 10 years of surgical experience. Injury 2009;40(6):652–6.
7. Heyman P, Gelberman RH, Duncan K, et al. Injuries of the ulnar collateral ligament of the thumb metacarpophalangeal joint. Biomechanical and prospective clinical studies on the usefulness of valgus stress testing. Clin Orthop Relat Res 1993;292:165–71.
8. Johnson JW, Culp RW. Acute ulnar collateral ligament injury in the athlete. Hand Clin 2009;25(3):437–42.
9. Lee AT, Carlson MG. Thumb metacarpophalangeal joint collateral ligament injury management. Hand Clin 2012;28(3):361–70, ix-x.
10. Ritting AW, Baldwin PC, Rodner CM. Ulnar collateral ligament injury of the thumb metacarpophalangeal joint. Clin J Sport Med 2010;20(2):106–12.
11. Tang P. Collateral ligament injuries of the thumb metacarpophalangeal joint. J Am Acad Orthop Surg 2011;19(5):287–96.
12. Edelstein DM, Kardashian G, Lee SK. Radial collateral ligament injuries of the thumb. J Hand Surg Am 2008;33(5):760–70.
13. Gerber C, Senn E, Matter P. Skier's thumb. Surgical treatment of recent injuries to the ulnar collateral ligament of the thumb's metacarpophalangeal joint. Am J Sports Med 1981;9(3):171–7.
14. Warme WJ, Feagin JA Jr, King P, et al. Ski injury statistics, 2981-1993, Jackson Hole Ski Resort. Am J Sports Med 1995;23:597–600.
15. Carr D, Johnson RJ, Pope MH. Upper extremity injuries in skiing. Am J Sports Med 1981;9:378–83.
16. Steedman DJ. Artificial ski slope injuries: a 1-year prospective study. Injury 1986; 17:208–12.

17. Campbell CS. Gamekeeper's thumb. J Bone Joint Surg Br 1955;37-B(1):148–9.

18. Mall NA, Carlisle JC, Matava MJ, et al. Upper extremity injuries in the National Football League, part I: hand and digital injuries. Am J Sports Med 2008; 36(10):1938–44.

19. Murray PM. Chapter 11: treatment of the osteoarthritic hand and thumb. In: Wolfe SW, Hotchkiss RN, Pederson WC, et al, editors. Greens operative hand surgery. 7th edition. Philadelphia: Elsevier; 2017. p. 359–60.

20. Posner MA, Retaillaud JL. Metacarpophalangeal joint injuries of the thumb. Hand Clin 1992;8(4):713–32.

21. Carlson MG, Warner KK, Meyers KN, et al. Anatomy of the thumb metacarpophalangeal ulnar and radial collateral ligaments. J Hand Surg Am 2012;37(10): 2021–6.

22. Bean CH, Tencer AF, Trumble TE. The effect of thumb metacarpophalangeal ulnar collateral ligament attachment site on joint range of motion: an in vitro study. J Hand Surg Am 1999;24(2):283–7.

23. Avery DM, Inkellis ER, Carlson MG. Thumb collateral ligament injuries in the athlete. Curr Rev Musculoskelet Med 2017;10(1):28–37.

24. Cooney WP, Chao EY. Biomechanical analysis of static forces in the thumb during hand function. J Bone Joint Surg Am 1977;59(1):27–36.

25. Smith RJ. Post-traumatic instability of the metacarpophalangeal joint of the thumb. J Bone Joint Surg Am 1977;59(1):14–21.

26. Yoshida R, House HO, Patterson RM, et al. Motion and morphology of the thumb metacarpophalangeal joint. J Hand Surg 2003;28A:753–7.

27. Le M, Lourie GM, Gaston G. Relationship of surgically repaired ulnar collateral ligament injury of the thumb to the morphology of the metacarpophalangeal joint of the thumb. J Hand Surg Eur Vol 2017;43(2):214–5.

28. Stener B. Displacement of the ruptured ulnar collateral ligament of the metacarpophalangeal joint of the thumb. J Bone Joint Surg Br 1962;44-B:869–79.

29. Derkash RS, Matyas JR, Weaver JK, et al. Acute surgical repair of the skier's thumb. Clin Orthop Relat Res 1987;216:29–33.

30. Palmer AK, Louis DS. Assessing ulnar instability of the metacarpophalangeal joint of the thumb. J Hand Surg Am 1978;3(6):542–6.

31. Coyle MP. Grade III radial collateral ligament injuries of the thumb metacarpophalangeal joint: treatment by soft tissue advancement and bony reattachment. J Hand Surg Am 2003;28(1):14–20.

32. Doty JF, Rudd JN, Jemison M. Radial collateral ligament injury of the thumb with a Stener-like lesion. Orthopedics 2010;33(12):925.

33. Melone CP, Beldner S, Basuk RS. Thumb collateral ligament injuries. An anatomic basis for treatment. Hand Clin 2000;16(3):345–57.

34. Schroeder NS, Goldfarb CA. Thumb ulnar collateral and radial collateral ligament injuries. Clin Sports Med 2015;34(1):117–26.

35. Mayer SW, Ruch DS, Leversedge FJ. The influence of thumb metacarpophalangeal joint rotation on the evaluation of ulnar collateral ligament injuries: a biomechanical study in a cadaver model. J Hand Surg Am 2014;39(3):474–9.

36. Cooper JG, Johnstone AJ, Hider P, et al. Local anaesthetic infiltration increases the accuracy of assessment of ulnar collateral ligament injuries. Emerg Med Australas 2005;17(2):132–6.

37. Malik AK, Morris T, Chou D, et al. Clinical testing of ulnar collateral ligament injuries of the thumb. J Hand Surg Eur Vol 2009;34(3):363–6.

38. McKeon KE, Gelberman RH, Calfee RP. Ulnar collateral ligament injuries of the thumb: phalangeal translation during valgus stress in human cadavera. J Bone Joint Surg Am 2013;95(10):881–7.
39. Hintermann B, Holzach PJ, Schutz M, et al. Skier's thumb – the significance of bony injuries. Am J Sports Med 1993;21(6):800–4.
40. Hergan K, Mittler C, Oser W. Ulnar collateral ligament: differentiation of displaced and nondisplaced tears with US and MR imaging. Radiology 1995;194(1):65–71.
41. Owings FP, Calandruccio JH, Mauck BM. Thumb ligament injuries in the athlete. Orthop Clin North Am 2016;47(4):799–807.
42. Hoglund M, Tordai P, Muren C. Diagnosis by ultrasound of dislocated ulnar collateral ligament of the thumb. Acta Radiol 1995;36(6):620–5.
43. Sollerman C, Abrahamsson SO, Lundborg G, et al. Functional splinting versus plaster cast for ruptures of the ulnar collateral ligament of the thumb. A prospective randomized study of 63 cases. Acta Orthop Scand 1991;62(6):524–6.
44. Catalano LW, Cardon L, Patenaude N, et al. Results of surgical treatment of acute and chronic grade III [corrected] tears of the radial collateral ligament of the thumb metacarpophalangeal joint. J Hand Surg Am 2006;31(1):68–75.
45. Goldfarb CA, Puri SK, Carlson MG. Diagnosis, treatment, and return to play for four common sports injuries of the hand and wrist. J Am Acad Orthop Surg 2016;24(12):853–62.
46. Landsman JC, Seitz WH, Froimson AL, et al. Splint immobilization of gamekeeper's thumb. Orthopedics 1995;18(12):1161–5.
47. Kuz JE, Husband JB, Tokar N, et al. Outcome of avulsion fractures of the ulnar base of the proximal phalanx of the thumb treated nonsurgically. J Hand Surg Am 1999;24(2):275–82.
48. Sorene ED, Goodwin DR. Non-operative treatment of displaced avulsion fractures of the ulnar base of the proximal phalanx of the thumb. Scand J Plast Reconstr Surg Hand Surg 2003;37(4):225–7.
49. Dinowitz M, Trumble T, Hanel D, et al. Failure of cast immobilization for thumb ulnar collateral ligament avulsion fractures. J Hand Surg Am 1997;22(6):1057–63.
50. Christensen T, Sarfani S, Shin AY, et al. Long-term outcomes of primary repair of chronic thumb ulnar collateral ligament injuries. Hand 2016;11(3):303–9.
51. De Giacomo AF, Shin SS. Repair of thumb ulnar collateral ligament with suture tape augmentation. Tech Hand Up Extrem Surg 2017;21:164–6.
52. Shin SS, van Eck CF, Uquillas C. Suture tape augmentation of the thumb ulnar collateral ligament repair: a biomechanical study. J Hand Surg Am 2018;43(9):868.e1–6.
53. Werner BC, Belkin NS, Kennelly S, et al. Injuries to the collateral ligaments of the metacarpophalangeal joint of the thumb, including simultaneous combined thumb ulnar and radial collateral ligament injuries, in National Football League Athletes. Am J Sports Med 2017;45(1):195–200.
54. Bernstein DT, McCulloch PC, Winston LA, et al. Early return to play with thumb spica gauntlet casting for ulnar collateral ligament injuries complicated by adjacent joint dislocations in collegiate football lineman. Hand 2018. https://doi.org/10.1177/1558944718788644.

Hand and Wrist Injuries in the Pediatric Athlete

Dan A. Zlotolow, MD[a,b,c,d,*], Scott H. Kozin, MD[a]

KEYWORDS

- Gymnast wrist • Scaphoid fracture • Galeazzi fracture • Salter-Harris fracture
- Wrist fracture • Distal radius fracture

KEY POINTS

- Children are increasingly susceptible to adult-type injuries as their sports participation intensifies.
- Intra-articular fractures are unlikely to remodel to within acceptable parameters, and should merit an anatomic or nearly anatomic reduction with stable fixation whenever possible.
- Avoid crossing the physes with anything other than a smooth pin, and avoid multiple passes with the pin.
- Intraphyseal fractures warrant an anatomic reduction within 7 days whenever possible.

INTRODUCTION

Gone are the days when children were allowed free play to develop their motor skills at their own pace. Today, children are being encouraged or even pushed to pursue sports at higher and higher levels at younger and younger ages. As a result, adult-type injuries have become the norm in the pediatric population. One example is scaphoid fractures, which a few decades ago were rare and mostly limited to the distal pole, but are now being seen more frequently and in the same configurations as adult injuries.[1]

The increasing rate of adult-type injuries are in addition to the pediatric-specific injuries more commonly seen, such as physeal injuries and ligamentous avulsions. Children are not just small adults. The growth plate serves as a stress riser in the distal radius and ulna, resulting in injuries that can impact overall growth, joint alignment, and/or differential ulnar/radial length. Ligamentous injuries in children usually present

[a] The Sidney Kimmel Medical College of Thomas Jefferson University, Shriners Hospital for Children Philadelphia, 3551 North Broad Street, Philadelphia, PA 19140, USA; [b] Shriners Hospital for Children Greenville, Greenville, SC, USA; [c] The Hospital for Special Surgery, New York, NY, USA; [d] The Philadelphia Hand to Shoulder Center, Philadelphia, PA, USA
* Corresponding author. The Sidney Kimmel Medical College of Thomas Jefferson University, Shriners Hospital for Children Philadelphia, 3551 North Broad Street, Philadelphia, PA 19140.
E-mail address: dzlotolow@yahoo.com

Clin Sports Med 39 (2020) 457–479
https://doi.org/10.1016/j.csm.2020.01.001
0278-5919/20/© 2020 Elsevier Inc. All rights reserved.

sportsmed.theclinics.com

as avulsion injuries rather than midsubstance tears. Special attention should be given to understanding the soft tissue attachments of any bony fleck seen on radiographs. In very young children with incompletely ossified epiphyses and carpal bones, avulsions may be purely cartilaginous, making radiographic diagnosis without an MRI or ultrasound impossible. Radiographs weeks to years later may reveal the true extent of the injury as the cartilaginous avulsion ossifies.

There is a bias among orthopedic surgeons to undertreat fractures in children, with the common refrain that "it will just remodel." There is an almost magical belief in the power of a child to erase any evidence of traumatic insult. However, joint dislocations and subluxations do not remodel. Ligamentous injuries likewise do not remodel. It is precisely those ligamentous and soft tissue attachments that may help to guide bony remodeling, and their loss can lead to worsening deformity as the child grows. Galeazzi fractures have been seen that worsen, rather than improve over time because the distal radius becomes untethered from and grows independent of the distal ulna (**Fig. 1**).

Remodeling occurs by two methods: periosteal remodeling and physeal, or Hueter-Volkmann, remodeling (**Fig. 2**). Periosteal remodeling allows straightening of the bone by laying down bone in the gap created by elevated periosteum, while removing bone where the bone no longer sees compressive load. This occurs in response to Wolff's law. Periosteal remodeling does nothing to change where the joint is in space; however. Hueter-Volkmann remodeling occurs at the physis because of the enhanced growth of a partially offloaded physis and the restricted growth of a partially overloaded physis. Ligamentous/tendinous tethering and joint motion work in concert to steer the joint back to where it was in space relative to the native axis of the bone. Lack of motion or, in the case of the wrist, disruption of the triangular fibrocartilage complex (TFCC) can minimize remodeling.

This review examines the most common problematic hand and wrist injuries in pediatric athletes. Special emphasis is placed not on just returning children to their sport quickly, but also on the long-term effects of their injuries and treatment on the long-term life goals of the child.

FINGER AND THUMB INJURIES

Finger and thumb fractures, sprains, and dislocations most commonly occur in ball sports, but is seen in nearly all contact and noncontact sports. Finger proximal

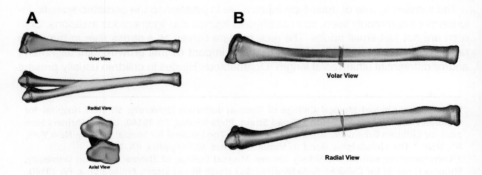

Fig. 1. Galeazzi fracture malunion. A child with a Galeazzi fracture malunion presented with worsening deformity and DRUJ instability. Three-dimensional computer modeling demonstrated the deformity (*A*) and allowed for surgical planning of the osteotomy (*B*). (*Courtesy of* Shriners Hospital for Children Philadelphia.)

A   **B**

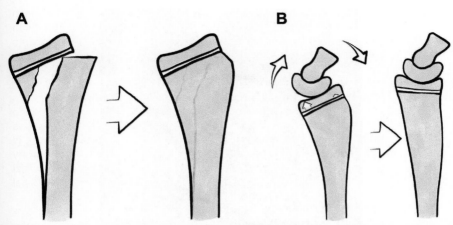

Fig. 2. Periosteal versus Hueter-Volkmann remodeling. Periosteal remodeling, whereby the intact periosteum fills in the gap between the periosteum and the cortical bone while the side with torn periosteum loses bone (A), occurs more quickly than Hueter-Volkmann remodeling, where the offloaded physeal cartilage grows faster than the compressed physeal cartilage (B). Periosteal remodeling is independent of joint motion, whereas Hueter-Volkmann remodeling requires joint motion and therefore has a greater impact in the direction of joint motion. (*Courtesy of* Dan A. Zlotolow.)

interphalangeal (PIP) joint sprains are perhaps the most common, often from a direct blow with another athlete, the ground, or a ball. The long finger is the most exposed and therefore the most likely to be injured. Examination of the PIP joints is fairly straightforward: (1) radiographs should always be obtained with any PIP joint injury before physical examination because fractures and sprains can look identical clinically, (2) the collateral ligaments and the volar plate should be tested gently for competence, and (3) the integrity of the central slip should be assessed with an Elson test.[2] If there is no fracture and the ligaments and tendons are intact, we buddy tape or strap the injured to its adjacent digit and begin early motion with no period of immobilization to prevent contractures. Ligament injuries require immobilization for up to 4 weeks. Central slip avulsions require at least 6 weeks of immobilization in PIP joint extension with the distal interphalangeal joint free. We use low-temperature plastic to quickly manufacture the splint in the office without the need for a therapist (**Fig. 3**).

Sprains of the distal interphalangeal joint are examined and treated in like manner, with the exception that the terminal tendon replaces the central slip. Acute mallet fractures and deformities without a fracture are treated equally. Late-presenting mallet deformities are also commonly well-managed with just immobilization. Late-presenting fractures require a takedown of the malunion site and pinning if the deformity is not tolerated.

The most common type II phalangeal neck fractures (**Fig. 4**) are most easily treated using the Strauch technique (**Fig. 5**) (https://youtu.be/2ADhL2AOYMU). In their series of four patients, all regained near full painless motion.[3] We attempt an osteoclasis[4] for late injuries up to 2 weeks old or if they remain tender and painful (**Fig. 6**). Older injuries are effectively healed and are mobilized after 4 weeks from injury. There is evidence that malunions remodel if more than 2 years of growth remain. All eight patients in one study regained full motion after 1 year.[5] Although the sagittal deformities completely remodeled in all patients, coronal deformities showed less remodeling potential, correcting only 7° on average.

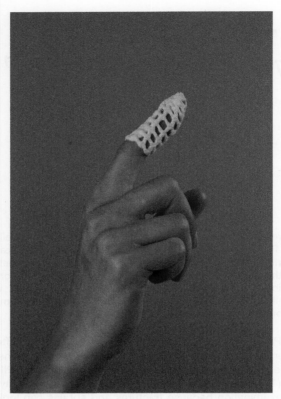

Fig. 3. Finger splinting. Finger splints are easily manufactured in the office using low-temperature thermoplastic material. (*Courtesy of* Steven J. Thompson and Dan A. Zlotolow.)

Intercondylar fractures are nearly always unstable and require fixation. Open treatment is risky because of the high risk of avascular necrosis of the condyles. Closed reduction and pinning is therefore recommended. A towel clamp or pointed reduction forceps is applied above the midaxial line to effect a reduction while minimizing neurovascular injury risk. Fingertrap traction also is helpful. There should be a minimum of

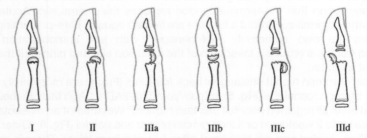

Fig. 4. Classification of phalangeal neck fractures. Type I fractures are nondisplaced. Type II fractures are displaced with some remaining cortical contact. Type III fractures are displaced with no cortical contact. (*From* Karl JW, White NJ, Strauch RJ. Percutaneous reduction and fixation of displaced phalangeal neck fractures in children. *J Pediatr Orthop*. 2012;32(2):156-161; with permission.)

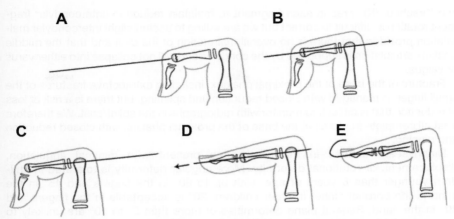

Fig. 5. Strauch pinning technique for phalangeal neck fractures. Engage the single K-wire on the reduced phalangeal head with the distal interphalangeal (DIP) joint maximally flexed (*A*). Drive the K-wire across the fracture and out skin through a flexed PIP joint (*B*). The reduction is adjusted at this time (*C*) before extending the DIP and directing the wire distally (*D, E*). (*From* Karl JW, White NJ, Strauch RJ. Percutaneous reduction and fixation of displaced phalangeal neck fractures in children. *J Pediatr Orthop.* 2012;32(2):156-161; with permission.)

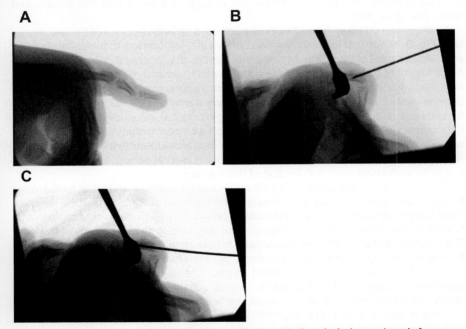

Fig. 6. Displaced phalangeal neck nascent malunion. Displaced phalangeal neck fractures that have begun to heal (*A*) are treated with osteoclasis (*B*) and pinning (*C*). (*Courtesy of* Shriners Hospital for Children Philadelphia.)

two Kirschner (K)-wires in each fragment to maintain reduction. Intercondylar fragment rotation is difficult to correct but we are willing to accept slight intercondylar malrotation provided that there is no overall malrotation of the digit and that the middle phalanx articulation is supported by the condyles and will not collapse into either varus or valgus.

Fracture of the base of the proximal phalanx, including extraoctave fractures of the small finger, is managed with closed reduction and splinting, but there is a risk of loss of reduction that is difficult to monitor with radiographs in the splint/cast. We therefore treat all complete fractures at the base of the proximal phalanx with closed reduction and pinning.

Diaphyseal fractures in the hand often present with minimal angulation, displacement, or rotational deformity. More angular deformity is tolerated in children younger than 8 years of age, with up to 30° in the fingers and 45° in the hand in the coronal plane. In older children, 20° is acceptable in the fingers and 30° in the hand. Sagittal plane deformities of more than 5° to 10° are unlikely to remodel. Shortening of up to 5 mm is also acceptable at any age. Rotational deformities are not well tolerated and do not remodel.[6–8] Phalangeal and metacarpal shaft fractures outside of acceptable parameters are best treated with closed reduction and pinning whenever possible. However, we always consent for open reduction and internal fixation, because reduction by closed means is not possible in all fractures. Care needs to be taken not to dissect through the perichondral ring or to otherwise damage or cross the physis. We use interfragmentary screws for long oblique or spiral fractures and small plates for transverse or short oblique fractures (**Fig. 7**). Metacarpal neck fractures, including boxer's fractures, are treated using the same criteria as adults, because these commonly occur near skeletal maturity. We prefer a single pin through the head and the physis and down the shaft (**Fig. 8**).

An often missed injury is the Seymour fracture, a physeal fracture of the distal phalanx (**Fig. 9**). Given that the nail plate and bed are the only barriers to the distal phalanx, any displacement of the nail plate that accompanies displacement or angulation of the distal fragment results in an open fracture. The nail bed and nail plate fragments can become interposed, leading to difficulty with reduction. Emergent irrigation and debridement is required as for any other open fracture. The nail bed needs to be tucked back under the eponychial fold. Pinning is optional, depending on stability after debridement. Delays in treatment risk malunion with permanent nail plate deformity, osteomyelitis, and in severe cases amputation. Subacute treatment includes nail plate removal, extrication of debris within the fracture, open reduction, wound culture followed by antibiotics, and stabilization of the fracture.

Thumb metacarpophalangeal joint injuries in a child usually manifest as avulsions of the ligament insertion onto the epiphysis of the proximal phalanx (**Fig. 10**). These are most commonly seen in skiers and football players. Any displacement of more than a few millimeters or rotation of the fragment can lead to long-term instability of the joint. The fragment tends to be larger than what is visible on radiographs and can make up a sizable percentage of the articular surface. We therefore opt for open reduction and fixation of the bony fragment in most cases. The approach is equivalent to the approach in adults for a metacarpophalangeal collateral ligament injury.[9] Branches of the radial sensory nerve always cross the field and can lead to a painful neuroma if overly retracted or cut. The fragment is reduced and fixed either with a K-wire, a small transepiphyseal screw (that does not cross the physis), or a suture anchor in the epiphysis. Depending on fixation, 4 to 6 weeks of postoperative immobilization is suggested.

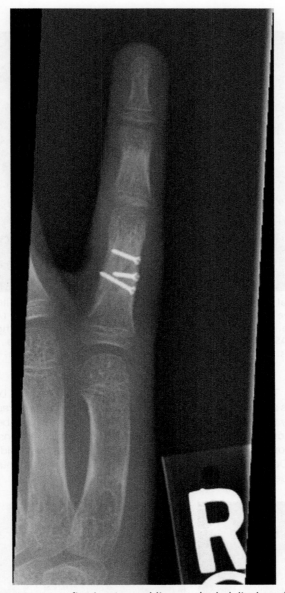

Fig. 7. Interfragmentary screw fixation. Long oblique and spiral diaphyseal fractures are unstable injuries usually treated with interfragmentary screw fixation. (*Courtesy of* Shriners Hospital for Children Philadelphia.)

SCAPHOID FRACTURES

The scaphoid is not fully ossified until approximately 15 years of age. It is the fifth carpal bone to begin to ossify, at between 4 and 6 years of age. The ossification center is distal, and ossification is retrograde following the blood supply. Fractures of the waist and proximal pole are therefore unlikely, and even less likely to be detected, before

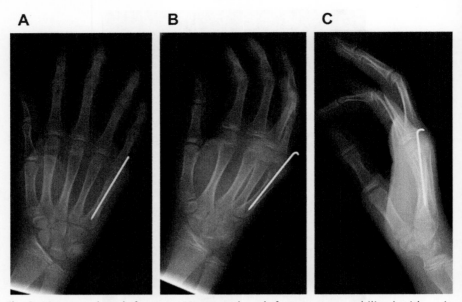

Fig. 8. Metacarpal neck fracture. Metacarpal neck fractures are stabilized with a single pin across the physis as long as there is no rotational deformity. (*A–C*) Posteroanterior, oblique, and lateral radiographs, respectively, of the pin configuration. (*From* Cassel S, Shah AS. Metacarpal Fractures. In Scott H. Kozin, Joshua Abzug, Dan A. Zlotolow, Editors. The Pediatric Upper Extremity. Springer, 2014. p. 982-1003; with permission.)

8 years of age. The so-called "bipartite" scaphoid (**Fig. 11**) has been previously described, and is a normal anatomic variant (Dormans).[10] The true atraumatic bipartite scaphoid is likely to be bilateral. A unilateral bipartite scaphoid may be the result of a cartilaginous fracture that went on to a nonunion, but this remains controversial. Regardless of congenital or traumatic cause, the bipartite scaphoid may not be a benign finding. Degenerative changes analogous to a scaphoid nonunion advanced collapse have been reported.[11]

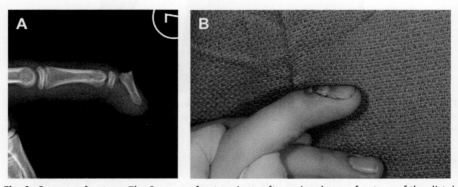

Fig. 9. Seymour fracture. The Seymour fracture is an often missed open fracture of the distal phalanx best seen on lateral radiographs (*A*). Clinical appearance can be underwhelming and contributes to the underdiagnosis (*B*). (*Courtesy of* Shriners Hospital for Children Philadelphia.)

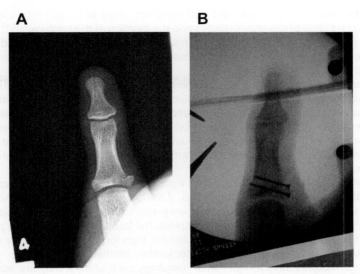

Fig. 10. Thumb metacarpophalangeal ligament avulsion. Thumb metacarpophalangeal ligament avulsion injuries are more common than ligament ruptures in children. (*A*) The fracture is usually a Salter-Harris IV injury with intra-articular involvement seen best on posteroanterior radiographs. (*B*) Treatment of displaced fractures is anatomic reduction and fixation. In this case, the physis was nearly closed, so screws traversing the physis were chosen for better fixation. (*Courtesy of* Shriners Hospital for Children Philadelphia.)

Scaphoid fractures are still uncommon in children, making up 0.34% of pediatric fractures, but are the most common carpal fracture.[12] Up until the turn of the century, most pediatric scaphoid fractures occurred at the distal pole. The benign location of scaphoid fractures historically has created a prevailing sense among orthopedic surgeons that all scaphoid fractures in children will heal if provided a course of immobilization.[13,14] More recent studies have shown not only that fracture patterns have

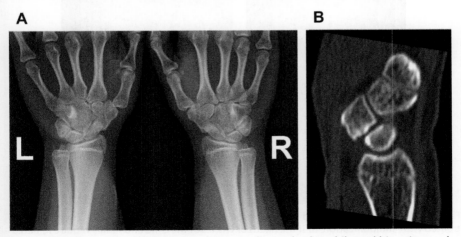

Fig. 11. Bipartite scaphoid. (*A*) Anteroposterior radiographs show bilateral bipartite scaphoids. (*B*) This is confirmed on sagittal computed tomography image. (*Courtesy of* Shriners Hospital for Children Philadelphia.)

changed to mirror adult injuries, but that nonunion rates approach those of adults depending on status of the growth plates and the location of the fracture.[1,15–17] In children with open physes, 68% of scaphoid fractures occurred at the waist and 17% of fractures occurred at the proximal pole. Acute nondisplaced waist fractures treated in a cast had a nonunion rate of 8%.[1]

Management of scaphoid fractures is therefore similar in children as in adults, with some notable exceptions. Acute, nondisplaced fractures are treated with either cast immobilization or percutaneous screw fixation. There are no convincing data in children to indicate whether a long- or a short-arm cast is optimal, or whether thumb immobilization is required. Because of the low risk of motion loss in a child or adolescent, we tend to favor a thumb spica long-arm cast for the first 6 weeks and short-arm cast thereafter.

Percutaneous screw fixation is achieved through either a volar or a dorsal approach, provided that the scaphoid is fully ossified. If the proximal pole is cartilaginous with incomplete ossification on the radiograph, we prefer to place a retrograde volar screw (**Fig. 12**).[18] Care should be taken not to displace the fracture when placing a percutaneous screw. The screw lengths are also shorter than for adults for obvious reasons but particularly short if the scaphoid is incompletely ossified.

Displaced fractures have a high risk of nonunion, particularly if they are across the proximal pole.[1] We treat all displaced fractures with open reduction and screw fixation. Using traction, the proximal pole of the scaphoid is brought distalward, obviating division and repair of the radioscapholunate ligament (**Fig. 13**H). Preservations of

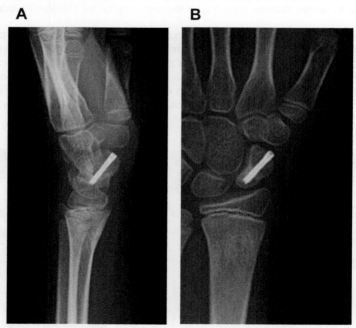

Fig. 12. Nondisplaced scaphoid fracture. Nondisplaced scaphoid fractures in children are treated with immobilization, or if the needs or wishes of the child and family require it, percutaneous screw fixation. Lateral (*A*) and posteroanterior (*B*) radiographs demonstrate a retrograde screw placed via an anterior approach because of incomplete ossification of the proximal pole in this 13-year-old boy. (*Courtesy of* Shriners Hospital for Children Philadelphia.)

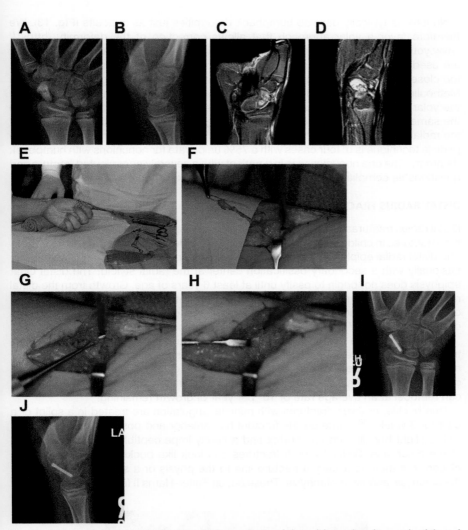

Fig. 13. Scaphoid fracture nonunion. Posteroanterior (*A*) and lateral radiographs (*B*) and coronal (*C*) and sagittal MRIs (*D*) confirmed a nonunion with a humpback deformity. The patient underwent open reduction and internal fixation using traction through the thumb using a fingertrap and a traction table (*E*). The superficial volar branch of the radial artery (*F*) was placed into the nonunion site and covered with cancellous bone graft from the distal radial metaphysis (*G*) with care not to injure the physis. A cortical fragment from the volar distal radius was then used to contain the bone graft and lend structural support to the volar scaphoid during screw compression (*H*). Six weeks later, the nonunion has healed on posteroanterior (*I*) and lateral radiographs (*J*). (*Courtesy of* Shriners Hospital for Children Philadelphia.)

carpal ligaments in children may be more important than in adults, because disruptions may change the kinematics and growth patterns of the wrist. We also routinely use a vascular pedicle from the superficial volar branch of the radial artery to inset into the fracture site.[19–21] This artery is otherwise sacrificed routinely during the approach.

Nonunions typically develop humpback deformities just as in adults (**Fig. 13**). We therefore favor a volar approach that allows correction of the deformity (https://www.youtube.com/watch?v=C43O3m6UzNM). Dorsal vascularized bone grafts that are used for adults are not an option in children, because the graft harvest site is too close or may cross the physis.[22] The volar vascularized bone graft described by Mathoulin and Haerle[23] is also not appropriate for children, because this removes the volar artery to the physis along the watershed line (**Fig. 14**). We therefore use the same vascular pedicle described previously from the superficial volar branch of the radial artery in cases of nonunion. The only published series on the vascularized pedicle technique is of four cases with a 75% union rate for nonunions with humpback deformity. The one nonunion was in a patient with a severely comminuted fracture and questionable compliance. The vascularity of the proximal pole was not defined.[20]

DISTAL RADIUS FRACTURES

Distal radius fractures are among the most common sports injuries and the most common fractures in children,[24,25] with an increasing incidence over the past 40 years.[26,27] The distal radial epiphysis does not begin to ossify until at least 6 months of age, occasionally with a secondary ossification center at the radial styloid. The distal ulnar epiphysis does not begin to ossify until at least 6 years of age. Growth from the distal radius and ulna contributes to approximately 80% of the length of the forearm. The distal ulnar physis closes typically 6 months ahead of the distal radius, at 16 years of age in girls and 17 years of age in boys.[28]

Although most are treated with closed reduction and immobilization, some undertreated injuries can result in lifelong deformity and disability. It is important to recognize and mitigate the sequelae of the "bad actors" of the pediatric wrist, while not overtreating fractures that will remodel. Angulation in the plane of motion of the wrist can remodel at an average rate of 10° per year of growth remaining.[29]

True buckle, or torus, fractures with minimal angulation are treated in a splint or a cast for 3 weeks.[30] A true buckle fracture has anterior and posterior cortices intact, with a slight buckling on one cortex and a nearly imperceptible plastic deformation of the other side. Salter-Harris II fractures can look like buckle fractures if nondisplaced, but there is usually a fracture line to the physis or a slight misalignment of the epiphysis and the metaphysis. These occult Salter-Harris II fractures can displace,

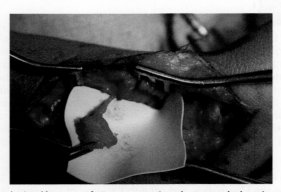

Fig. 14. Volar vascularized bone graft. Intraoperative photograph showing the volar vascularized bone graft described by Mathoulin and Haerle.[23] Note that the pedicle is the volar blood supply to the physis and the bone is adjacent to the physis, and therefore cannot be used in skeletally immature children. (*Courtesy of* Shriners Hospital for Children Philadelphia.)

so a well-molded plaster short-arm cast and close observation with weekly radiographs is recommended.

More displaced Salter-Harris type II fractures generally require a reduction. The best scenario is a timely closed reduction and either plaster sugar-tong splint or long-arm cast on the day of injury. However, because many emergency departments are not able to provide this service, patients typically present with still displaced fractures in a tightly bandaged poorly made splint[31] many days after injury. Initial evaluation includes orthogonal radiographs before splint removal to evaluate for any further displacement. If the splint is adequate, retain the splint. If not, the splint has to be changed. Before splint removal, we prefer to place the child in linear traction via the thumb only with the elbow bent 90° and 5 lb of weight on the brachium, which is parallel to the floor (**Fig. 15**).[18,32] Traction reduces the risk of further fracture displacement and minimizes the number of assistants required for the splint change.

If the Salter-Harris II fracture is less than 7 days old, we take the child to the operating room for a closed reduction and casting (**Fig. 16**). Fractures older than 7 days old are best left unreduced. It is better to have a deformity than a physeal arrest. Large Thurston-Holland fragments render fractures unstable and usually require percutaneous pinning for stability. Fractures with smaller metaphyseal fragments are usually

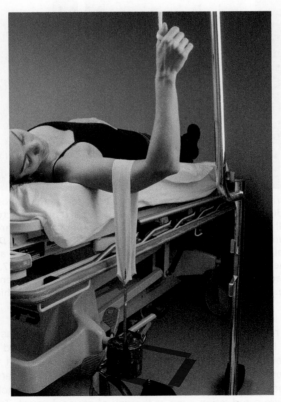

Fig. 15. Traction for distal radius fracture. Both a cast or splint change and a closed reduction are most easily achieved using elbow flexion and traction across only the thumb to neutralize the primary deforming force of the brachioradialis. (*Courtesy of* Steven J. Thompson and Dan A. Zlotolow.)

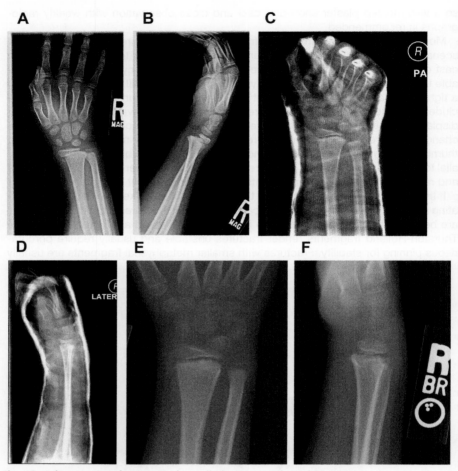

Fig. 16. Salter-Harris II fracture with small Thurston-Holland fragment. Posteroanterior (*A*) and lateral (*B*) radiographs demonstrate a displaced Salter-Harris II fracture of the distal radius with a small Thurston-Holland fragment. These injuries typically are treated with a closed reduction and casting in a well-molded plaster long-arm cast (*C, D*). Note that the plaster has no visible onion-skinning (layering) and that the mold is deep and in the appropriate location. The padding is minimal and the cast index is less than 0.7. Posteroanterior (*E*) and lateral (*F*) radiographs 4 weeks later confirmed union and the patient was nontender at the fracture site. (*Courtesy of* Shriners Hospital for Children Philadelphia.)

stable and rarely require fixation. However, every fracture must be assessed individually for stability. Long-arm, well-molded plaster casts are preferred if no fixation is used because there is no opportunity for rereduction. Follow-up is 1 week later with radiographs. If there is any redisplacement, the incidence of physeal arrest is too great to attempt a rereduction in most cases. Salter-Harris III and IV fractures are intra-articular and require a reduction even at the risk of physeal arrest. Type III fractures develop a bar if not anatomically reduced. Type IV fractures also have a high risk of growth arrest, regardless of reduction. Physeal injuries of the distal radius carry a 5% risk of growth arrest. By contrast, ulnar physeal injuries carry a 50% risk.

Extra-articular, extraphyseal fractures in the metaphysis are unlikely to go on to physeal arrest, but associated ligamentous and/or distal ulnar fractures can lead to long-term instability. It is difficult to define an acceptable reduction, because so many factors play a role, including the risk of loss of reduction. A quarter of all complete metaphyseal fractures in children redisplace after closed reduction and immobilization. The risk is greater if initial angulation was greater than 30° in the sagittal plane or the fracture was more than 50% displaced.[33–35] Associated ulnar fractures increase the risk of redisplacement. We therefore attempt a closed reduction and cast/splint in children younger than 10 years of age regardless of initial angulation if there is no ulnar fracture and there is minimal displacement, so long as the fracture does not have a long oblique orientation. Given that these long oblique shear fractures are inherently unstable, we rigidly fix any displaced fracture that has a shear component (**Fig. 17**). Transverse metaphyseal fractures are stable once reduced and merit at least an attempt at closed management. Risk factors for redisplacement of metaphyseal fractures include greater than 50% initial translation and poor cast technique. We recommend minimal padding, plaster sugar-tong splint or below the elbow cast with a good mold, and a cast index of less than 0.7.[18,32] Despite evidence of the success of short-arm cast, we do not hesitate to place a long-arm cast if rotational stability is in question. In children younger than 5, a long-arm cast with the elbow at 90° is usually required to keep the cast on.

If there is evidence of distal radioulnar ligamentous injury, such as initial or persistent distal radioulnar joint (DRUJ) subluxation on radiographs, a large ulnar styloid fracture fragment, or intraoperative instability of the DRUJ, we advocate for rigid fixation and anatomic reduction. Although most metaphyseal fractures are not true Galeazzi injuries,[36] a high index of suspicion should be maintained.

Follow-up for metaphyseal fractures treated with closed reduction without fixation should be reimaged weekly to assess reduction. Rereduction in the operating room is recommended if angulation exceeds 20° of dorsal tilt or 10° loss of inclination in children with more than 2 years of growth remaining. Less angulation is tolerated in older children and adolescents.

GYMNAST WRIST

Humans are the only primate to walk on their hands, and we only do it regularly as gymnasts. Our closest relatives, the other great apes, walk on their forelimbs but weight bear either across their middle phalanges or proximal phalanges, with the wrist in neutral. They rarely place all of their weight on a single forelimb. High-level gymnasts are expected not only to repeatedly walk on their hands, but also to bear loads at multiples of body weight on a daily basis, and to do so on the palm of the hand with the wrist in terminal extension. This highly nonphysiologic loading pattern causes concentration of supraphysiologic load across the wrist. Because this type of weight bearing begins at a young age in girls, and particularly because puberty is delayed in this demographic, the physis of the distal radius responds with hypertrophy, edema, and eventually arrest.

Wrist pain in a gymnast, particularly a young girl, should merit at least radiographs of the wrist regardless of the examination (**Fig. 18**). Contralateral comparison film may be necessary. Any widening of the physis on radiograph requires cessation of gymnastics training and splinting or, if severe, immobilization in a cast until the pain resolves. The athlete may return to gymnastics once the radiographs normalize, the patient is pain free, and there is no tenderness about the distal radius. The timing can vary greatly but 6 weeks is minimal.

Longstanding or severe physiolysis can lead to complete or, more commonly, partial physeal arrest (**Figs. 19** and **20**). This is difficult to manage in the young girl who still

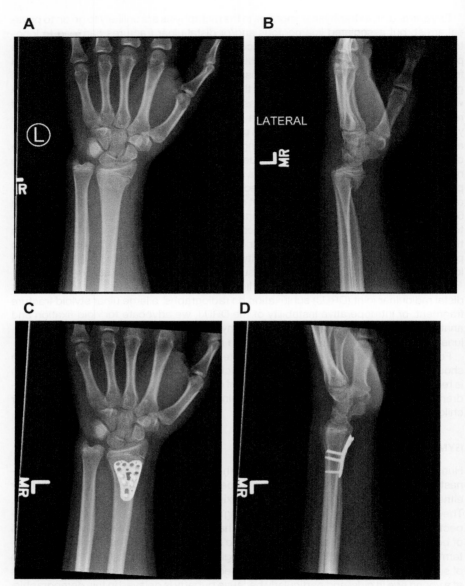

Fig. 17. Salter-Harris II fracture with large oblique Thurston-Holland fragment. Posteroanterior (*A*) and lateral (*B*) radiographs demonstrate a displaced Salter-Harris II fracture of the distal radius with a large oblique Thurston-Holland fragment. These fractures are inherently unstable and require buttress plating. Posteroanterior (*C*) and lateral (*D*) radiographs 6 weeks later confirmed union and the patient was nontender at the fracture site. (*Courtesy of* Shriners Hospital for Children Philadelphia.)

has many years of growth remaining. Girls generally reach skeletal maturity 2 years after menarche, usually around 14 years of age. Boys reach skeletal maturity around 16 years of age. Partial growth arrest of the distal radius results in angular deformity and ulnar-positive variance. Bowing of the radial and ulnar diaphyses is common.

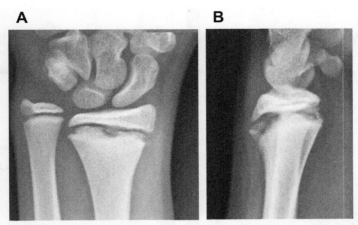

Fig. 18. Gymnast wrist. Posteroanterior (*A*) and lateral (*B*) radiographs of a gymnast with wrist pain demonstrate widening of the physis with irregular calcification. There is already evidence of radial growth arrest or slowing with a markedly ulnar-positive variance. (*Courtesy of* Shriners Hospital for Children Philadelphia.)

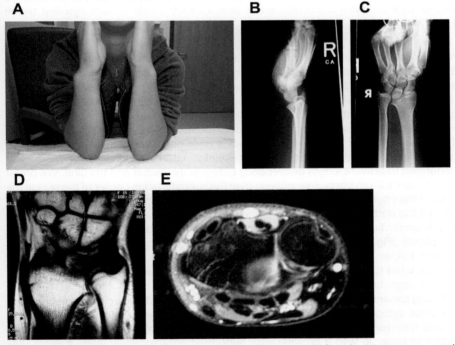

Fig. 19. Chronic gymnast wrist with physeal arrest. A 16-year-old female gymnast presented with wrist deformity (*A*) and pain. Radiographs showed a "Madelung" type deformity with growth arrest of the distal radial volar/ulnar corner in a skeletally mature wrist (*B, C*). MRI did not show a Vicker ligament (*D, E*), consistent with her history. The absence of a Vicker ligament confirms that her etiology was not a true Madelung case, but rather most likely the result of repetitive trauma or acute injury to the physis. (*Courtesy of* Shriners Hospital for Children Philadelphia.)

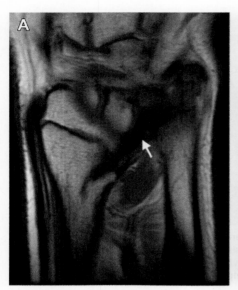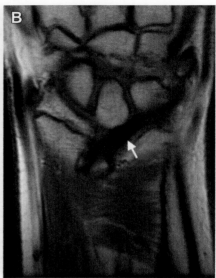

Fig. 20. (A and B) demonstrate sequential coronal T1 weighted MRI images of the wrist in a patient with Leri-Weill Dischondrosteosis with a clearly visible Vicker's ligament (*white arrows*).

An MRI is used to determine the percentage of remaining open physis. Anything less than 70% of the physis remaining is highly unlikely to respond to bar resection. In our experience, even if 85% of the physis remains open by MRI criteria, physeal bar resection may recover a year or 2 of growth but eventually the physis closes prematurely and radioulnar growth discrepancy remains.

Complete growth arrest leads to early ulnar-positive variance and late ulnar bowing if the ulna is allowed to grow while the radius does not. Caught early, before positive ulnar variance is noted, and in a child near skeletal maturity, an ulnar epiphyseodesis is performed to prevent length discrepancy between the radius and the ulna. We prefer to use a small 2-cm transverse incision over the subcutaneous border of the ulna at the level of the physis. Blunt dissection is performed down to the capsule to identify and protect the dorsal sensory branch of the ulnar nerve. A guidewire is inserted into the physis under fluoroscopic guidance and a 1.7-mm cannulated drill is used to enter the physis (**Fig. 21**). We then use a small curette to remove the physeal cartilage without further violating the perichondral ring. Fixation is not required. A short arm splint is used for 2 weeks and the child is allowed to return to sports when bridging bone is seen, typically 6 weeks after surgery.

Young patients with an arrest that is picked up before radioulnar length discrepancy becomes symptomatic are difficult to manage. The patient and the family need to decide between two treatment strategies: serial radial lengthenings with an external fixator to keep up with a growing ulna performed approximately every 2 years until skeletal maturity; or ulnar epiphyseodesis with the acceptance of a potentially very short forearm at skeletal maturity. This is a difficult decision, and both likely result in cessation of athletic competition.

Radial lengthening is more complicated to perform than ulnar lengthening, because there is no subcutaneous border of the radius. We prefer a Thompson approach[37] to the midshaft radius with use of a monoplanar external fixator (**Fig. 22**). In two case

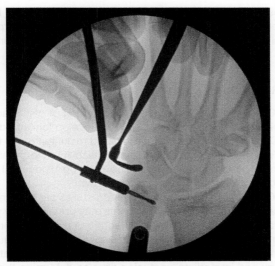

Fig. 21. Epiphyseodesis. Epiphyseodesis is performed with a 1.7-mm cannulated drill (shown) and expanded with a curette. (*Courtesy of* Shriners Hospital for Children Philadelphia.)

series of four patients each, radial lengthening showed good clinical outcomes with a postoperative DASH score of 11 and 2 and a Mayo wrist score of 76 and 89. Length of distraction was not reported in either study. A circular frame was used in both studies for a total of 106 and 150 days, respectively.[38,39]

Patients who present late or are underdiagnosed initially that already have a radio-ulnar length discrepancy require either a radial lengthening, ulnar shortening, or both. Again the decision to either undergo potentially multiple complex operations or to live with a short forearm is highly personal and has long-term consequences. Correction of any ulnar deformity, when present, is performed at the same time with a closing wedge osteotomy. For complex deformities, computed tomography–based computer modeling may be used.

If the radiographs are normal, a period of 2 weeks of immobilization in a cast or splint is recommended. If the pain is resolved, gradual return to full activities is permitted. If

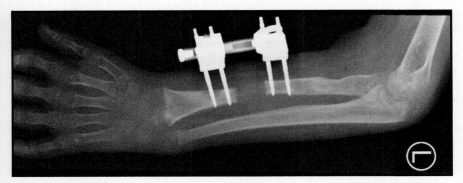

Fig. 22. Radial lengthening. The radius is lengthened with a monoplanar external fixator via the Thompson approach. (*Courtesy of* Shriners Hospital for Children Philadelphia.)

the pain continues, MRI examination of the wrist may be necessary. Early changes in the physis are seen on MRI, and occult fractures, stress fractures, carpal avascular necrosis, ulnocarpal impaction, TFCC tears, and redundancy of the dorsal capsule with synovitis.

ULNAR-SIDED WRIST PAIN

Injuries to the TFCC of the wrist can occur in the setting of distal radial and/or ulnar fractures or in isolation.[40,41] It is rare for a child to develop longstanding DRUJ instability from a TFCC tear unless there is an associated malunion of the forearm or wrist. However, true DRUJ instability can lead to pain, disability, and potentially erosion of the growing sigmoid notch. Children may also develop ulnocarpal impaction as a result of radial growth arrest/delay or ulnar overgrowth.

Traumatic TFCC injuries with associated wrist fractures are uncommon[36] and typically heal if the bony anatomy is restored. Patients may present many years after injury with a history of fracture but no evidence of a fracture or a malunion on radiographs. In these patients, remodeling will have erased the evidence, but the sequelae of the fracture malunion remain with malalignment of the DRUJ. In these patients, it is important to assess the injury and immediate postunion films to determine the degree of malunion. MRI has been shown to have a 50% false-negative rate for diagnosing a TFCC tear in children.[41] In our practice, we perform diagnostic/therapeutic steroid injections after rest, splinting, and activity modification have failed to relieve symptoms. If the pain improves immediately after injection of the TFCC but recurs, an arthroscopy is recommended.

Oftentimes, restoration of the bony alignment without a soft-tissue procedure is sufficient to stabilize the DRUJ.[42] Patients with persistent DRUJ instability after a fracture are difficult to treat because even a small degree of malunion, which is often the case with any initially displaced or angulated pediatric wrist fracture not treated with an open reduction, can lead to symptomatic DRUJ microinstability and subtle but clinically significant sigmoid notch dysplasia. We agree with Miller and colleagues[42] that restoration of bony anatomy is necessary and sufficient for stabilization of the DRUJ in children. Likewise, in the absence of a fracture, DRUJ instability is rare. There may be a history of trauma leading to an undiagnosed fracture or plastic deformation.

The typical adult DRUJ ligament reconstruction using volar and dorsal constructs passed through the ulnar head[43] is not possible in children because it crosses the distal ulnar physis. We have performed delayed TFCC repairs in adolescents after restoration of bony anatomy did not stabilize the DRUJ, with good results in a limited number of patients. Most tears are Palmer 1B. Both open and arthroscopic repair techniques have yielded good results. Out of 22 open repairs, all but 7 had complete resolution of their symptoms.[41] In another series of 12 patients with an average of 16 years, patients treated with an arthroscopically assisted TFCC repair for Palmer 1B tears decreased their pain score from an average of 7 to less than 2, and had a DASH of 16 at final follow-up.[44] If a repair is not possible or fails, delayed ligament reconstruction after skeletal maturity is recommended.

Another common source of ulnar-sided wrist pain in athletes is ulnocarpal or stylocarpal impaction. Most commonly there is a history of a wrist injury that likely resulted in either a growth disruption of the distal radius or an overgrowth of the ulna. However, idiopathic ulnar-positive variance can occur. Contralateral true posteroanterior radiographs in idiopathic cases often reveal identical variance on the symptomatic and nonsymptomatic sides, raising the question of why only one side hurts.

Regardless of cause, restoring a neutral to slightly negative variance has worked well in our practice. There is currently no study on ulnar shortening in children, with or without arthroscopic TFCC debridement, so the optimal treatment remains controversial. In skeletally immature patients who are near the end of growth but have open physes at the radius and the ulna, epiphyseodesis of the ulna is considered, allowing the radius to grow longer than the ulna. Regular interval follow-ups with radiographs every 4 to 6 months are required to ensure that the radius does not overgrow. If the radius reaches the desired length but growth remains, an epiphyseodesis is performed.

In younger patients, it may be best to wait and observe with interval follow-up again every 4 to 6 months. The variance may self-correct with time, and ulnar epiphyseodesis in a young child's arm leads to a tethering of the distal radius and potentially risks excessive radial inclination and bowing, and radial head dislocation. The forearm also remains short. If the radius and ulna seem to be growing at the same rate and the variance has not changed after a year, consider ulnar shortening without an epiphyseodesis and continue to observe the patient until skeletal maturity. Overcorrection of the variance by a few millimeters may be performed, because the osteotomy may lead to acceleration of growth at the ulna.

SUMMARY

The hand and wrist of the pediatric athlete merit special considerations for the remodeling potential of fractures and the long-term sequelae of malunited fractures, growth arrest, early joint degeneration, and ligamentous instability. The success of remodeling cannot be overestimated, because not all fractures remodel. However, the tolerance for malunion must be higher in children with growth remaining than in adults, unless joint instability, articular incongruity, or physeal malalignment are at risk.

REFERENCES

1. Gholson JJ, Bae DS, Zurakowski D, et al. Scaphoid fractures in children and adolescents: contemporary injury patterns and factors influencing time to union. J Bone Joint Surg Am 2011;93(13):1210–9.
2. Elson RA. Rupture of the central slip of the extensor hood of the finger. A test for early diagnosis. J Bone Joint Surg Br 1986;68(2):229–31.
3. Karl JW, White NJ, Strauch RJ. Percutaneous reduction and fixation of displaced phalangeal neck fractures in children. J Pediatr Orthop 2012;32(2):156–61.
4. Waters PM, Taylor BA, Kuo AY. Percutaneous reduction of incipient malunion of phalangeal neck fractures in children. J Hand Surg Am 2004;29:707–11.
5. Puckett BN, Gaston RG, Peljovich AE, et al. Remodeling potential of phalangeal distal condylar malunions in children. J Hand Surg Am 2012;37(1):34–41.
6. Egol KA, Koval KJ, Zuckerman JD. Pediatric wrist and hand. Handbook of fractures. 4th edition. Philadelphia: Lippincott Williams and Wilkins; 2010. p. 660–80.
7. Feller R, Kluk A, Katarincic J. Pediatric phalanx fractures: evaluation and management. In: Kozin SH, Abzug J, Zlotolow DA, editors. The pediatric upper extremity. New York: Springer; 2014. p. 962–78.
8. Cassel S, Shah AS. Metacarpal fractures. In: Kozin SH, Abzug J, Zlotolow DA, editors. The pediatric upper extremity. New York: Springer; 2014. p. 982–1003.
9. Heyman P. Injuries to the ulnar collateral ligament of the thumb metacarpophalangeal joint. J Am Acad Orthop Surg 1997;5:224–9.
10. Doman AN, Marcus NW. Congenital bipartite scaphoid. J Hand Surg 1990;15(6): 869–73.

11. Richards RR, Ledbetter WS, Transfeldt EE. Radiocarpal osteoarthritis associated with bilateral bipartite carpal scaphoid bones: a case report. Can J Surg 1987; 30(4):289–91.

12. Hove LM. Epidemiology of scaphoid fractures in Bergen, Norway. Scand J Plast Reconstr Surg Hand Surg 1999;33:423–6.

13. Mussbichler H. Injuries of the carpal scaphoid in children. Acta Radiol 1961;56: 361–8.

14. Vahvanen V, Westerlund M. Fracture of the carpal scaphoid in children. A clinical and roentgenological study of 108 cases. Acta Orthop Scand 1980;51:909–13.

15. Stanciu C, Dumont A. Changing patterns of scaphoid fractures in adolescents. Can J Surg 1994;37:214–6.

16. Toh S, Miura H, Arai K, et al. Scaphoid fractures in children: problems and treatment. J Pediatr Orthop 2003;23:216–21.

17. Louis DS, Calhoun TP, Garr SM, et al. Congenital bipartite scaphoid: fact or fiction? J Bone Joint Surg Am 1976;58A:ll08–12.

18. Zlotolow DA, Knutsen E, Yao J. Optimization of volar percutaneous screw fixation for scaphoid waist fractures using traction, positioning, imaging, and an angiocatheter guide. J Hand Surg Am 2011;36:916–21.

19. Fernandez DL, Eggli S. Non-union of the scaphoid. Revascularization of the proximal pole with implantation of a vascular bundle and bone-grafting. J Bone Joint Surg Am 1995;77(6):883–93.

20. Tang P, Fischer CR. A new volar vascularization technique using the superficial palmar branch of the radial artery for the collapsed scaphoid nonunion. Tech Hand Up Extrem Surg 2010;14(3):160–72.

21. Hori Y, Tamai S, Okuda H, et al. Blood vessel transplantation to bone. J Hand Surg Am 1979;4(1):23–33.

22. Kakar S, Bishop AT, Shin AY. Role of vascularized bone grafts in the treatment of scaphoid nonunions associated with proximal pole avascular necrosis and carpal collapse. J Hand Surg Am 2011;36(4):722–5.

23. Mathoulin C, Haerle M. Vascularized bone graft from the palmar carpal artery for treatment of scaphoid nonuinion. J Hand Surg Br 1998;23B(3):318–23.

24. Nellans KW, Kowalski E, Chung KC. The epidemiology of distal radius fractures. Hand Clinics 2012;28(2):113–25.

25. Solvang HW, Nordheggen RA, Clementsen S, et al. Epidemiology of distal radius fracture in Akershus, Norway, in 2010-2011. Journal of Orthopaedic Surgery and Research 2018;13(1):199–7.

26. Khosla S, Melton LJ, Dekutoski MB, Achenbach SJ, Oberg AL, Riggs BL. Incidence of childhood distal forearm fractures over 30 years: a population-based study. JAMA 2003;290(11):1479–85.

27. de Putter CE, van Beeck EF, Looman CWN, Toet H, Hovius SER, Selles RW. Trends in Wrist Fractures in Children and Adolescents, 1997–2009. Journal of Hand Surgery 2011;36(11):1810–5.e1812.

28. Waters PM, Bae DS, Montgomery KD. Surgical management of posttraumatic distal radial growth arrest in adolescents. Journal of Pediatric Orthopaedics 2002;22(6):717–24.

29. Bae DS, Waters PM. Pediatric distal radius fractures and triangular fibrocartilage complex injuries. Hand Clinics 2006;22(1):43–53.

30. Davidson JS, Brown DJ, Barnes SN, et al. Simple treatment for torus fractures of the distal radius. J Bone Joint Surg Br 2001;83:1173–5.

31. Abzug JM, Schwartz BS, Johnson AJ. Assessment of splints applied for pediatric fractures in an emergency department/urgent care environment. J Pediatr Orthop 2019;39(2):76–84.
32. Thompson SJ, Zlotolow DA, editors. Handbook of splinting and casting. Philadelphia: Elsevier; 2011.
33. Miller BS, Taylor B, Widmann RF, et al. Cast immobilization versus percutaneous pin fixation of displaced distal radius fractures in children; a prospective, randomized study. J Pediatr Orthop 2005;25:490–4.
34. McQuinn AG, Jaarsma RL. Risk factors for redisplacement of pediatric distal forearm and distal radius fractures. J Pediatr Orthop 2012;32(7):687–92.
35. Zamzam MM, Khoshhal KI. Displaced fracture of the distal radius in children: factors responsible for redisplacement after closed reduction. J Bone Joint Surg Br 2005;87(6):841–3.
36. Ring D, Rhim R, Carpenter C, et al. Isolated radial shaft fractures are more common than Galeazzi fractures. J Hand Surg Am 2006;31(1):17–21.
37. Jockel CR, Zlotolow DA, Butler RB, et al. Extensile surgical exposures of the radius: a comparative anatomic study. J Hand Surg 2013;38(4):745–52.
38. Page WT, Szabo RM. Distraction osteogenesis for correction of distal radius deformity after physeal arrest. J Hand Surg Am 2009;34(4):617–26.
39. Gundes H, Buluc L, Sahin M, et al. Deformity correction by Ilizarov distraction osteogenesis after distal radius physeal arrest. Acta Orthop Traumatol Turc 2011;45(6):406–11.
40. Andersson JK, Lindau T, Karlsson J, et al. Distal radio-ulnar joint instability in children and adolescents after wrist trauma. J Hand Surg Euro Vol 2014;39(6): 653–61.
41. Terry CL, Waters PM. Triangular fibrocartilage injuries in pediatric and adolescent patients. J Hand Surg Am 1998;23(4):626–34.
42. Miller A, Lightdale-Miric N, Eismann E, et al. Outcomes of isolated radial osteotomy for volar distal radioulnar joint instability following radial malunion in children. J Hand Surg Am 2018;43(1):81.e1–8.
43. Adams BD, Berger RA. An anatomic reconstruction of the distal radioulnar ligaments for posttraumatic distal radioulnar joint instability. J Hand Surg Am 2002; 27(2):243–51.
44. Farr S, Zechmann U, Ganger R, et al. Clinical experience with arthroscopically-assisted repair of peripheral triangular fibrocartilage complex tears in adolescents: technique and results. Int Orthop 2015;39(8):1571–7.

Therapy Considerations for Getting Athletes to Return to Play

Jane M. Fedorczyk, PT, PhD, CHT

KEYWORDS

- Rehabilitation • Return to play • Protective gear • Taping • Orthoses • Hand • Wrist
- Sports medicine

KEY POINTS

- The rehabilitation considerations of athletes depend on the nature of the injury, sport, and level of play.
- The use of protective orthoses is established by sports-specific regulations, level of play, and position played, and may ultimately be determined by sport officials on the day of competition.
- The rehabilitation plan of care should not only focus on rapid, safe return to sport but should include strategies to optimize overall performance and to prevent future injuries.
- A team approach engaging in close communication between the athlete, surgeon, therapist, coaches, and trainers optimizes recovery and safe return to competition.

INTRODUCTION

The primary role of occupational therapists (OTs) or physical therapists (PTs) in the rehabilitation of athletes that have sustained a wrist or hand injury is to restore function and optimize performance for safe return to play (RTP) as quickly as possible. This article uses therapists to represent both OTs and PTs. Ideally, therapists possess specialized training in hand and wrist conditions consistent with the Certified Hand Therapist (CHT) credential.[1]

The access points to treatment following sports-related injury vary depending on age of the athlete, level of play, time of season, and nature of the injury. Therapists may be the initial point of entry into the health care system for injury, but this does vary by the credential in the practice location (registration or licensure), clinic setting, years of experience, and age of patient.[2,3] For this reason, therapists are trained to

Center for Hand and Upper Limb Health and Performance, Jefferson College of Rehabilitation Sciences, Thomas Jefferson University, 901 Walnut Street, Suite 600, Philadelphia, PA 19107, USA
E-mail address: Jane.Fedorczyk@jefferson.edu

Clin Sports Med 39 (2020) 481–502
https://doi.org/10.1016/j.csm.2019.12.009
0278-5919/20/© 2019 Elsevier Inc. All rights reserved.

sportsmed.theclinics.com

perform screening examinations to determine whether the nature of injury is suitable for therapy management alone or whether the athlete requires further medical or surgical examination and treatment.[4,5] For example, an athlete with radial-sided wrist pain with a history of a fall on an outstretched hand (FOOSH) may make an appointment in a therapy clinic and state that the wrist is sprained. Based on the velocity associated with the FOOSH, and the presenting symptoms, the therapist may determine that imaging is needed to rule out a wrist fracture or ligament injury and, therefore, a referral to a hand surgeon is indicated.

Rehabilitation education emphasizes movement analysis and treatment strategies to assist patients to optimize their performance for everyday life, work, and play. Promoting health and wellness is a key component in the plan of care for all patients, including athletes, to maximize the patient's experience, outcome, and overall health.[6,7]

ATHLETES AS PATIENTS OR PATIENTS AS ATHLETES

It is frequently stated that rehabilitating injured athletes can be a challenge, especially if they are unrealistic or anxious to RTP. However, RTP depends on many factors, and few standards for clinical decision making have been established.[8–11] **Box 1** provides a list of the common factors that influence RTP. The managing hand surgeon is typically the primary decision maker in determining RTP; however, the physician usually works collaboratively with the other members of the team.[9] Team members may include the family physician, team physician, therapist, trainer, coach, agent, parent, league officials, and the athlete. The coordination of medical resources for injury management, rehabilitation, and determination of RTP varies based on the athlete's level of play: professional, collegiate, high school, and youth.[9–11]

Athletes are considered to be highly motivated patients because of their dedication to their sports, competitive attitude, high level of fitness, and efficiency with learning novel movements or tasks. However, athletes are often risk takers and an overaggressive attitude (no pain no gain) may lead to premature stress on healing injured tissues. During the protective phase of rehabilitation, the therapist spends the most time with the athlete, so it is the therapist's responsibility to control the athlete throughout all phases of rehabilitation, and emphasize the need to respect the biology of tissue healing.

Regardless of the mechanism of injury, the rehabilitation principles are the same for all patients and the nuances specific to individual patients, including how they occupy their time, are considered when the plan of care is established. These considerations include activities of daily living, as well as education, occupation, and recreational tasks. Some of the unique considerations for sports rehabilitation are an emphasis on the cause of the sports injury, incorporating sport-specific activities, optimizing skills required for the sport, and providing a holistic conditioning program to improve or maintain the level of fitness, while safely protecting the healing injury.

REHABILITATION PHASES

The rehabilitation outcome is to return the athlete back to optimum performance as safely and rapidly as possible.[8–14] Therefore, none of the aspects of rehabilitation should be skipped, especially once clinical healing of the injured tissue is determined. Downtime during the protective phase of therapy may lead to impairments in strength and endurance of the involved upper limb, and the nature of the injury may decrease the overall level of fitness, including impairments in strength and endurance in the noninvolved limbs and core. Premature RTP may put the athlete at risk for repeat injury

Box 1
Factors that influence return to play

General
- All team members bound to ethical considerations within their professional standards.
- Parents have a voice in all athletes less than 18 years of age.
- If clear guidelines are not available regarding the use of protective gear, consult sports officials.
- For K–12 (kindergarten to grade 12) athletes, consult National Collegiate Athletic Association (NCAA) guidelines, league rules, and state boards of education.

Nature of hand/wrist injury:
- Traumatic injury may require complete healing to use the hand.
- Traumatic injury may be sufficiently protected with an orthosis to allow use of hand.
- Overuse injury may be sufficiently protected with an orthosis to allow use of hand.
- Overuse injury may lead to more significant injury if not handled immediately.
- Overuse injury may be sufficiently managed during season to delay further treatment to after the season.

Timing in the season:
- Injury may be season ending because of the severity of the injury.
- Minor injuries may be protected to delay care until end of season.

Level of play:
- Elite (regulations, legal, contractual)
  Professional athletes: legal or contractual factors associated with sports association/league
  Collegiate: NCAA regulations; impact on scholarship or eligibility
  High school: not regulated by NCAA; impact on scholarship or college recruitment; resources provided by AAOS, ACSM, NFHS, AAHPERD; generally accepted that full healing of injury should occur
- Nonelite (less regulated; note from physician may be required to return to participation)
  Leisure: not regulated at any age; athletes 18 years of age and older make independent decisions regarding their care; athletes less than 18 years of age must have parental permission
  Intramural/club: not regulated by NCAA at collegiate level; K–12 school may have some policies within school district or state board of education
  Community youth leagues: league or state specific if tied to board of education

Sport
- Some sports have limited or no NCAA guidelines or resources.

Position play
- NCAA guidelines may vary with regard to the use of protective gear for a particular position within a sport

Abbreviations: AAOS, American Academy of Orthopaedic Surgeons; ACSM, American College of Sports Medicine; NFHS, National Federation of State High School Associations; AAHPERD, American Alliance for Health, Physical Education, Recreation, and Dance.
   Data from Refs.[8–11]

to the wrist or hand, as well as increasing the potential for a new injury to another part of the body.

Protective Phase: Managing the Acute Injury

Postinjury and postoperative protocols vary with the specific injury. However, the overall therapy objective in this phase of care is to provide a careful balance between protecting the injured or repaired tissues and applying controlled stress. This delicate balance facilitates increases in tensile strength of healing structures, restores motion, modulates pain, decreases edema, and prevents the ill effects of immobilization, such as joint stiffness and muscle atrophy. Although the healing time varies by condition and severity of the injury, athletes generally have an accelerated program because of their general health status, level of fitness, and low incidence of comorbidities that may delay healing.

Surgeons may choose to protect hand or wrist conditions with splints, casts, or commercial braces or they may refer the athlete to a therapist skilled in custom orthotic fabrication to make a protective orthosis. The custom orthosis may be the standard for the specific injury provided the athlete is unable to RTP. Modifications to the standard custom orthosis may be required to allow the athlete to RTP, if appropriate, during the protective phase. The complexity of the injury determines the amount of time needed to control the activity level of the athlete as this phase is initiated.

Controlled therapeutic exercises specific to moving the hand and wrist are emphasized during this phase, but the quality of the exercise may depend on the patient's willingness to move. Other therapy interventions typically incorporated into the plan of care for patients during the protective phase include interventions that focus on reduction of pain, edema, and inflammation, including physical agents such as electrical stimulation or ultrasonography, therapeutic taping, pain science education, graded mental imagery, and activity modification.[12-18] General patient education about the scope of injury and expected therapy outcomes are ongoing throughout the episode of care.

Therapists are encouraged to use a biopsychosocial approach when establishing the individualized plan of care for all patients.[19,20] This approach ensures the therapist can assist in the identification of red flags that affect the athlete's recovery. High pain scores and psychological factors, such as anxiety or depression caused by the impact of injury, have been associated with poor recovery outcomes and chronic pain.[21] Although specific guidelines for hand and wrist injuries may not list therapy as a primary treatment of acute pain, the use of therapy for chronic pain management has been established as an alternative to opioids in prescribing guidelines.[22,23] Future investigations regarding therapy during the acute protective phase of rehabilitation may show a reduction in the use of opioids, especially in athletes eager to RTP.

A conditioning program that focuses on maintaining premorbid fitness level should be developed in a safe and controlled manner to minimize risk to the healing tissues. The specifics of a conditioning program depend on the complexity of the hand or wrist condition, but the program should include aerobic exercise and lower extremity (LE) strengthening exercises to maintain muscle strength, power, and endurance. A strengthening program for the noninvolved upper extremity (UE) and the noninvolved muscle groups of the injured hand and wrist should be tailored to the athlete without risking further injury. The athlete may need to wait 4 to 12 weeks before vigorous sports-specific activities can be resumed.

It is beyond the scope of this article to address the specifics of postoperative protocols for flexor/extensor tendon repairs, carpal ligament injuries, and intra-articular phalangeal fractures. This information can be found elsewhere.[24] During the protective phase, the acute management of hand and wrist injuries does not vary much between athletes.

Postprotection Phase: Preparing for Safe Return to Play

Following the protective phase of rehabilitation and the clinical healing or union of injured structures, athletes progress to strengthening exercises, proprioceptive training, and sport-specific activities simulated in the clinic under the supervision of the therapist. If relevant, the athlete is asked to bring in equipment used for the sport. Although the hand and wrist might be the primary site of injury, the functional use of the involved upper limb or both upper limbs may have been discouraged. Total arm strengthening exercise programs, commonly used for shoulder and elbow conditions, benefit athletes with a wrist or hand injury.[25] Recognizing that the tensile strength of the injured tissues is not fully restored at this phase, care must be taken to progressively increase the resistance to not overload the muscles of the injured limb.

UE weight-bearing tolerance is another essential component in the postprotection phase. Athletes, especially those involved in leisure, club, or intramural sports, usually ask their therapists when they can return to their sport-related activities. If the patient has sustained a fracture, ligament, or tendon injury of the hand and wrist, weight-bearing through the involved upper limb may be prohibited for about 4 to 12 weeks during the protective phase. Because the FOOSH is a protective mechanism associated with loss of balance and falls, before RTP, the athletes must be able to tolerate UE weight-bearing during high-level conditioning activities such as running on uneven surfaces. Fig. 1A–F shows an UE weight-bearing sequence used by this author.

In general, the athletes participate in some low-level strengthening and conditioning during the protective phase. Depending on the restrictions placed on the athlete during the protective phase, the level of fitness, LE conditioning, and core strength may also be diminished. The emphasis during the postprotection phase is to reduce kinesiophobia, restore neuromuscular control, improve the components of muscle performance (strength, power, endurance), and restore the athletes' confidence in their performance levels.[26] Once cleared to resume total body strengthening and conditioning, it is best to refer the athlete to a physical therapist, athletic trainer, and/or coaches. The therapist that has been managing the hand and wrist injury should continue to consult with these team members to address any lifting or weight-bearing restrictions.

The final part of this phase involves a collaborative effort between athlete, therapist, athletic trainer, and coaching staff. All of the activities in this phase are involved in restoring the athlete's work capacity without causing stress to the healing injury. Work capacity is defined as the athlete's ability to perform repetitive technically proficient sports skills and exercise without the onset of excessive fatigue.[26] High-level sports-specific activities to optimize performance and safe RTP are progressed as

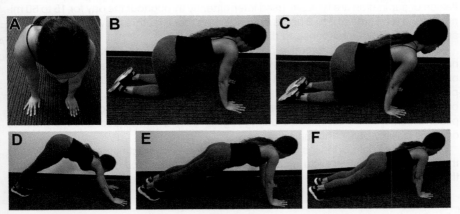

Fig. 1. UE weight-bearing positions to progress tolerance. (*A*) Quadruped (front view) requires full wrist and finger extension with full forearm pronation. (*B*) Quadruped; wrists aligned with shoulders. (*C*) Quadruped leaning into hands; shoulders forward to wrists, requiring maximum end-range wrist extension. (*D*) Downward dog position requires increased weight-bearing tolerance but not maximum wrist extension. (*E*) Plank; wrists aligned with shoulders. (*F*) Plank, shoulders forward to wrists, requiring maximum end-range wrist extension and weight-bearing tolerance.

strength and endurance improve. However, there are no specific guidelines available for hand or wrist injuries in any sport; therefore, team communication is essential to optimize the athletes' recovery. Sometime during this final phase, the need for hand therapy will decrease to consultation to address tissue reactivity (**Box 2**) while performance is building, and determining the need and value of protective orthoses, braces, or supportive taping.

ORTHOTIC INTERVENTION

Orthosis is the term used by therapists to describe an externally applied device fitted to the hand or wrist. It may be custom fabricated by a therapist or prefabricated from commercial distributors but fitted and/or adjusted by the therapist. The application of the orthosis includes patient education for use, wearing schedule, hygiene care, and review of precautions. The therapist evaluates the need for the orthosis and determines whether the selected orthosis achieves the intended purpose. Orthoses may be used to protect an injury or repaired tissues, provide support to reduce pain, provide mobilizing forces to improve passive motion, and provide substitution for impaired muscle function following peripheral nerve injury. The variable nature of sports-related injuries may require the use of an orthosis for any of these purposes through the rehabilitation process.

Mobilizing orthoses are typically indicated following required, prolonged immobilization for complex hand injuries. Adhesion formation and limited mobility may cause joint contracture or tendon tightness that restrict joint range of motion (ROM). When therapeutic exercises, especially passive stretching, fail to resolve the limitation in motion, a mobilizing orthosis can be applied to provide a low-load prolonged stretch. Mobilizing orthoses are commonly used to improve limitations in passive flexion, extension, or supination. The wearing schedules vary by the degree and direction (flexion, extension) of limited motion, the end feel of the passive limitation, and the joints involved. For example, to improve extension of a joint, the mobilizing orthosis may be worn during sleeping (6–8 hours). Orthoses that are fabricated to improve flexion or supination are typically used intermittently throughout the day for 15 to 60 minutes for a total time of 2 to 8 hours depending on those factors previously mentioned, as well as the joint's response to the stress application.[27]

As mentioned in the protective phase, the use of standard orthoses for wrist and hand injuries is common. If the athlete is able to participate in practice, a duplicate orthosis can be fabricated. When it is fitted to the athlete before practice, extra strapping, taping, and padding are used to protect vulnerable structures. After practice and bathing, the practice orthosis is removed and the original standard orthosis is reapplied, which ensures compliance during regular daily activities because the practice orthosis is likely bulky and malodorous.

Rigid or semirigid orthoses intended for use during competition must comply with the rules and regulations of the applicable regulatory agency. For collegiate athletes, this is the National Collegiate Athletic Association (NCAA). The NCAA has established

---

Box 2
Signs of tissue reactivity

Signs of inflammation (pain, edema) at rest

Increased pain with motion or activity

Decrease in motion caused by pain

guidelines for both mandatory protective equipment and special protective equipment for many sports.[28] In general, if the orthosis may harm another athlete, it is prohibited. Some sports, such as football, permit the use of rigid orthoses that are covered in padding. The orthosis must be covered on all exterior sides and edges with foam padding, 12.7-mm (0.5-inch) thickness (**Fig. 2**A–C) Not all football players, such as the quarterback or wide receiver, are able to wear padded rigid orthoses on their hands or wrists because of the bulky nature and the hand function needed for their playing positions. Therapists need to be aware of participation regulations. They also need to be realistic and creative to identify the best options to protect the injury but permit skillful use of the hand when needed.[29,30]

The availability of prefabricated orthoses and braces has increased to meet the demands of active lifestyles. Marketed to manage simple musculoskeletal disorders of the hand and wrist, physicians and therapists have identified indications for their use with their patients, especially athletes. Many of these braces are fabricated from low-profile durable materials suited for sports-related activities. Commercially available devices are typically less expensive than custom orthoses, so, if the prefabricated orthosis addresses the clinical goal for the athlete, it may be a wise investment to purchase 2; one to wear when the other is washed. Commercial orthoses provide options for therapists not skilled in custom orthotic fabrication and for athletes with limited insurance coverage for custom braces.[29] However, prefabricated orthoses are not available for some of the most vulnerable hand injuries that require full-time protection during the healing phase, such as repaired flexor tendons.

THERAPEUTIC TAPING AND COMPRESSION GARMENTS

Taping techniques are commonly used by athletes to prevent or manage soft tissue injuries. Athletic trainers are skilled in the use of common taping techniques for the hand and wrist to provide joint stability and restrict movement.[31] For decades, standard white cloth tape, such as Coach (Johnson and Johnson, New Brunswick, NJ) and Elastikon (Johnson and Johnson, New Brunswick, NJ) were the only taping products available, and they are still available.

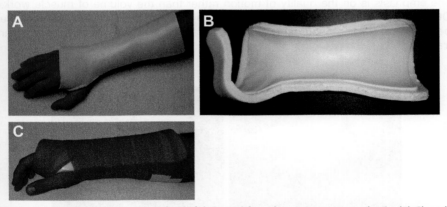

Fig. 2. (A) Custom dorsal wrist orthosis fabricated from low-temperature plastic. (B) Closed-cell slow-recovery foam padding covering all exposed sides of the orthosis. (C) Padded orthosis secured to hand and forearm with self-adherent wrap to be used for practice or competition.

Because of the popularity of elastic therapeutic tape, therapists are also using taping techniques to modulate pain, reduce edema, support weak muscles, and control motion.[16,17] This highly elasticized tape is applied to the skin with variable stretch over muscles to control specific movements and may be useful for athletes returning to sport after an injury. Although taping techniques for the hand and wrist are theorized to assist with injury recovery and provide support during play, there is a paucity of peer-reviewed evidence showing the value of its intended use.[16] Tape selection is largely determined by the preference and experience of therapists, athletic trainers, and athletes. The support offered by tape decreases with functional use; therefore, reapplication during play may be necessary. **Figs. 3**A, B and **4**A, B show examples of therapeutic taping.

Compression garments or sleeves may provide light support to enhance comfort following minor soft tissue injuries such as tendinopathies or after immobilization from injury or surgery. A recent study using a made-to-measure pressure garment on patients with distal radius fractures showed statistically significant improvements in pain, ROM, and function score on the patient-rated wrist evaluation.[32] Compression gloves may be a reasonable form of light protection, especially for athletes that are not working with therapists or athletic trainers.

PROPRIOCEPTION TRAINING

A rehabilitation program that includes proprioception training facilitates motion, muscle performance, joint stability, agility, and coordination. Proprioception involves the conscious and unconscious ability to detect position in space, movement precision, and dynamic stability of a joint.[33] There is no single, definitive definition for proprioception, but it may be considered as the ability of the body to use position sense to respond, consciously or unconsciously, to perturbations imposed on the body by altering posture and movement.[34] Injury interrupts the neuromuscular feedback between the peripheral afferent input and central nervous system (CNS) efferent output that facilitates motor activity, control, and coordination.[35] Proprioceptive exercises are progressed in terms of skill complexity rather than muscle overload for strengthening. The objective is to perform gradually more challenging skills, tasks, or actions while sustaining movement accuracy. The emphasis is on the quality of motion rather than the volume of muscle work. Other rehabilitation terms widely accepted to include proprioceptive training are perturbation training, neuromuscular reeducation, and reactive neuromuscular training.[33,36]

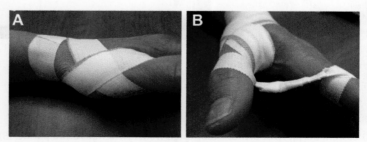

Fig. 3. (*A*) Thumb metacarpophalangeal (MCP) support taping (initial layer) using standard cloth athletic tape. At least 3 layers should be applied, as shown in (*B*). (*B*) Check-rein strap applied to limit thumb abduction or extension.

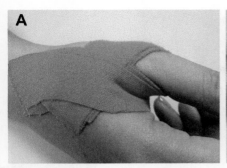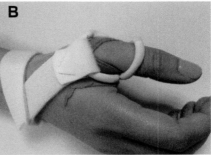

Fig. 4. (*A*) Thumb MCP support taping using elastic therapeutic tape. (*B*) A custom figure-8 orthosis offers more stabilization to prevent MCP joint hyperextension.

Mechanoreceptors in ligaments, tendons, muscles, and joint capsules provide the somatosensory input to the CNS.[33,37] Ligaments that provide static constraints to joint motion are loaded with Ruffini endings, Pacinian corpuscles, Golgi-like receptors, free nerve endings, and unclassified joint receptors that translate the mechanical stimuli associated with pressure, pain, stretch, and motion, including amplitude and velocity.[37] Widely accepted to be present in larger joints,[33–35] mechanoreceptors in wrist and hand ligaments have recently been identified.[38–44] This discovery has increased the interest in using proprioceptive training in the rehabilitation of hand and wrist injuries.[37]

Proprioception training begins during the protective phase of injury rehabilitation, focusing on early controlled motion. Pain and edema may inhibit movement, so interventions to address these impairments are necessary to facilitate motion. Mirror therapy and implicit motor imagery may promote conscious joint control and proprioception awareness.[37] Active and/or passive motion exercises should be incorporated as the tolerance to motion increases or tissue healing allows a larger arc of motion or increased vigor of exercise. Global movement of the upper limb as well as refined motions of the wrist and hand should be used in both the open and closed chain, depending on weight-bearing status. Proprioceptive neuromuscular facilitation (PNF) techniques for the upper limb can be used to increase motion in functional movement patterns, promoting cocontraction, synergistic muscle activity, and coordination.[45] Light purposeful prehension activities should also be encouraged (**Fig. 5**).

Neuromuscular control, conscious and unconscious, is emphasized primarily in the postprotection phase, although isometric strengthening exercises may be used during the protective phase depending on the nature of the injury. The proprioceptive training focuses on strengthening exercises, which increase not only strength but also power, endurance, and speed. Reactive muscle activation is designed to restore synchronous muscle firing patterns around the involved joint, which are required for dynamic joint stability and fine motor control. Proprioceptive training allows therapists to link the achievement of clinical-based goals and RTP.[36]

There is growing evidence that proprioceptive training can yield clinically meaningful improvements in cortical reorganization, somatosensory, and sensorimotor function.[46,47] However, studies specific to hand and wrist injuries are limited.[48–50] The Birmingham Wrist Instability Program provides a guideline for acute partial scapholunate ligament injury[49]; however, more research is needed to establish treatment guidelines for other hand and wrist injuries. **Table 1** provides an overview of the components of proprioception training with recommendations for types of exercise and outcome assessment.

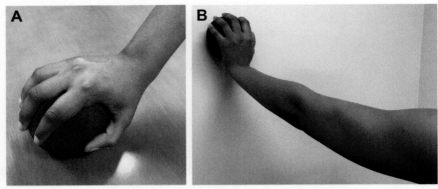

Fig. 5. Examples of light proprioception exercises to be used during the protective phase. (A) Tabletop ball rolling for movement awareness and partial weight-bearing. (B) Ball movements on the wall engaging the entire upper limb.

Specific training programs and assessment tools to evaluate proprioception and RTP are limited to knee and shoulder injuries.[33–35] There are no specific assessment tools for wrist and hand injuries, but there are some UE measures developed primarily for the shoulder that might be useful to assess upper limb performance to determine RTP.[52–55] The seated medicine ball throw assesses muscle power, coordination, and agility.[52] The modified pull-up test examines upper arm strength.[53] The closed kinetic chain (CKC) UE stability test is essentially a push-up test that addresses strength and weight-bearing tolerance.[54] The Y Balance Test evaluates UE weight-bearing, balance, and proprioception.[55] This author has not had the opportunity to evaluate the clinical utility of these tests with athletes.

SPORTS-SPECIFIC TRAINING METHODS
Periodization

Periodization is a model of sports conditioning that is used in the rehabilitation of athletes.[13,56] Essentially, the periodization program changes the workout plan at regular intervals, manipulating variables such as intensity, duration, frequency, and skill training. The training program is divided into cycles with specialized training and specific goals for each cycle. The goal is the development of sport-specific skill and performance that takes into consideration the demands of the specific sport. Progressive changes in training prevent a plateau in progress from occurring and continually challenge the athlete to achieve peak performance. The training program may vary based on time of year for the sport: preseason, in season, or postseason.

The periodization model has 3 cycles: the macrocycle, mesocycle, and microcycle. Training priorities may shift within the cycles to prevent overtraining and optimize performance. For example, sport-specific activities may be included in one cycle and then shift to exercises that are not sport-specific in the next cycle. In the conventional periodization program, the intensity may gradually progress over time (linear) or it can fluctuate the load and volume of core exercises (nonlinear).

Another approach is called block periodization. This model takes into account that there is not just 1 peak season. Athletes in some sports now typically continue competitive play throughout the year and the convention model only accounts for one peak season per year. The block approach is also sport specific in that, if 1 component of training (eg, endurance) is not needed for the sport, it is not included

Table 1
Proprioception training for hand and wrist injuries

	Proprioception: the conscious and unconscious ability to detect position, movement precision, and dynamic stability of a joint					
	Conscious proprioception Somatosensory function: afferent input contributes to motion awareness and precision Emphasized during the protective phase of rehabilitation			Unconscious proprioception Neuromuscular function: efferent response to afferent input that creates dynamic stability and reactive muscle activation Emphasized during the postprotective phase of rehabilitation Before RTP		
Component	Kinesthesia	Joint position sense	Neuromuscular rehabilitation	Agility	Balance UE Weight-bearing Tolerance	Coordination
Purpose	To sense movement without visual cues	To replicate a predetermined joint angle	To restore muscle performance to enhance joint movement and stability	To control the direction of the body or body part during rapid movements	To prevent loss of balance and facilitate UE weight-bearing tolerance	To enhance the smoothness of skilled movements
Exercises	Active and passive motion with or without mirror therapy	Blinded active and passive motion to reproduce joint angle on involved and uninvolved hands	Isometric Isotonic (concentric, eccentric) Isokinetic PNF techniques[45]	Throwing, catching, bouncing drills using balls of various sizes and weights Rapid reaching Plyometrics Sports-specific skills	LE and trunk strengthening UE weight-bearing exercises or drills	Agility ball drills Right-left hand manipulation tasks Rhythmic movements Plyometrics Sports-specific skills
Assessment	Threshold to detection of passive movement	Accuracy of joint motion, measured with goniometer	Muscle strength Joint stability during muscle activation	Athletic agility assessment tools[52] Sports-specific skill performance Work capacity	Athletic agility assessment tools[52,53] Sports-specific skill performance Work capacity	Athletic agility assessment tools[51,52] Sports-specific skill performance Work capacity

in the training cycles. There is limited evidence on how to incorporate periodization into rehabilitation, but recommendations and guidelines are available.[56,57]

Plyometrics

Plyometric exercise has become an integral component of the later part of the post-protection phase of rehabilitation as the athlete nears RTP.[13,58] It is theorized that plyometrics assist in the development of power, a foundation from which the athlete can refine the skills of the sport. Because of the high overload forces involved in plyometrics, therapists reserve this type of exercise for the late phase of rehabilitation to avoid contraindications such as inflammation, joint instability, mobility limitations, muscle weakness, and healing repaired structures that may not possess the tensile strength to withstand applied forces.[58]

Plyometrics training involves the quick stretching of muscle from an eccentric contraction to a concentric contraction. There are 3 phases of a plyometric exercise: eccentric prestretch, amoritization (rebound), and concentric shortening. The prestretch phase involves elastic loading and generates forces to transfer kinetic energy to the shortening cycle. The resultant force production in the performance pattern facilitates power by maximizing explosive shortening. The rebound or amoritization phase refers to the time delay between the eccentric and concentric phases. A shorter time delay generates a more powerful concentric contraction in the movement. If this time delay is prolonged, then the stretch reflex is not activated and the resultant concentric muscle contraction is not as powerful. Therefore, a key goal of plyometric training is to decrease the time delay between eccentric and concentric phases to result in improved muscle performance.[58]

Compared with the large number of studies on lower limb plyometrics, there are fewer studies that address plyometric training within the upper limb. Most of these studies have been focused on the shoulder and elbow in overhead athletes. Plyometric exercises for the UE may be performed in either the CKC or open kinetic chain (OKC). When initiating UE plyometrics in rehabilitation, the exercises are usually performed in a limited arc of motion to allow the athlete to begin working on power without compromising healing structures. Specific guidelines and recommendations have been described in a recently published clinical commentary.[58]

The Upper Extremity Kinetic Chain

The UE kinetic chain includes the shoulder, elbow, wrist, and hand. Kinetic chain exercises translate to focus on functional and/or sport-specific movements. By using multiple body segments in the exercise, adjacent segments can facilitate the activation of the involved muscles to develop appropriate patterns of movement and stabilization. Both open and closed chain exercises may be used to meet the treatment goals of the athlete depending on the nature of the injury and the sport.[13]

CKC exercises are performed with the distal segment (hand/wrist) fixed. OKC exercises involve a freely moving wrist and hand, although the hand may be fixed to a load, such as a free weight or weighted ball. Although typical UE functions take place using the OKC, UE weight-bearing is required for some everyday activities and is an integral component in sports such as gymnastics[59] or other activities such as breakdancing or yoga. All athletes need to tolerate UE weight-bearing to withstand a FOOSH if the sport has a loss of balance or falls risk. CKC exercises involve coactivation of agonist and antagonist muscles across the joints in the chain, which facilitates proximal joint stability (shoulder) in the upper limb. Therapists use CKC exercises with caution in the rehabilitation of hand and wrist injuries and only after the athlete has been cleared for UE weight-bearing.

Table 2
General therapy guidelines for hand and wrist injuries by phase of rehabilitation

Injury	Protective Phase	Postprotection Phase	RTP
Hand/wrist tendinopathies[63]	Taping/braces/orthoses to abate acute resting pain Interventions to reduce acute inflammation ROM, isometrics, and isotonic (eccentrics) exercises Conditioning to maintain preinjury fitness levels with activity modification for involved hand	Taping or compression garments to provide support and comfort Grip and forearm strengthening emphasis on eccentrics Progressive strengthening and fitness conditioning: core, LE, total arm (OKC, CKC) Proprioception training Plyometrics Address physical factors associated with sports technique/skills, equipment, or training schedule that may contribute to symptoms (activity/skill modification)	Athlete not likely to be pulled from play except when symptom severity warrants full rest or surgical management Muscle-tendon unit is strong but painful Athlete does not need to be pain free to progress program or RTP,[63] but pain with activity should not exceed VRS = 5/10 to reduce chance of further injury caused by impaired muscle performance caused by pain level
Hand/wrist fractures[12,63–72]	Cast/splints/braces/orthoses for fracture stabilization and soft tissue support Interventions to reduce acute inflammation Early pain-guided active motion for stable fractures AROM/PROM to uninvolved joints AROM/PROM to minimize loss of joint mobility and facilitate conscious proprioception Conditioning to maintain preinjury fitness levels without or limited use of involved hand	Cast/splints/braces/orthoses, taping or compression garments to provide support Address impairments associated with immobilization: decreased motion (joint stiffness) and strength deficits (grip, pinch, forearm) Address UE weight-bearing tolerance Progressive strengthening and fitness conditioning: core, LE, total arm (OKC, CKC) Proprioceptive training Plyometrics Higher-level conditioning to restore preinjury fitness levels Advanced proprioception activities Sports-specific skills	Timing depends on severity of fracture, sport, position played, and regulations regarding protective gear Protective cast/brace/orthosis may allow safe RTP during fracture healing for elite or collegiate athletes 3–6 wk for simple, nonoperative hand/ wrist fractures without protection 8–24 wk for complex, surgically managed hand/wrist fractures including thumb ROM should be pain free and within 10° of the noninvolved side[70] Grip strength should be 80%–90% of the noninvolved side and pain free[69,70] For wrist fractures, tolerates UE weight bearing for at least 30 s in downward dog (see **Fig. 1D**)

(continued on next page)

Table 2
(continued)

Injury	Protective Phase	Postprotection Phase	RTP
Extensor tendon injuries[12,63,72]	Custom extension orthosis for 4–8 wk depending on zone of injury Early motion protocol may be initiated depending on zone Interventions to reduce acute inflammation AROM/PROM to minimize loss of joint mobility and facilitate conscious proprioception Conditioning to maintain preinjury fitness levels without or limited use of involved hand	Splints/braces/orthoses, taping or compression garments to provide support Address impairments associated with immobilization: decreased motion (joint stiffness) and strength deficits Progressive strengthening and fitness conditioning: core, LE, total arm (OKC, CKC) Proprioceptive training Plyometrics Higher-level conditioning to restore preinjury fitness levels Advanced proprioception activities Sports-specific skills	RTP at 4–12 wk depending on zone of injury and surgical management Protective cast/orthosis may allow safe RTP during tendon healing; buddy taping fingers together to provide additional protection Timing depends on zone of injury, sport, position played, and regulations regarding protective gear
Flexor tendon injuries[63,72,73]	Custom forearm-based dorsal block orthosis for 4–6 wk Early active/passive motion to promote tendon gliding, prevent joint stiffness, and promote healing Interventions to reduce inflammation AROM/PROM to minimize loss of joint mobility and facilitate conscious proprioception Conditioning to maintain preinjury fitness levels without or limited use of involved hand	Taping or compression garments to provide support Address impairments associated with immobilization: decreased motion (joint stiffness) and strength deficits Progressive strengthening and fitness conditioning: core, LE, total arm (OKC, CKC) Proprioceptive training Plyometrics Higher-level conditioning to restore preinjury fitness levels Advanced proprioception activities Sports-specific skills	Because of nature of this injury and position-specific hand use, early RTP is not common to avoid rupture of repaired tendon 12–24 wk typical without protective orthosis depending on hand use in the sport Tests and measures for ROM and strength should be 80%–90% of the noninvolved side before RTP 4–6 mo is recommended for sports that use forceful gripping

| Flexor tendon pulley injuries[74,75] | Single/multiple pulley repairs follow similar postoperative guidelines for flexor tendon repairs; use hand-based dorsal block orthosis and/or thermoplastic pulley ring
Symptomatic pulley/tendon strains may benefit from finger orthoses, taping, or compression sleeves to provide support and abate symptoms
Controlled active and passive motion to promote tendon gliding and prevent joint stiffness
Interventions to reduce inflammation
Conditioning to maintain preinjury fitness levels with activity modification for involved hand | Finger orthoses, taping, or compression sleeves to provide support
Address impairments associated with immobilization: decreased motion (joint stiffness) and strength deficits
Progressive strengthening and fitness conditioning: core, LE, total arm (OKC, CKC)
Proprioceptive training
Plyometrics
Higher-level conditioning to restore preinjury fitness levels
Advanced proprioception activities
Sports-specific skills | Injuries common in rock climbers
RTP depends on the type of climbing
Return to easy climbing in 2 mo if pulley injury managed with therapy and 4 mo if surgically repaired[74]
Most climbers can resume unrestricted climbing in 6 mo[74]
Climbing in rock gyms may be easier and more controlled than in outdoor settings; this type of climbing is repetitive, so climbing time should be gradually increased
Premature return to climbing with symptoms may result in chronic problems with pain and hand mobility[75] |

(continued on next page)

Table 2
(continued)

Injury	Protective Phase	Postprotection Phase	RTP
Carpal instabilities[49,59,63,76–79] SLIL LTIL Palmar midcarpal instability	Therapy depends on severity of the ligament injury and surgical intervention Casts/braces/orthoses, forearm based, used to abate pain and to protect injured or repaired ligament for 4–8 wk Interventions to reduce inflammation (after injury or postoperatively) ROM to uninvolved joints if wrist immobilized; avoid UE weight-bearing activities AROM/PROM in a protected range to minimize loss of joint mobility and facilitate conscious proprioception[49] ROM in the dart thrower's plane within protected range for scapholunate (SLIL) injuries[78] Targeted muscle reeducation for the ECRL, FCR, and APL; avoid ECU activation (SLIL)[78,79] Targeted muscle reeducation for ECU; avoid ECRL, FCR, and APL activation (LTIL)[79] Targeted muscle reeducation for palmar MC instability[79] Conditioning to maintain preinjury fitness levels with activity modification for involved hand or no use of involved hand	Rehabilitation specifics as outlined in protection phase may still be used Cast/braces/orthoses, taping or compression garments to provide support as weight-bearing and RTP activities progress Address impairments associated with immobilization: decreased motion (joint stiffness) and strength deficits as tolerated Initiate and progress UE weight-bearing as tolerated Progressive strengthening and fitness conditioning: core, LE, total arm (OKC, CKC) Proprioceptive training Plyometrics Higher-level conditioning to restore preinjury fitness levels Advanced proprioception activities Sports-specific skills Therapy precautions focus on avoidance of pain or perception of joint instability at the wrist Address physical factors associated with sports technique/skills, equipment, or training schedule that may contribute to symptoms (activity/skill modification)	RTP 2–6 mo depending on severity of instability, use of surgical intervention, period of immobilization[76,77] Protective brace or orthosis may be used indefinitely depending on sport Because of nature of this injury and position-specific hand use, early RTP is not common to avoid further damage to injured or repaired ligament Tolerates UE weight-bearing for at least 30 s in downward dog (see **Fig. 1D**) Tests and measures for ROM and grip strength should be 75% of the noninvolved side before RTP

Injury	Acute Phase	Protection Phase	Rehabilitation	Return to Play
Ulnar-sided wrist pain[59,80-83] TFCC DRUJ ECU	Therapy depends on severity of injury, use of surgical intervention, and length of immobilization Casts/braces/orthoses, forearm based, used to abate pain and to protect injured or repaired structures for 4-8 wk; forearm rotation and/or wrist motion are avoided Interventions to reduce inflammation (after injury or postoperatively) ROM to uninvolved joints if wrist immobilized; avoid UE weight-bearing activities AROM/PROM in a protected range to minimize loss of joint mobility and facilitate conscious proprioception[49]	Interventions to reduce inflammation (after injury or postoperatively) ROM to uninvolved joints Conditioning to maintain preinjury fitness levels with activity modification for involved hand or no use of involved hand	Rehabilitation specifics as outlined in protection phase may still be used Braces, orthoses, taping or ulnar compression wraps to provide support as weight-bearing and RTP activities progress Address impairments associated with immobilization: decreased motion (joint stiffness) and strength deficits as tolerated Initiate and progress UE weight-bearing as tolerated Progressive strengthening and fitness conditioning: core, LE, total arm (OKC, CKC) Proprioceptive training Plyometrics Higher-level conditioning to restore preinjury fitness levels Advanced proprioception activities Sports-specific skills Therapy precautions focus on avoidance of pain or perception of joint instability at the wrist Address physical factors associated with sports technique/skills, equipment, or training schedule that may contribute to symptoms (activity/skill modification)	RTP 2-6 mo depending on severity of instability, use of surgical intervention, period of immobilization[59,81-83] Protective brace or orthosis may be used indefinitely depending on sport Because of nature of this injury and position-specific hand use, early RTP is not common to avoid further damage to injured or repaired ligament Tolerates UE weight-bearing for at least 30 s in downward dog (see **Fig. 1D**) Tests and measures for ROM and grip strength should be 75% of the noninvolved side before RTP

Abbreviations: APL, abductor pollicis longus; AROM, active ROM; DRUJ, distal radioulnar joint; ECRL, extensor carpi radialis longus; ECU, extensor carpi ulnaris; FCR, flexor carpi radialis; LTIL, lunotriquetral interosseous ligament; MC, midcarpal; PROM, passive ROM; SLIL, scapholunate interosseous ligament; TFCC, triangular fibrocartilage complex.

MENTAL IMAGERY

Mental imagery or visualization involves imagining the performance of a task without any physical movement. In sports, athletes see themselves performing the movements of their sport. The imagery can be imagined (visualized internally) or they can watch videos, if available, of their past performances.[60–62] The use of mental practice comes from functional MRI research, which shows similar cortical activation for actual and imagined motor repetitions in the premotor areas of the brain. It is theorized that, when an athlete repeatedly visualizes sports-specific activities, the muscle memory is maintained as it would be with physical activities.[60] This process may help athletes maintain their fundamental skills and facilitate RTP during the postprotection phase of rehabilitation. Mental imagery assists the rehabilitation effort of the athlete by reducing pain, increasing motivation, and enhance coping skills.[61] Consistent with many therapy interventions, further investigations are needed.[62]

SUMMARY

Therapy for hand and wrist injuries in athletes is similar to the plan of care provided to all patients during the protective phase. The nuances in the care provided to athletes become apparent as clinicians transition to the postprotective phase of rehabilitation and focus on RTP. The therapy program should be tailored to the individual needs of the athletes in their everyday lives, including work and/or school, and should consider the specifics of their training routines, sports-specific activities, and preparation for competition or RTP. **Table 2** summarizes general therapy guidelines for conditions covered in this issue. More detailed rehabilitation guidelines for each of the conditions presented in the table is available in this issue and elsewhere.[12,23,49,59,63–83] These guidelines are based on the clinical expertise of this author. Further study is recommended to increase the level of evidence and establish clinical practice guidelines. As a collaborative member of the team, the therapist progresses the athlete to an optimal recovery and health, which it is hoped will prevent future injury, enhance the patient experience, and achieve a positive outcome.

DISCLOSURE

The author has nothing to disclose.

REFERENCES

1. The CHT credential. Available at: https://www.htcc.org/consumer-information/the-cht-credential. Accessed March 1, 2019.
2. OT state statutes and regulations. Available at: https://www.aota.org/Advocacy-Policy/State-Policy/Licensure/StateRegs.aspx. Accessed March 1, 2019.
3. Direct access at the state level. Available at: http://www.apta.org/StateIssues/DirectAccess/. Accessed March 1, 2019.
4. 2018 Accreditation Council for Occupational Therapy Education (ACOTE®) standards and interpretive guide. Available at: https://www.aota.org/~/media/Corporate/Files/EducationCareers/Accredit/StandardsReview/2018-ACOTE-Standards-Interpretive-Guide.pdf. Accessed March 1, 2019.
5. Standards and required elements for accreditation of physical therapist education programs. Available at: http://www.capteonline.org/uploadedFiles/CAPTEorg/About_CAPTE/Resources/Accreditation_Handbook/CAPTE_PTStandards Evidence.pdf. Accessed March 1, 2019.

6. About AOTA. Vision statement 2025. Available at: https://www.aota.org/AboutAOTA.aspx. Accessed March 1, 2019.

7. Vision statement for the physical therapy profession and guiding principles to achieve that vision. Available at: http://www.apta.org/Vision/. Accessed March 1, 2019.

8. Coppage JM, Carlson MG. Expediting professional athletes' return to competition. Hand Clin 2017;33:9–18.

9. Shrier I, Safai P, Charland L. Return to play following injury: whose decision should it be? Br J Sports Med 2014;48:394–401.

10. Elbanna AM, Spindler KP, Schickendantz M. Care of athletes at different levels: from pee wee to professional. In: Madden CC, Putukian M, McCarty EC, et al, editors. Netter's sports medicine. 2nd edition. St Louis (MO): Elsevier; 2018. p. 104–7.

11. Clover J, Wall J. Return to play criteria following sports injury. Clin Sports Med 2010;29:169–75.

12. Ng CY, Hayton M. Management of acute hand injuries in athletes. Orthopedics and Trauma 2012;27:25–9.

13. Bertini T, Laidig T, Pettit N, et al. Management of common sports injuries. In: Skirven TM, Osterman AL, Fedorczyk JM, et al, editors. Rehabilitation of the hand and upper extremity. 6th edition. St Louis (MO): Elsevier; 2011. p. 1706–13.

14. Gart MS, Weidrich TA. Therapy and rehabilitation for upper extremity injuries in athletes. Hand Clin 2017;33:207–20.

15. Priganc VW, Stralka SW. Graded motor imagery. J Hand Ther 2011;24:164–8.

16. Williams S, Whatman C, Hume PA, et al. Kinesio taping in treatment and prevention of sports injuries: a meta-analysis of the evidence for its effectiveness. Sports Med 2012;44:153–64.

17. Poretto-Loehrke A. Taping techniques for the wrist. J Hand Ther 2016;29:213–6.

18. Louw A, Puentedura E, Zimney K. Teaching patients about pain: it works, but what should we call it? Physiother Theory Pract 2016;32:328–31.

19. Raman J, Walton D, MacDermid JC, et al. Predictors of outcomes after rotator cuff repair- a meta-analysis. J Hand Ther 2017;30:276–92.

20. Carpenter NR, Breeden KL. Opioid guidelines and their implications for occupational therapy. AOTA CE Article 2018. Available at: https://www.aota.org/~/media/Corporate/Files/Publications/CE-Articles/CE-Article-August-2018.pdf. Accessed February 26, 2019.

21. Mehta SP, MacDermid JC, Richardson J, et al. Baseline pain intensity is a predictor of chronic pain in individuals with distal radius fracture. J Orthop Sports Phys Ther 2015;45:119–27.

22. Mintkin PE, Moore JR, Flynn TW. Physical therapists' role in solving the opioid epidemic. J Orthop Sports Phys Ther 2018;48:349–53.

23. CDC guideline for prescribing opioids for chronic pain. 2019. Available at: https://www.cdc.gov/drugoverdose/prescribing/guideline.html. Accessed February 26, 2019.

24. Skirven TM, Osterman AL, Fedorczyk JM, et al, editors. Rehabilitation of the hand and upper extremity. 6th edition. St Louis (MO): Mosby; 2011.

25. Wilk KE, Arrigo CA, Hooks TR, et al. Rehabilitation of the overhead throwing athlete: there is more to it than just external/internal rotation strengthening. PM R 2016;8:S78–90.8.

26. Totlis T, Panariello RA, Oliver-Welsh L. Rehabilitation and postrehabilitation performance enhancement training and injury prevention following surgery for common

sports injuries: a process from surgery to return to play – preface. Oper Tech Sports Med 2017;25:129–31.

27. McKee P, Rivard A. Foundations of orthotic intervention. In: Skirven T, Osterman L, Fedorczyk J, et al, editors. Rehabilitation of the hand and upper extremity. 6th edition. Philadelphia: Elsevier; 2011. p. 1565–80.

28. NCAA publications: rule manuals. Available at: http://www.ncaapublications.com/. Accessed March 30, 2019.

29. Russell CR. Therapy challenges for athletes: splinting options. Clin Sports Med 2015;34:181–91.

30. Singletary S, Geissler WB. Bracing and rehabilitation for wrist and hand injuries in collegiate athletes. Hand Clin 2009;25:443–8.

31. NATA: athletic training services: an overview of skills and services provided by certified athletic trainers. 2010. Available at: https://www.nata.org/sites/default/files/GuideToAthleticTrainingServices.pdf. Accessed March 30, 2019.

32. Miller-Shahabar I, Schreuer N, Katsevman H, et al. Efficacy of compression gloves in the rehabilitation of distal radius fractures: randomized controlled study. Am J Phys Med Rehabil 2018;97:904–10.

33. Wilk K, Hooks TR. Neuromuscular training after anterior cruciate ligament reconstruction. In: Noyes FR, editor. Noyes' knee disorders: surgery, rehabilitation, clinical outcomes. 2nd edition. St Louis (MO): Elsevier; 2017. p. 330–42. https://doi.org/10.1016/B978-0-323-32903-3.00012-3.

34. Houglum PG. The ABCs of proprioception. In: Houglum PG, editor. Therapeutic exercise for musculoskeletal injuries. 3rd edition. Champaign (IL): Human Kinetics; 2010. p. 255–70.

35. Lephart SM, Pincivero DM, Giraldo JL, et al. The role of proprioception in the management and rehabilitation of athletic injuries. Am J Sports Med 1997;25:130–7.

36. Guido JA, Stemm J. Reactive neuromuscular training: a multi-level approach to rehabilitation of the unstable shoulder. N Am J Sports Phys Ther 2007;2:97–103.

37. Hagert E. Proprioception of the wrist joint. A review of current concepts and possible implications on the rehabilitation of the wrist. J Hand Ther 2010;23:2–17.

38. Hagert E, Lee J, Ladd AL. Innervation patterns of thumb trapeziometacarpal joint ligaments. J Hand Surg 2012;37:706–14.e1.

39. Hagert E, Forsgren S, Ljung BO. Differences in the presence of mechanoreceptors and nerve structures between wrist ligaments may imply differential roles in wrist stabilization. J Orthop Res 2005;23:757–63.

40. Hagert E, Garcia-Elias M, Forsgren S, et al. Immunohistochemical analysis of wrist ligament innervation in relation to their structural composition. J Hand Surg 2007;32:30–6.

41. Rein S, Semisch M, Garcia-Elias M, et al. Immunohistochemical mapping of sensory nerve endings in the human triangular fibrocartilage complex. Clin Orthop Relat Res 2015;473:3245–53.

42. Chikenji T, Berger RA, Fujimiya M, et al. Distribution of nerve endings in human distal interphalangeal joint and surrounding structures. J Hand Surg 2011;36:406–12.

43. Chen YG, McClinton MA, DaSilva MF, et al. Innervation of the metacarpophalangeal and interphalangeal joints: a microanatomic and histologic study of the nerve endings. J Hand Surg Am 2000;25:128–33.

44. Ludwig A, Mobargha N, Okogbaa J, et al. Altered innervation pattern in ligaments of patients with basal thumb arthritis. J Wrist Surg 2015;4:284–91.

45. Adler S, Beckers D, Buck M. PNF in practice: an illustrated guide. 3rd edition. Berlin: Springer-Verlag; 2008. p. 19–35.
46. Karagiannopoulos C, Michlovitz S. Rehabilitation strategies for wrist sensorimotor control impairment: from theory to practice. J Hand Ther 2016;29:154–65.
47. Hagert E, Lluch A, Rein S. The role of proprioception and neuromuscular stability in carpal instabilities. J Hand Surg Eur 2016;41:94–101.
48. Karagiannopoulos C, Sitler M, Michlovitz S, et al. Responsiveness of the active wrist joint position sense test after distal radius fracture intervention. J Hand Ther 2016;29:474–82.
49. Hincapie OL, Elkins JS, Vasquez-Welsh L. Proprioception retraining for a patient with chronic wrist pain secondary to ligament injury with no structural instability. J Hand Ther 2016;29:183–90.
50. Holmes MK, Taylor S, Miller C. Early outcomes of 'the Birmingham wrist instability programme':a pragmatic intervention for stage one scapholunate instability. Hand Ther 2017;22:90–100.
51. Borms D, Maenhout A, Cools AM. Upper quadrant field tests and isokinetic upper limb strength in overhead athletes. J Athl Train 2016;51:789–96.
52. Harris C, Wattles AP, DeBeliso M, et al. The seated medicine ball throw as a test of upper body power in older adults. J Strength Cond Res 2011;25:2344–8.
53. Westrick RB, Miller JM, Carow SD, et al. Exploration of the Y-balance test for assessment of upper quarter closed kinetic chain performance. Int J Sports Phys Ther 2012;7:1139–47.
54. Tucci HT, Martins J, Sposito G, et al. Closed kinetic chain upper extremity stability test (CKCUES test): a reliability study in persons with and without shoulder impingement syndrome. BMC Musculoskelet Disord 2014;15:1474–2474.
55. Negrete RJ, Hanney WJ, Kolber MD, et al. Reliability, minimal detectable change, and normative values for tests of upper extremity function and power. J Strength Cond Res 2010;24:3318–25.
56. Lorenz D, Morrison S. Current concepts in periodization of strength and conditioning for the sports physical therapist. Int J Sports Phys Ther 2015;10:734–47.
57. Harris-Love MO, Seamon BA, Gonzales TI, et al. Eccentric exercise program design: a periodization model for rehabilitation applications. Front Physiol 2017; 23:1–16.
58. Davies G, Riemann BL, Manske R. Current concepts of plyometric exercise. Int J Sports Phys Ther 2015;10:760–86.
59. Wolf MR, Avery D, Wolf JM. Upper extremity injuries in gymnasts. Hand Clin 2017; 33:187–97.
60. McDuff DR. Mental preparation. In: Sports psychiatry: strategies for life balance & peak performance. Washington, DC: American Psychiatric Publishing, Inc; 2012. p. 29–52.
61. Sardoni C, Hall C, Forwell L. The use of imagery by athletes during injury rehabilitation. J Sport Rehabil 2000;9:329–38.
62. Zach S, Dobersek U, Filho E, et al. A meta-analysis of mental imagery effects on post-injury functional mobility, perceived pain, and self-efficacy. Psychol Sport Exerc 2018;34:79–87.
63. Jaworski C, Krause M, Brown J. Rehabilitation of the wrist and hand following sports injury. Clin Sports Med 2010;29:61–80.
64. Halim A, Weis A. Return to play after hand and wrist fractures. Clin Sports Med 2016;35:597–608.
65. Bansal A, Carlin D, Moley J, et al. Return to play and complications after hook of the hamate fracture surgery. J Hand Surg Am 2017;42:803–9.

66. Morse KW, Hearns KA, Carlson MG. Return to play after forearm and hand injuries in the National Basketball Association. Orthop J Sports Med 2017;5:1–4.
67. Kadow TR, Fowler JR. Thumb injuries in athletes. Hand Clin 2017;33:161–73.
68. Rossenwasser MP. Proximal interphalangeal joint fracture dislocations in professional baseball players. Hand Clin 2012;28:417–20.
69. Belsky MR, Leibman MI, Ruchelsman DE. Scaphoid fracture in the elite athlete. Hand Clin 2012;28:269–78.
70. Winston MJ, Weiland AJ. Scaphoid fractures in the athlete. Curr Rev Musculoskelet Med 2017;10:38–44.
71. Beleckas C, Calfee R. Distal radius fractures in the athlete. Curr Rev Musculoskelet Med 2017;10:62–71.
72. Elzinga KE, Chung KC. Finger injuries in football and rugby. Hand Clin 2017;33:149–60.
73. Neumann JA, Leversedge FJ. Flexor tendon injuries in athletes. Sports Med Arthrosc Rev 2014;22:56–65.
74. King EA, Lien JR. Flexor tendon pulley injuries in rock climbers. Hand Clin 2017;33:141–8.
75. McDonald JW, Henrie AM, Teramoto M, et al. Descriptive epidemiology, medical evaluation and outcomes of rock climbing injuries. Wilderness Environ Med 2017;28:186–96.
76. Morrell NT, Moyer A, Quinlan N, et al. Scapholunate and perilunate injuries the athlete. Curr Rev Musculoskelet Med 2017;10:45–52.
77. Williams A, Ng CY, Hayton MJ. When can a professional athlete return to play following scapholunate ligament delayed reconstruction? Br J Sports Med 2013;47:1071–4.
78. Wolf AL, Scott W. Rehabilitation for scapholunate injury: application of scientific and clinical evidence to practice. J Hand Ther 2016;29:146–53.
79. Esplugas M, Garcia-Elias M, Lluch A, et al. Role of muscles in ligament-deficient wrists. J Hand Ther 2016;29:166–74.
80. Altman E. The ulnar side of the wrist: clinically relevant anatomy and biomechanics. J Hand Ther 2016;29:111–22.
81. Graham TJ. Pathologies of the extensor carpi ulnaris tendon and its investments in the athlete. Hand Clin 2012;28:345–56.
82. Conroy C, Ruchelsman DE, Vitale MA. Extensor carpi ulnaris instability in athletes- Diagnosis and treatment. Oper Tech Sports Med 2016;24:139–47.
83. Fram B, Wall LB, Gelbermanm RH, et al. Surgical transposition for chronic instability of the extensor carpi ulnaris tendon. J Hand Surg Eur 2018;43:925–30.